School Discipline and Self-Discipline

The Guilford Practical Intervention in the Schools Series
Kenneth W. Merrell, Series Editor

This series presents the most reader-friendly resources available in key areas of evidence-based practice in school settings. Practitioners will find trustworthy guides on effective behavioral, mental health, and academic interventions, and assessment and measurement approaches. Covering all aspects of planning, implementing, and evaluating high-quality services for students, books in the series are carefully crafted for everyday utility. Features include ready-to-use reproducibles, lay-flat binding to facilitate photocopying, appealing visual elements, and an oversized format.

Recent Volumes

Helping Students Overcome Depression and Anxiety, Second Edition: A Practical Guide
Kenneth W. Merrell

Inclusive Assessment and Accountability: A Guide to Accommodations for Students with Diverse Needs
Sara E. Bolt and Andrew T. Roach

Bullying Prevention and Intervention: Realistic Strategies for Schools
Susan M. Swearer, Dorothy L. Espelage, and Scott A. Napolitano

Conducting School-Based Functional Behavioral Assessments, Second Edition: A Practitioner's Guide
Mark W. Steege and T. Steuart Watson

Evaluating Educational Interventions: Single-Case Design for Measuring Response to Intervention
T. Chris Riley-Tillman and Matthew K. Burns

Collaborative Home/School Interventions:
Evidence-Based Solutions for Emotional, Behavioral, and Academic Problems
Gretchen Gimpel Peacock and Brent R. Collett

Social and Emotional Learning in the Classroom: Promoting Mental Health and Academic Success
Kenneth W. Merrell and Barbara A. Gueldner

Executive Skills in Children and Adolescents, Second Edition:
A Practical Guide to Assessment and Intervention
Peg Dawson and Richard Guare

Responding to Problem Behavior in Schools, Second Edition: The Behavior Education Program
Deanne A. Crone, Leanne S. Hawken, and Robert H. Horner

High-Functioning Autism/Asperger Syndrome in Schools: Asessment and Intervention
Frank J. Sansosti, Kelly A. Powell-Smith, and Richard J. Cowan

School Discipline and Self-Discipline: A Practical Guide to Promoting Prosocial Student Behavior
George G. Bear

Response to Intervention, Second Edition: Principles and Strategies for Effective Practice
Rachel Brown-Chidsey and Mark W. Steege

School Discipline and Self-Discipline

A Practical Guide to Promoting Prosocial Student Behavior

GEORGE G. BEAR

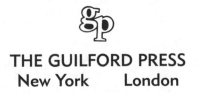

THE GUILFORD PRESS
New York   London

© 2010 The Guilford Press
A Division of Guilford Publications, Inc.
72 Spring Street, New York, NY 10012
www.guilford.com

Printed in the United States of America

This book is printed on acid-free paper.

Last digit is print number: 9 8 7 6 5 4 3 2 1

Library of Congress Cataloging-in-Publication Data

Bear, George G.
  School discipline and self-discipline: a practical guide to promoting prosocial student behavior / by George G. Bear.
    p. cm. — (The Guilford practical intervention in the schools series)
  Includes bibliographical references and index.
  ISBN 978-1-60623-681-9 (pbk.: alk. paper)
  1. School discipline.   2. Classroom management.   3. Problem children—Behavior modification.   I. Title.
  LB3012.B318 2010
  371.5—dc22

                                                              2010009740

IN MEMORIAM

Susan A. Golia (1949–2008; colon cancer)—my daughter-in-law's mother and recipient of The Washington Post Distinguished Educational Leadership Award as an elementary school principal in Howard County Public Schools, Maryland. You touched the lives of tens of thousands of children and demonstrated what social and emotional learning is all about. We thank you. You live in your daughter, Melissa, in your son, Mark, and in your grandchildren.

Kimberly Cottrell Hughes (1979–2008; melanoma)—my cousin and the assistant research director of the Effective Schoolwide Discipline initiative in Virginia, at Old Dominion University. You were only months away from finishing your dissertation and never got the chance to prove to me that schoolwide positive behavior support was as effective as you believed. You live in your children, Vivian and Evan.

About the Author

George G. Bear, PhD, is Professor of School Psychology at the University of Delaware. Formerly a school psychologist in Iowa and Virginia, he continues to work in the schools one day weekly as a practitioner. For the past 8 years he has been a consultant to the state of Delaware's Positive Behavior Support (PBS) Initiative, devoting much of this time to evaluating the impact of PBS on school climate and student behavior. Dr. Bear has published over 60 journal articles, book chapters, and books, most of which focus on school discipline and the social, emotional, and moral development of children. He is coeditor of the bestselling *Children's Needs: Development, Prevention, and Intervention;* author of *Developing Self-Discipline and Preventing and Correcting Misbehavior,* a textbook on classroom management; and an associate editor of the *School Psychology Review.*

Acknowledgments

Consistent with the schoolwide positive behavior support (SWPBS) approach, I would like to acknowledge, recognize, praise, or reward the following people. First, I acknowledge the valuable input from teachers and other educators who read drafts: Eileen Baker, Rachel Burwell, Debby Boyer, Casey Wharton, Melissa Simpson, Pamala Change, Jessica Blank, and Michael Partie (I didn't expect such nice comments from an ardent applied behavior analyst). I also would like to acknowledge that without the secretarial support of Doris Davidson, this book never would have been done on time. Happy retirement, Doris!

Next, I would like to recognize the substantial influence that teachers and SWPBS leaders in Delaware had on my thinking about schoolwide discipline and school reform. They include Eileen Baker, Rachel Burwell, Susan Corey, Sarah Hearn, Kathy Minke, Linda Smith, and Brian Touchette; Jeanne Geddes-Keye (the best principal I've ever worked with); and the truly exceptional teachers at The College School in Newark, Delaware. Three superb graduate students working with the Delaware PBS Initiative also deserve special recognition: Jessica Blank, Megan Pell, and Cecilia Till. Those deserving of the greatest praise are Debby Boyer and Brian Touchette. Thank you for your patience and respect for diverse viewpoints as well as your statewide leadership for many years. Each of these educators and leaders forced me to try to reconcile the differences between the SWPBS and social and emotional learning approaches. This book is my attempt to do so.

I am grateful to Series Editor Kenneth Merrell at the University of Oregon and to Editors Natalie Graham and Craig Thomas at The Guilford Press for believing that a book on the topic of self-discipline is greatly needed and for providing encouragement and support throughout the writing and publishing process. The largest rewards, however, will go to those family members with whom I missed spending as much time as I would have liked during the past year: my wife, Patti (she and her co-teacher, Robin, practice *every* good thing in this book), Brian, Adam, Melissa, Katie, and especially the grandkids, Madison, Susan, and Jackson. We'll have more fun now.

Contents

CHAPTER 1

Classroom Management and School Discipline
Punishment and Its Positive Alternatives

The most important issue confronting educators and educational theorists is the choice of ends of the educational process. Without clear and rational educational goals, it becomes impossible to decide which educational programs achieve objectives of general import and which teach incidental facts and attitudes of dubious worth. Although there has been a vast amount of research comparing the effects of various educational methods and programs on various outcome measures, there has been very little empirical research designed to clarify the worth of these outcome measures themselves.
—KOHLBERG (1981, p. 49)

TWO COMMON AIMS OF DISCIPLINE: MANAGING STUDENTS AND DEVELOPING SELF-DISCIPLINE

Since the 19th century, two general approaches to classroom management and school discipline have existed in U.S. schools. They are consistent with the two contrasting meanings of the term *discipline* (Bear, 2005). The first approach is consistent with the meaning of discipline as the *use* of a wide range of techniques to manage, govern, control, or correct student behavior. In practice, this translates into the use of *teacher-centered* strategies; rules, behavioral expectations, and the consequences of misbehavior, either punitive or positive, receive primary, if not exclusive, attention. The use of punitive strategies and techniques is commonly seen in schools that adopt a pervasive zero tolerance approach to school discipline, characterized by the frequent use of suspension and expulsion for managing behavior problems. In contrast, an emphasis on the use of positive techniques to manage student behavior is seen in the more recently popular schoolwide positive behavioral supports (SWPBS) approach (also often referred to in the literature as schoolwide positive behavioral interventions and supports [SWPBIS] and effective behavioral supports [EBS]; Horner, Sugai, Todd, & Lewis-Palmer, 2005; Sugai & Horner, 2002, 2009; Sugai, Horner,

1

& McIntosh, 2008). As in the zero-tolerance approach, in many SWPBS programs the most valued student outcomes and indicators of effectiveness are compliance and safety, typically as measured by reduced office disciplinary referrals. Whether punishment or positive reinforcement is the primary means of schoolwide discipline, the aim of those schools adopting the teacher-centered approach is similar—to manage or control student behavior and bring about student compliance with rules and behavioral expectations (Center for Mental Health in Schools, 2008; Freiberg, 1999; Kohn, 1996, 1999).

The second meaning of the term *discipline* refers to developing self-discipline—developing *within* students the cognitions, emotions, and behaviors associated with self-control, self-regulation, character, autonomy, and social and moral responsibility. Although it often has been overshadowed by the more immediate aim of *using* discipline to manage students, most educators have viewed the long-term aim of developing self-discipline as critical to American democracy grounded in individual rights and self-governance (McClellan, 1999). Although strategies and techniques to help develop self-discipline certainly include those that are teacher-centered, greater emphasis is placed on the use of *student-centered* strategies and techniques. Their use reflects an understanding that students must guide themselves, especially when teachers, rewards, and the fear of punishment are no longer salient. Thus, in addition to student behavior, the thoughts and emotions that underlie self-discipline are developed. As discussed in Chapter 3, student-centered strategies and techniques for developing self-discipline are best found in programs referred to as social and emotional learning (SEL; Collaborative for Academic, Social, and Emotional Learning, 2005; Zins & Elias, 2006). SEL includes character education (Berkowitz & Schwartz, 2006; Character Education Partnership, 2004) and programs based on positive psychology (Bear, 2009).

To be sure, and as emphasized throughout this book, both aims of school discipline—*using* discipline to manage student behavior and *developing* self-discipline—are equally important. The most effective classroom teachers and schools strive to balance both aims while using a combination of teacher- and student-centered strategies and techniques. They recognize that when adult supervision and management is not present, students must manage their own behavior (and hopefully would do so when adults *are* present). Likewise, they

> **Traditionally, discipline has referred to (a) the *management of student behavior*, with an emphasis on the use of teacher-centered strategies and techniques, both punitive and positive, and (b) the *development of self-discipline*, with an emphasis on the use of student-centered strategies.**

recognize that it would be naïve and utopian to dismiss the value, importance, and need to manage student behavior. They understand that occasionally nearly all students misbehave and that some students even engage in serious acts of misbehavior that threaten the safety of others. Thus, effective teachers and schools realize that there are times when teacher-centered external techniques of behavior management are necessary and appropriate. Moreover, they understand that when these techniques are used wisely, they help promote the development of self-discipline, but that, when used alone, they simply are not sufficient for achieving that important aim.

THE NEED FOR
A BALANCED AND COMPREHENSIVE APPROACH

Unfortunately, too many educators adopt an "either–or" perspective toward school discipline. They adopt *either* the aim of managing students with external rewards or punishment, as often found in the SWPBS and zero tolerance approaches, respectively, or they adopt the aim of developing self-discipline with student-centered strategies and techniques, as found in SEL. In adopting one aim or the other, educators fail to offer a balanced and comprehensive approach to classroom and schoolwide discipline. As described later in this chapter and presented throughout this book, a balanced and comprehensive approach strives to achieve *both* aims while integrating a combination of evidence-based strategies and techniques that comprise four critical components of comprehensive school discipline. These key components are (1) developing self-discipline, (2) preventing behavior problems, (3) correcting behavior problems, and (4) addressing the needs of students with serious and chronic behavior problems (Bear, 2005, 2008).

The first three components apply primarily at the classroom level but also schoolwide at the universal level of prevention (i.e., Tier 1 in many universal-level prevention programs). They benefit *all* students. The fourth component is specific to what is commonly referred to as Tier 2 (secondary or selective level) and Tier 3 (tertiary or indicated level) of prevention and intervention. The strategies and techniques at those two tiers go beyond what is typically provided to all students, either in regular classrooms or schoolwide. Because the focus of this book is on discipline at the universal level, Component 4 receives little attention. It should be noted, however, that all of the strategies and techniques under the first three components—*developing* self-discipline and *preventing* and *correcting* misbehavior—certainly apply to the fourth component. Indeed, strategies and techniques that are effective for students who are at risk or who currently exhibit serious and chronic behavior problems are largely the same ones used at the universal level. The difference is that those strategies and techniques are used more frequently, intensely, and in a more structured and systematic manner that often requires supports and resources outside of the regular classroom.

In arguing the need for a balanced and comprehensive approach to classroom and schoolwide discipline, this chapter begins with a discussion of the zero tolerance approach and its emphasis on punishment. The many limitations to punishment are examined, but, to be fair, its advantages also are noted. Its advantages help explain why punishment is the most common technique used in classroom management and school discipline (Brophy, 1996). Next, brief overviews are presented of two popular alternatives to the zero tolerance approach—SWPBS and SEL. SWPBS is discussed in greater detail in Chapter 2 and SEL in Chapter 3. As will be seen, both of those approaches offer numerous evidenced-based strategies and techniques for comprehensive classroom management and schoolwide discipline. Each approach has its strengths—but also its limitations. Fortunately, when elements of both approaches are combined, the limitations of each are largely offset by the other's strengths. This fortunate aspect is discussed briefly in this chapter and will become more evident in later chapters.

WHY PUNISHMENT IS OFTEN USED TO MANAGE STUDENT BEHAVIOR

Punishment *is* effective, and generally necessary, for the schoolwide management of student behavior. This statement may sound overly strong to some readers, but not when *punishment* is defined—as it is in psychology—as any unpleasant or undesired event or consequence that follows a behavior and decreases its future occurrence (Landrum & Kauffman, 2006; Martens, Witt, Daly, & Vollmer, 1999). The subsequent event or consequence can range in harshness from a principal spanking or suspending a student to a teacher simply making eye contact or moving toward the student (indicating that an undesired consequence is likely to follow if the behavior continues). If the event or consequence succeeds in decreasing occurrence of the behavior, then by definition it constitutes punishment. Teachers routinely use the "evil eye," proximity control, verbal warnings and reprimands, response cost (e.g., taking away privileges or points earned), and time out—techniques that students generally find unpleasant and that decrease student misbehavior. Each technique has been shown to be effective and thus to be part of nearly every teacher's repertoire of classroom management techniques (Brophy, 1996; Doyle, 1986). Likewise, at the schoolwide level, research shows that fair and consistent behavioral expectations and sanctions against misbehavior characterize the most effective schools (Arum, 2003; Catalano, Berglund, Ryan, Lonczak, & Hawkins, 2004; Gottfredson, Gottfredson, & Hybl, 1993; Gottfredson, Gottfredson, & Skroban, 1996). Thus, it is understandable that to some extent all models of classroom management and school discipline include the use of punishment. Often, however, it is called something more appealing, such as *consequences* (e.g., Dreikurs & Grey, 1968; Nelsen, Lott, & Glenn, 2000). The use of such a euphemism makes the approach seem more attractive to educators, avoids the risk of equating punishment with corporal punishment, and leads educators to believe that punishment is neither necessary nor desirable (Bear, 2005).

> It would be naïve and utopian to think that punishment, ranging from verbal reprimands to suspension, should never be used in schools. However, it would be foolish and unethical to ignore its many limitations.

There are multiple reasons why punishment is the most common technique of classroom management and school discipline, with the following among the primary ones:

- Punishment is effective in decreasing behavior problems (Landrum & Kauffman, 2006).
- Punishment often serves as an effective deterrent of misbehavior. When children see that others are punished for their behavior, they are less likely to act the same (Bandura, 1986). Likewise, at the school level, clear rules, expectations, and sanctions help deter behavior problems (Gottfredson, 2001; Mayer & Leone, 1999). (As discussed later, however, harsher forms of punishment are generally *less* effective than milder forms.)
- Educators often have no choice in the use of punishment. That is, codes of conduct in

nearly all schools, as well as state and federal laws, *require* that students be punished following certain behaviors.

- Even the most effective teachers cannot prevent all behavior problems from occurring. Few, if any, students *never* misbehave. As noted previously, effective teachers recognize the need and usefulness of mild forms of punishment and apply them judiciously and in combination with other techniques of classroom management (Brophy, 1996; Brophy & McCaslin, 1992).
- Although certainly not sufficient for developing self-discipline, punishment can help foster self-discipline when used in an authoritative, as opposed to authoritarian, manner (i.e., not overly harsh and in a fair, caring, and guiding fashion) (Baumrind, 1996).

BEHAVIOR MANAGEMENT WITH PUNISHMENT: THE ZERO TOLERANCE APPROACH

For centuries, and continuing today, punishment has been used too frequently and harshly, with little recognition of its multiple limitations. In the past the use of discipline most often meant the use of corporal punishment to correct misbehavior. The number of lashes with a stick, or strikes from a paddle, was contingent upon the severity of the offense. Although many professional organizations, including the National Education Association, National Association of School Psychologists, and American Psychological Association, strongly discourage its use, corporal punishment continues to be allowed in schools in 21 states, most of which are in the South (Center for Effective Discipline, 2009). Most schools, however, have replaced corporal punishment with noncorporal forms of punishment. School suspension, both in school and out of school, has been the most common replacement. Indeed, each year over 3 million children are suspended from school (Planty et al., 2009).

Just as corporal punishment has been roundly criticized as overly harsh and ineffective, so too has the use of school suspension and expulsion. The particular focus of such criticism has been a zero tolerance approach to behavior problems in which school removal is automatic, dictated by lengthy school codes of conduct, or "sentencing manuals" (Curtis, Batsche, & Mesmer, 2000). Students are removed irrespective of the circumstances involved, their previous histories of behavior, or the likelihood that doing so reduces future occurrence of the behavior (or improves school engagement or academic learning). In schools with a zero tolerance approach, student behavior is closely monitored and managed by teachers, administrators, and school resource officers, typically assisted by surveillance cameras, metal detectors, identification badges, and locker searches. Rule violations are dealt with swiftly and harshly, often resulting in "criminalizing" behaviors that police were rarely, if ever, involved with in the past (Skiba & Noam, 2002; Wald & Losen, 2003). Students are removed from school not only for serious rule violations, such as possessing drugs or weapons and fighting, but also for relatively minor acts of misbehavior such as not completing homework, not complying with a teacher's request, being tardy, or simply bothering the teacher (Advancement Project/Civil Rights Project, 2000). In the words of Kauffman and Brigham (2000, p. 278), too often zero tolerance "now means something stupid—getting tough on little things without allowing discretion in what to do about them."

Schools that adopt the zero tolerance approach ignore research demonstrating the overall negative impact of harsh and unfair punishment on the school's climate, or environment (Arum, 2003; Hyman & Perone, 1998). As noted by Mayer and Leone (1999), "Creating an unwelcoming, almost jail-like, heavily scrutinized environment, may foster the violence and disorder school administrators hope to avoid" (p. 349). Zero tolerance schools also tend to ignore research questioning the effectiveness of the approach in preventing school violence and showing that a frequent outcome of a zero tolerance approach is the disproportionate number of school removals of African American males (Advancement Project/Civil Rights Project, 2000; American Psychological Association Zero Tolerance Task Force, 2008; Gregory & Weinstein, 2008).

Zero Tolerance Approach versus Reasonable Zero Tolerance Policies

It is important to distinguish a pervasive and overly harsh zero tolerance *approach*, as described above, from more reasonable zero tolerance *policies* adopted by many schools pertaining to serious behavior problems, especially among older children and adolescents, that may truly harm or threaten the safety of others or seriously disrupt learning. Those behavior problems would include possession of weapons or drugs, serious bodily injury, and seriously disruptive behavior that is resistant to evidence-based interventions. When used judiciously (i.e., with fairness and discretion, including consideration of the circumstances involved, the student's age, intentions, and prior history), zero tolerance policies have their place as part of a comprehensive schoolwide discipline program (Bear, 2005); that is, they help ensure school safety by removing students who are truly a threat to the safety of others. They also often help improve the learning of others by removing those who are chronically disruptive. However, to benefit not only other students but also those who are removed, all removals should result in placement in an alternative educational setting with appropriate interventions and supports to prevent behavior problems from recurring (Bear, Quinn, & Burkholder, 2002).

Reasonable zero tolerance policies also can function as social sanctions that transmit clear expectations and standards of behavior. In this sense, they help deter serious crimes and conduct problems that impede the learning of others. They lose their effectiveness, however, when they are perceived by students as overly harsh and unfair (Arum, 2003). This distinction then, is the major difference between a pervasive zero tolerance approach and reasonable zero tolerance policies: when most students believe the social sanctions are fair, and when they are only one part of a school's comprehensive approach to school discipline that includes an emphasis on caring and supportive relations, sanctions become powerful deterrents against misbehavior.

Another important reason why reasonable zero tolerance policies should be part of every school's comprehensive disciplinary program is that, to some extent, they are mandated by either the federal or state government or the local school board. For example, the federal Gun-Free Schools Act (1994) mandates that schools expel for at least 1 year any student who possesses a gun on school property (administrators are given some discretion, however). Zero tolerance policies governing other criminal acts also exist in nearly all schools. As such, schools and teachers often have no choice in the matter. Where they do have a choice, however, is in limiting their zero tolerance policies to certain criminal acts that harm others or expanding them to include nearly all acts of noncompliance and misbehavior, as seen in the pervasive zero tolerance approach to school discipline.

Limitations to Punishment

Reasonable zero tolerance policies that entail the judicious use of noncorporal forms of punishment to correct student misbehavior are a necessary and important component of comprehensive schoolwide discipline. However, it is critical that schools recognize the many limitations to the use of punishment. Primary among those limitations are the following (Bear, 2005).

- *Punishment teaches students what not to do and not to get caught.* Almost 40 years ago, Winett and Winkler (1972) noted that the greatest limitation to the use of punishment is that it teaches students to perform the same behaviors that can be performed by a dead person. That is, they are taught to avoid punishment by being quiet, docile, and compliant: "Don't get out of your seat," "Don't talk," "Don't run in the halls," and so forth. Indeed, when used alone and not in combination with other positive techniques, punishment simply teaches students *what not to do.* Because such punishment is external, coming from adults, students learn to either demonstrate compliance or avoid getting caught. Punishment does not teach prosocial behaviors or behaviors that should replace those that led to punishment. Likewise, punishment does not teach cognitions and emotions that often underlie prosocial behavior and the inhibition of antisocial behavior, such as an understanding of the value of rules, respect for others, empathy, and responsibility for one's own behavior (especially in the absence of getting caught).

- *Punishment's effects are short-term and are often dependent on the presence of adults.* For most problem behaviors, students cease the behaviors as soon as punishment is applied, whether it be the use of a verbal warning, the "evil eye," physical proximity, or other actions that students find unpleasant. Although the punishment achieves its short-term objective, the objectionable behavior often continues when the likelihood of being punished is no longer salient, such as when adults are not watching or when students decide that engaging in the misbehavior is worth the risk of getting caught (e.g., "So what if I get caught. Getting yelled at or sent to the office isn't that bad"). As such, the effectiveness of punishment is largely dependent on the constant surveillance and monitoring of student behavior, the perceived risk of getting caught among students, and often their calculation of whether the misbehavior is worth the risk of getting caught, given the severity of the punishment.

- *Punishment teaches students to be aggressive toward and punish others.* Through the process of observational or incidental learning, students learn that punishment is an effective and legitimate means of power and control. That is, they learn to use punishment by observing adults who control students with threats, sarcasm, ridicule, and even physical punishment (in the 21 states where the laws permit it). Modeling is a powerful means of teaching behavior, especially when the behavior is modeled by someone in a position of respect and recognized authority and when the modeled behavior is effective in obtaining desired outcomes, such as control of or compliance from others (Bandura, 1986).

- *Punishment fails to address the multiple factors that typically contribute to a student's misbehavior.* When students violate school rules, it is rarely because they were unaware of the rules and their consequences (*if* they get caught), especially beyond early elementary school or after the first few days of each school year. Rather than a lack of knowledge or social skills being the cause of their misbehavior, multiple other factors typically are involved. While the use of punishment may well stop the behavior in the short run, it does not address these factors. For example, punishment does little to curtail the impulsivity and hyperactivity of a child with attention-deficit/hyperactivity disorder (ADHD), the noncompliant attitude and behavior of an adolescent who hates school or is emotionally distraught, the inattentive and disruptive behavior of a student reading 3 years below grade level, the intention among students in a class when instruction is boring and nonmotivating, or the inappropriate behaviors of students that are reinforced by peers.

- *Use of punishment can be reinforcing to those who use it.* Because punishment often *works*, or stops a behavior (at least in the short term), people continue to use it. That is, those who mete out the punishment often are reinforced for doing so, typically in one of three ways: negative reinforcement, positive reinforcement, and self-reinforcement. First, the use of punishment might be reinforced by cessation of the undesired behavior, which is referred to as negative reinforcement. For example, a student is noncompliant and argues with a teacher; the teacher raises her voice and threatens to send the student to the office; and the student then stops arguing and becomes compliant. In such common cases, punishment works in stopping something aversive to teachers. When a similar behavior occurs in the classroom in the future, the teacher uses the same strategy after having learned that it worked before. In this case the use of punishment (both raising one's voice and threatening to send the student to the office) is reinforced by the student's compliance and cessation of arguing.

A second way that the use of punishment is often reinforced is by positive reinforcement, which happens when adults who use punishment are actually praised, recognized, or otherwise reinforced for doing so. For example, the school principal praises teachers for maintaining orderly classroom environments and for controlling their students, and the teachers believe that it was their use of punishment that resulted in achieving the school's aim of order and control. The principal might also be recognized by the school board and community for the school's zero tolerance approach, and such recognition is shared with all teachers and staff.

Finally, the use of punishment also can be *self-reinforcing*. For example, when meting out punishment, such as yelling or sending a student to the office, adults often feel a sense of control and power. Although the actual effectiveness of the punishment is likely to strengthen feelings of power and control, this outcome is not necessary for the teacher to keep using it. That is, even if students remain noncompliant either in the immediate situation or thereafter, the teacher might still experience a sense of power and authority when using punishment and thus continue to use it.

• *Punishment is likely to produce undesirable side effects.* Few people like to be punished by others, largely because punishment often generates negative emotions of frustration, anger, fear, and shame. When intense and unregulated, each of those emotions is related not only to problems of behavior, as discussed below, but also to problems of learning. The latter is seen in poor attention, concentration, and memory. Punishment generates frustration by interfering with, or precluding, the achievement of a student's goals, such as wanting to talk to peers or avoiding work. Once induced, frustration can easily turn to anger, especially when the punishment is viewed as unfair, overly harsh, or attributed to others (Weiner, 2006). In turn, anger can lead to retaliation or revenge, either direct (e.g., verbal or physical) or indirect (noncompliance, or attempts to undermine authority). Punishment, especially corporal punishment, yelling, and public ridicule, also can generate anxiety and fear. In turn, anxiety and fear often lead to avoidance behavior—avoiding the source of the anxiety and fear.

In addition to generating frustration, anger, and fear, punishment can generate the emotions of guilt and shame. When mild and regulated, such emotions can be constructive (especially guilt), but when these are experienced frequently or intensely, or are unregulated, they can be harmful (Izard, 1991). Punishment is an affront to one's perceptions of self. It sends the message "What I did was bad" or, much worse, "I am a bad person." Whereas behavior-specific feelings of guilt often result from the first message, more pervasive feelings of shame result from the second. When frequent, intense, and unregulated, guilt and shame can interfere with learning and trigger either avoidance or aggression. To be sure, both feelings are uncomfortable, but it is shame that can be most harmful with respect to learning and mental health and more likely to lead to blaming, anger, and retaliation (Tangney, Stuewig, & Mashek, 2007).

Whether considering anxiety, frustration, anger, fear, or shame, students commonly *dislike* what they perceive to be the source of those negative emotions, including teachers, peers, or school in general. In turn, such disliking often leads to acts of aggression, noncompliance, or avoidance, as seen among many delinquents (Gottfredson, 2001; Hirischi, 1969) and adolescents who fail to complete school (Reschly & Christenson, 2006).

• *Punishment creates a negative school climate.* A final negative side effect of punishment, especially when its use is perceived by students as unfair and overly harsh, is that it harms the school climate, or atmosphere (Arum, 2003; Cohen, McCabe, Michelli, & Pickeral, 2009). When the school climate is poor, students suffer academically, socially, and emotionally. In schools with a positive school climate, however, students tend to be more engaged academically and experience less bullying, crime, general discipline problems, school avoidance, and other social and emotional problems.

POSITIVE ALTERNATIVES
TO ZERO TOLERANCE AND PUNISHMENT

In recognition of these limitations to punishment, many schools have adopted one of two alternative approaches: the SWPBS approach or the SEL approach (Osher, Bear, Sprague, & Doyle, 2010). Each of these popular approaches is described briefly below, and more thoroughly in the following two chapters.

Schoolwide Positive Behavior Supports

As in the zero tolerance approach, the primary aim of the SWPBS approach is the management of student behavior. However, while the zero tolerance approach focuses on the use of punishment to reduce or correct behavior problems, SWPBS focuses on use of *positive* behavioral techniques, particularly external rewards and the direct training of social skills, to prevent behavior problems. Both approaches emphasize rules and behavioral expectations, but—in contrast to the zero tolerance approach—SWPBS devotes much greater time and resources to "catching kids being good" rather than bad.

Additional key features of SWPBS, as reviewed in Chapter 2, include (1) three tiers of interventions and supports (i.e., universal; selective, or secondary; and indicated, or tertiary), (2) an emphasis on student outcomes (i.e., with reduced disciplinary referrals being the most common outcome measured), (3) use of research-validated procedures (e.g., making rules and expectations clear, using positive reinforcement, teaching social skills), (4) supportive systems (e.g., a SWPBS planning team, coaches, budgetary and administrator supports), and (5) the ongoing collection and use of data for decision making (typically, office disciplinary referrals). Educators should find many of those key features attractive, and indeed they should incorporate them into their comprehensive schoolwide discipline programs.

> Whereas the zero tolerance approach focuses on the use of punishment to reduce or correct behavior problems, SWPBS focuses on use of *positive* behavioral techniques, particularly external rewards and the direct training of social skills, to prevent behavior problems.

As is discussed in depth in the next chapter, there are limitations to the SWPBS approach of Sugai and Horner (2009), which is grounded in behaviorism and particularly applied behavior analysis (ABA). Foremost among the limitations is its reliance on the use of teacher-centered techniques aimed primarily, if not exclusively, at managing student behavior, and its neglect of student-centered techniques to develop social, emotional, and moral competencies, or self-discipline. Although this is a major limitation if one's aim to develop self-discipline, the strategies and techniques of ABA are major strengths of the SWPBS approach if one's aim is to manage student behavior, while at times is a worthwhile aim, particularly over the short term.

Social and Emotional Learning

In contrast to SWPBS, the primary aim of the SEL approach is to develop social, emotional, and moral qualities, strengths, and assets commonly associated with self-discipline (Osher et al., 2010). These include respect, resilience, bonding with others, resolving conflicts appropriately, caring, honesty, seeking social justice, spirituality, self-efficacy, and a positive self-concept (including moral identity and self-perceptions of competence, self-worth, and happiness). Each quality is viewed as important in its own right but also important to positive mental health, academic achievement, and the prevention of various problem behaviors, including bullying, aggression, and school violence. As discussed in Chapter 3, SEL incorporates character education and positive psychology. It also includes positive youth development programs (Berkowitz, Sherblom, Bier, & Battistich, 2006; Catalano et al., 2004; Damon, 2004) that aim to develop self-discipline rather than manage student behavior.

> The SEL approach focuses on developing social and emotional competencies that underlie self-discipline, while emphasizing the use of a variety of student-centered strategies and techniques.

The SEL approach is grounded in social learning and social cognitive theories that view learning and development as multidimensional, transactional, and reciprocal (Bandura, 1986, 2001). The environment alone is not seen as determining behavior. As noted by Bandura (2001), if external events were the sole determinants of behavior, "as a crude functionalism would suggest...people would behave like weather vanes, constantly shifting direction to conform to whatever influence happened to impinge upon them at the moment" (p. 7). All students in a given classroom would respond similarly and immediately to environmental antecedents and consequences manipulated by the teacher. The motivations, attitudes, beliefs, goals, values, reasoning, and emotions of students would not matter. From the perspective of the SEL approach, these factors *do* matter, and although the school environment certainly influences student behavior, so too do the behaviors, attitudes, and beliefs of students influence the classroom and school environment—that is, the influences are not unidirectional.

In seeking to develop self-discipline and other social and emotional competencies, the SEL approach focuses on the use of student-centered strategies and techniques and places great emphasis on the importance of teacher–student relationships. To be sure, teacher-centered strategies and techniques also are employed, but they receive less emphasis, especially relative to the SWPBS approach. With the SEL's more student-centered approach to learning, students actively participate in learning and practice self-discipline, as may be observed in planned opportunities for students to apply, practice, and further develop their social, emotional, and moral competencies. As in SWPBS, rewards are used to reinforce positive behavior, but praise is preferred over rewards and rewards are used much less frequently and systematically than in SWPBS; moreover, they are used to reinforce cognitions and emotions related to self-discipline.

Different, Yet Compatible

Although there are fundamental differences between the SWPBS and SEL approaches, the two have much in common. Both focus on prevention. Both emphasize a variety of strategies and techniques—albeit, often different ones—that are effective in preventing and correcting behavior problems and helping to develop self-discipline. Both also recognize the importance of home–school communications and motivating academic instructions and curricula. The two are largely compatible (Osher et al., 2010), and (as discussed below), the strengths of one largely complement the weaknesses of the other. Nevertheless, differences in their epistemological roots, their primary aims (managing behavior versus developing self-discipline), and the strategies and techniques that receive the greatest emphasis (or neglect) make it difficult to implement both approaches without encountering inconsistencies and contradictions in theory and practice. This dilemma is especially pointed in schools that aim to develop students' self-discipline but rely primarily, if not entirely, on external techniques to do so.

> The SWPBS and SEL approaches differ in important ways, but they are compatible. Together, they offer the full range of strategies and techniques needed for effective classroom management and schoolwide discipline.

COMPREHENSIVE CLASSROOM AND SCHOOLWIDE DISCIPLINE AT THE UNIVERSAL LEVEL

When combined, the SWPBS and SEL approaches provide a combination of evidence-based strategies and techniques that can be effective in achieving the dual aims of managing student behavior and developing self-discipline. They must be used wisely, however—as described in this book—if both aims are to be achieved. Together the two approaches provide the full range of strategies and techniques needed for comprehensive school discipline, consisting of four necessary components (Bear, 2005, 2008): (1) developing self-discipline, (2) preventing behavior problems, (3) correcting behavior problems, and (4) addressing the needs of students who currently exhibit (or who are at risk of exhibiting) serious and chronic behavior problems. As noted previously and illustrated in Figure 1.1, only the first three apply to the classroom level and the universal level of schoolwide prevention (Tier 1—and thus are the focus of this book. I describe each of these components briefly below while noting the strategies and techniques of the SWPBS and SEL approaches that fit best under each component.

Component 1: Developing Self-Discipline

What self-discipline consists of and why it is important are discussed in Chapter 3. As will be seen, strategies and techniques for developing the social, emotional, and moral competencies associated with self-discipline are the primary strength of the SEL approach.

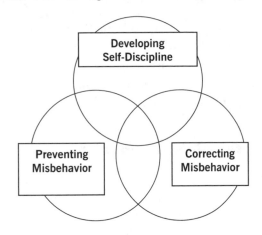

FIGURE 1.1. Components of schoolwide discipline at the universal level.

Ironically, this component is also the primary shortcoming of the SWPBS approach. That is, developing social, emotional, and moral competencies is specifically *not* an aim of the SWPBS approach. However, there is no reason why many of the behavioral strategies and techniques of ABA cannot be combined with SEL strategies and techniques to help develop self-discipline. Doing so is not an easy task and requires considerable reflection and planning. While adequately managing students' behavior is a critical consideration in the short term, it should not be accomplished at the cost of also developing their capacity for self-discipline. This undersirable result can be avoided by assuring that developing self-discipline is not only targeted as a specific separate component of comprehensive classroom and schoolwide discipline but also is included in strategies and techniques for preventing and correcting behavior problems—as, indeed, it is throughout this book.

Component 2: Preventing Behavior Problems

This is the one component of comprehensive school discipline that both the SEL and SWPBS approaches recognize as being of critical importance. Both approaches recognize that devoting increased time and energy to *preventing* behavior problems often results in decreased time and energy that has to be devoted to *correcting* behavior problems. They also recognize that it is easier to prevent behavior problems in school than outside of school, and that the best prevention programs do both. The SEL and SWPBS approaches have many preventive strategies and techniques in common: use of praise and rewards; modeling desired behavior; clear expectations, rules, procedures, and routines; respectful, supportive teacher–student relationships and student relationships; a physical environment conducive to learning and safety; academic instruction that engages and motivates learning; home–school communications and intervening early when problem behavior first appears.

There are differences, however, in how those strategies and techniques are used and which ones receive primary emphasis. For example, in SWPBS programs the emphasis is placed on teachers and other adults directly teaching rules or expectations and social skills and administering rewards schoolwide in a systematic manner to reinforce desired behaviors. In contrast, to accomplish the same goal of preventing behavior problems, the SEL approach favors having teachers use praise much more than tangible rewards, while focusing on developing SEL competencies rather than managing student behavior, and emphasizes the role of the teacher–student relationship in prevention.

Component 3: Correcting Behavior Problems

As described at length in Chapter 5, research shows that the greatest difference between effective and ineffective classroom managers is that the former prevent most behavior problems from ever occurring. Unfortunately, however, even the most effective teachers find it necessary now and then to correct behavior problems. This observation also holds true for the most efficacious schools: they simply cannot prevent all behavior problems and thus have to use corrective techniques. These may include punishment to reduce the future occurrence of behavior problems but also behavioral techniques for minimizing undesired behavior by either teaching or reinforcing desired behavior. ABA offers a variety of proven ways of reducing or eliminating misbehavior by individual students (Alberto & Troutman, 2007), which is clearly an advantage of the SWPBS approach. This emphasis on reducing misbehavior is the one component of comprehensive classroom and school discipline that tends to receive the least emphasis in SEL programs (especially in respect to the specific reductive techniques). By contrast, techniques for teaching and developing replacement behaviors, including cognitions and emotions supporting these behaviors, are not lacking in SEL programs. Most SEL programs target such cognitive and emotional skills as empathy, emotion regulation, social problem solving, and moral reasoning. Indeed, such techniques offer a healthy balance to the emphasis in ABA on social skills training and the positive reinforcement of replacement behavior. By combining social cognitive and behavioral techniques when correcting misbehavior, one not only enhances the likelihood of bringing about short-term compliance but also helps to develop long-term self-discipline in students.

Caution: Developing Self-Discipline Is Not the Same as Preventing and Correcting Behavior Problems

Developing self-discipline, preventing misbehavior, and correcting misbehavior are interrelated components of comprehensive classroom school discipline that build upon and support one another. For example, effectiveness in preventing behavior problems lessens the time and energy educators and others have to devote to correcting behavior problems. It also helps create an environment that promotes the development of self-discipline. Similarly, effectiveness in developing self-discipline lessens not only the need for correction but also the need to use external methods of preventing behavior problems, such as close adult supervision and the frequent use of praise and rewards. The components also are interrelated in that they use many of the same strategies and techniques. For example, supportive teacher–student relationships and the strategic use of praise are important in each component, although used for different purposes and applied in a different manner across components.

One of the biggest mistakes educators make with respect to school discipline is believing that by preventing and correcting behavior problems they are thereby developing self-discipline. Educators can be very effective in preventing and correcting behavior problems

> **One of the biggest mistakes educators make with respect to school discipline is believing that by preventing and correcting behavior problems they are therefore developing self-discipline.**

while doing little to develop self-discipline. This phenomenon is clearly seen in the most harsh and controlling zero tolerance facilities, such as juvenile correction facilities and prisons, in which surveillance cameras, clear rules, armed guards, and immediate and consistent consequences are very effective in both preventing and correcting behavior problems. However, whereas those techniques are effective for managing and controlling behavior in the short term, and in maintaining order and safety, they do little or nothing to help develop self-discipline. Such failure is reflected in the high recidivism rates of U.S. prisoners, with some two-thirds of all prisoners eventually being rearrested following their release (U.S. Department of Justice, 2006). Although an extreme example is used here to make the point, it is not uncommon for teachers and administrators to make a similar mistake in thinking that by preventing or correcting behavior problems, with either punitive or positive techniques, they are therefore necessarily inculcating self-discipline.

INTEGRATING STRATEGIES AND TECHNIQUES OF SEL AND SWPBS FOR COMPREHENSIVE CLASSROOM AND SCHOOLWIDE DISCIPLINE

As noted above, and shown in Table 1.1, the SEL and the SWPBS approaches have their strengths, and each has a specific weakness. If the strategies and techniques of both approaches are properly coordinated or integrated, the strengths of one approach can largely offset the weaknesses of the other. Educators would be wise to draw heavily from SEL to achieve the aim of developing self-discipline and from SWPBS to correct and manage student behavior *when needed*. Proper integration does not mean simply combining the

TABLE 1.1. Strengths and Weaknesses of SWPBS and SEL as Approaches to Comprehensive Classroom and School Discipline at the Universal Level

Components of comprehensive schoolwide discipline	Approach to school discipline	
	SWPBS (ABA)	SEL
Developing the social and emotional competencies of self-discipline	Weakness	Strength
Preventing behavior problems	Strength	Strength
Correcting behavior problems	Strength	Weakness

strategies and techniques of both approaches without reflecting upon one's aim. When one does so, inconsistencies and contradictions in the aims of different strategies and techniques are likely to emerge. For example, a school district's administrators that seek to combine the two without serious reflection and modification may find themselves disseminating tokens for good behavior to all students from elementary to high school in the mistaken belief that they are thereby developing self-discipline. More likely, the result will be self-centered students who are motivated by external rewards but lacking in intrinsic motivation. Self-discipline is not developed by relying on strategies and techniques that are best suited for correcting behavior problems. Equally well, the strategies and techniques for developing self-discipline in SEL are not necessarily the most effective ones for correcting behavior problems. In integrating strategies and techniques from both approaches, school officials must keep in mind the critical importance of *all* three components of classroom and school-wide discipline at the universal level: developing self-discipline, preventing behavior problems, and correcting behavior problems.

OVERVIEW OF THIS VOLUME

Consistent with the view that comprehensive classroom and schoolwide discipline at the universal level of prevention consists of developing self-discipline, preventing misbehavior, and correcting misbehavior, chapters are devoted to each of these components. Before presenting the specific strategies and techniques of each component, I critique the SWPBS approach in Chapter 2. Chapter 3 addresses the major shortcoming of most SWPBS programs, namely, neglect of the social and emotional competencies associated with self-discipline. What self-discipline is and why it is important are discussed, and the SEL approach to developing self-discipline is described in detail. How self-discipline relates to school climate also is discussed. The succeeding seven chapters (4–10) present evidence-based strategies and techniques for developing self-discipline, preventing misbehavior, and correcting misbehavior. Throughout those chapters I note that, in achieving these three goals, schools also simultaneously foster a positive school climate. Given that developing self-discipline is the particular strength of the SEL approach, evidence-based strategies and techniques of SEL for developing self-discipline and promoting a positive school climate are presented in Chapter 4.

Chapter 5 draws from both SWPBS and SEL in presenting evidence-based strategies and techniques for preventing behavior problems (and helping to develop self-discipline) in the classroom and schoolwide. Chapter 6 presents strategies and techniques that focus more specifically on developing self-discipline. Chapters 6, 7, and 8 focus on the use of praise and rewards in both preventing misbehavior and developing self-discipline (and to a lesser extent in the correction of misbehavior). In these chapters, the strategies and techniques of SWPBS and SEL are integrated in such a way that that praise in particular and rewards to a lesser extent are both targeted at student behavior and the cognitions and emotions that often underlie student behavior.

Chapters 9 and 10 focus on correction, and again the strategies of SWPBS and SEL are integrated such that their aim is not only a short-term improvement in behavior but also the long-term development of self-discipline. Finally, in Chapter 11 I discuss the key issues of school change or reform while presenting concrete steps, drawn from research and practice, for implementing comprehensive schoolwide discipline efforts, including measures that schools can use to assess their strengths, needs, and overall climate.

SUMMARY

The most important question educators should ask themselves with respect to school discipline is not "What works?" but "What is the primary aim (or aims) of school discipline?" It is only after answering that question that educators should ask "What works?" Two traditional aims of school discipline were discussed: to manage or correct student behavior and to develop self-discipline. Both aims are equally important. For managing or correcting behavior, schools have tended to adopt one of two approaches—the punishment-oriented zero tolerance approach or the reward-oriented approach of SWPBS. Punishment has many limitations, as reviewed in this chapter, and largely in response to them two alternative "positive" approaches have become popular, namely, SWPBS and SEL. Both approaches are discussed and dissected more thoroughly in the following chapters.

The SWPBS and SEL approaches have both strengths and weaknesses. The primary limitation of SWPBS, especially the ABA approach of Sugai and Horner (2009), is its lack of emphasis on self-discipline. Its primary strength is that it provides multiple techniques that are effective in managing and correcting behavior, which is needed at times, more so in certain classrooms and schools than in others. The opposite is true of SEL in that its key strength is developing self-discipline, and its relative weakness is providing techniques for managing and correcting behavior problems, especially serious and chronic ones. Both approaches share the strength of providing educators with a variety of evidence-based techniques for preventing misbehavior. Together, the two approaches offer strategies and techniques that, if properly implemented, can provide comprehensive classroom and school discipline at the universal level in all three of its guises: developing self-discipline, preventing misbehavior, and correcting misbehavior.

CHAPTER 2

Managing Student Behavior with the Positive Behavioral Techniques of Schoolwide Positive Behavior Supports

A rapidly growing number of schools, an estimated 9,000 in early 2009, have adopted the SWPBS approach to school discipline (Horner, 2009). The growth in SWPBS was sparked by inclusion of the term *positive behavior interventions and supports* in the 1997 and 2004 amendments to the Individuals with Disabilities Education Act (IDEA). The 2004 amendments require that a child's individualized education program (IEP) team *consider* the use of *positive behavioral interventions and supports* in cases in which the behavior of a child with a disability exhibits behavior that impedes the child's learning or the learning of others. *Where appropriate*, such behavioral interventions and supports are to be included in the child's individualized education plan.

Perhaps the greatest impetus for SWPBS, however, was the earmarking of federal funding in IDEA for "training for administrators, teachers, related services personnel, behavioral specialists, and other school staff in positive behavioral interventions and supports, behavioral intervention planning, and classroom and student management techniques" and for "developing or implementing specific curricula, programs, or interventions aimed at addressing behavioral problems." The specific purpose of such training and staff development is "to reduce the need to label children as disabled in order to address the learning and behavioral needs of such children." With funding for the schoolwide training of staff, and for the purpose of prevention, positive behavior supports (PBS) for individual children with disabilities evolved into SWPBS for *all* children.

Neither PBS nor SWPBS is defined in IDEA. As such, IDEA does not require one specific approach to SWPBS. Common definitions proposed by authorities in the field vary along a continuum from those that emphasize the application of behavior modification or applied behavioral analysis to those that are very broad, encompassing almost any technique that is "positive." The most popular approach to SWPBS (and it is often stated in the literature that it is the only one) was developed at the University of Oregon by Rob Horner and George Sugai (Horner et al., 2005; Sugai & Horner, 2009) with ample funding from the U.S. Department of Education's Office of Special Education Programs. With much less funding and visibility, other approaches to SWPBS (e.g., Project Achieve; Knoff, 2005, 2008) are less well known and have been adopted by far fewer schools. Because of its relative popularity and common use, the Horner and Sugai approach to SWPBS is the one referred to throughout this book whenever the term *SWPBS* (unless otherwise stated) is used.

The SWPBS approach is teacher-centered, its primary aim being to manage, control, or modify student behavior by manipulating the school environment. It is firmly grounded in behavior modification—or, more correctly, applied behavior analysis (Horner et al., 2005; Sugai & Horner, 2009). As noted by Horner (2000), "There is no

> **From the perspective of SWPBS, the school environment and particularly the actions of teachers and school staff are the primary causes of behavior problems in school.**

difference in theory or science between positive behavior support and behavior modification. These are the same approach with different names" (p. 99). In other articles (e.g., Sugai & Horner, 2009), however, it is made clear that SWPBS is grounded more in applied behavior analysis than in behavior modification per se. Although behavior modification and ABA are similar in many respects, applied behavior analysis emphasizes not only the modification of behavior but also the *analysis* of the principles of learning that cause observed changes in behavior (Alberto & Troutman, 2006; Baer, Wolf, & Risley, 1968). From the perspective of ABA, all behavior serves a given function, as discussed later in this chapter. According to the Sugai and Horner approach, an understanding of the functions of behavior is deemed necessary to bring about behavior change most effectively.

It is understood that the school environment, and particularly the actions of teachers and school staff, are the primary causes of behavior problems in school. Thus, in order to modify or control student behavior, the school environment and particularly the actions of teachers must be modified. SWPBS entails the process and techniques by which this occurs. The techniques are not new to classroom management (Bear, 2007; Osher et al., 2010). They consist primarily of positive reinforcement, punishment, and direct instruction, but with an emphasis on the first of these. Indeed, the techniques differ little from those in basic textbooks on the behavioral approach to classroom management (e.g., Canter & Canter, 2001) and changing individual behavior (Alberto & Troutman, 2006). What is different, however, is applying those techniques *schoolwide*—as opposed to solely with individual students or classes—and the process by which this is done.

KEY FEATURES OF THE SWPBS APPROACH

In addition to being grounded in applied behavior analysis, SWPBS is characterized by five key features, or elements, that are frequently cited in the literature (Horner et al., 2005;

Sugai & Horner, 2009): (1) a three-tiered model of prevention, interventions, and supports; (2) direct instruction; (3) evidence- or research-based behavioral practices; (4) supportive systems; and (5) the ongoing collection and use of data for decision making.

Three-Tiered Model of Prevention, Interventions, and Supports

Perhaps the most widely recognized feature of SWPBS is its three-tier model that offers a continuum of prevention and intervention strategies, techniques, and supports for all children. Adapted from the public mental health model of prevention (Adelman & Taylor, 2006), the three tiers are:

- Tier 1, primary, or universal, prevention, consisting of a system of positive supports provided schoolwide to all children and staff and in all classrooms and other school settings for the purpose of preventing future behavior problems.
- Tier 2, secondary prevention, also called selective prevention, consisting of a system of support for small groups of children at risk of exhibiting serious behavior problems and/or experiencing negative outcomes due to the presence of risk factors. Small-group social skills training receives particular emphasis at this tier.
- Tier 3, tertiary prevention, also frequently referred to as indicated or intensive intervention. This level is designed for individual students who exhibit chronic and serious behavior problems requiring intensive, comprehensive, and individualized interventions and services.

Tier 1, universal prevention, is the focus of this book. The four other key features of SWPBS, as discussed below, are found in each of the three tiers (Horner et al., 2005). Although each feature is generally found in other approaches to schoolwide discipline, the SWPBS approach is clearly reflected in the techniques, procedures, and measures characterizing the next two features, namely, direct instruction and evidence or research-based behavioral practices.

Direct Instruction

Although academic achievement is recognized as an important outcome, social skills receive the greatest attention. Consistent with the principles of applied behavior analysis, social skills are directly taught and are expected to be observable, measurable, and clearly defined. School officials are advised to focus on a small number of behavioral expectations and rules that teachers and staff believe are of greatest importance, to teach specific social skills directly related to those expectations and rules, and to reinforce those skills systematically and positively throughout all classrooms and school settings. Commonly taught social skills are "Follow directions," "Be respectful," and "Be responsible." Typically, being respectful and responsible means following school rules and obeying those in positions of authority; which is seen in the following example of the teaching of responsibility (Horner et al., 2005, p. 369):

In the classroom: Bring books and pencils to class. Do homework.
In gym: Participate. Wear appropriate shoes.
In the hallway: Keep books, belongings, litter off floor.
On the playground: Stay within the recess area.
In the bus area: Keep your books and belongings with you.

Behavioral expectations, such as those cited above, are posted throughout classrooms and other school settings. Student behavior is monitored closely by adults schoolwide throughout the day, with students exhibiting those social skills reinforced with verbal praise and often with tokens exchangeable for tangible rewards or privileges. Positive reinforcement is used much more frequently than punishment to teach social skills and prevent and discourage problem behavior. However, a broad range of clear and fair punitive consequences for inappropriate behavior also is firmly in place for the same purposes.

Evidence- or Research-Based Behavioral Practices

Evidence-based or research-based behavioral practices entail the curriculum, classroom management, instructional procedures, use of rewards and consequences, and an emphasis on the schoolwide application of prevention and positive techniques. Among the behavioral practices most commonly seen in SWPBS schools, the direct teaching of behavioral expectations and social skills and the use of positive reinforcement receive primary attention. As previously noted, at the core of the SWPBS approach is the systematic application of techniques of applied behavior analysis (Sugai & Horner, 1994, 2009; Sugai et al., 2000, 2008). As discussed later in this chapter, techniques of ABA have been found to be quite effective in changing the behavior of individual students, particularly in bringing about short-term changes in their behavior (Alberto & Troutman, 2006; Stage & Quiroz, 1997).

Supportive Systems

In emphasizing the importance of systems that support and sustain effective practices, SWPBS recommends that the following be in place: (1) team-based implementation, including the SWPBS team's developing a positive statement of purpose, completing a needs assessment, and implementing an action plan based on the needs assessment and consistent with the positive statement of purpose; (2) administrative leadership (e.g., direct and ongoing participation of the school principal); (3) the documented commitment of at least 80% of school staff members to actively participate and support the SWPBS program; (4) adequate personnel and time; (5) budgeted support; and (6) an adequate information system (e.g., newsletters, meetings).

Ongoing Collection and Use of Data for Decision Making

Recognizing the critical importance of data-based decision making, SWPBS schools collect data on an ongoing basis and use the data to guide decision making. Office disciplinary referrals provide the most common form of data used in SWPBS schools to assess student outcomes (e.g., Lohrmann-O'Rourke et al., 2000; Luiselli, Putnam, & Sunderland, 2002; Sadler, 2000; Taylor-Greene & Kartub, 2000). As recommended by Horner et al. (2005), SWPBS schools should organize and analyze disciplinary data "(1) per day and per month, (2) per type of problem behavior, (3) per location in the school, (4) per time of day, and (5) per child" (p. 374). Consistent with the ABA framework, such data are viewed as if one were conducting a functional behavioral assessment, except that a group of students rather than the individual child is the level of analysis (Scott & Caron, 2005; Sugai & Horner, 2002). For example, in understanding why a large number of office referrals tend to result from behavior on school buses, the SWPBS team might hypothesize that misbehavior on the bus serves the function of gaining attention. The team would then brainstorm developing a plan by which students would receive attention for more appropriate behavior on the bus.

KEY FEATURES
AS MEASURED BY THE SCHOOLWIDE EVALUATION TOOL

Perhaps the best representation of the key features of the SWPBS approach is seen in the School-wide Evaluation Tool (SET; Sugai, Lewis-Palmer, Todd, & Horner, 2001). The SET is widely used in both research and practice to document that schools have the key features of the SWPBS approach in place (Horner et al., 2004). The applied behavior analysis perspective of SWPBS is made clear in the following seven practices and systems measured by the 28 items of the SET. Note that each of the items is evaluated during brief individual interviews with students, staff members, and administrators and through a review of manuals, handbooks, and curriculum materials pertaining to schoolwide discipline.

1. *Expectations defined.* Two items assess whether the school has five or fewer "rules/behavioral expectations" that are positively stated and posted throughout the building.

2. *Behavioral expectations taught.* Five items assess the extent to which the rules or behavioral expectations are directly taught. Evidence that this system is in place is to be found in the students and staff being able to cite the school rules or behavioral expectations when interviewed.

3. *System of rewards.* Three items assess the school's "on-going system of rewarding behavioral expectations," which is observable through school materials and revealed that over 50% of students who are interviewed state that they have received a reward other than praise during the preceding 2 months and that 90% of staff members interviewed state that they have given rewards to students for behavior consistent with the school's rules and expectations.

4. *System for correcting behavior.* Four items measure the school's "system for responding to behavioral violations," which consists of a combination of positive and punitive techniques and the school's crisis management plan. Evidence is gleaned from the school's policy manuals.

5. *System for office disciplinary referrals.* Although this four-item section is called "monitoring, evaluating, and decision making," the only type of data addressed consists of office disciplinary referrals. Office disciplinary referral (ODR) forms are to include certain detailed information, and administrators and staff members are to report how ODR data are used. For example, the administrator is expected to "clearly define a system for collecting and summarizing discipline referrals."

6. *System of management.* Eight items target the management process the school uses to organize and oversee student behavior. Evidence that the school has an effective process or system in place should be found in the school's improvement or action plan, and in reports by the school's administrators and members of the PBS team on the composition of the team and how often it meets.

7. *System of district-level support.* Two items focus on budgetary support and whether or not there is a PBS liaison for the district or state.

The Benchmarks of Quality (BoQ; Cohen, Kincaid, & Childs, 2007) is another common tool used by many SWPBS programs to evaluate the extent to which key elements, or benchmarks, of SWPBS are in place. Items are very similar to those on the SET, but include a greater number (i.e., 50 benchmarks). Differing from the SET however, the BoQ is designed to be completed by staff within the school, thus not requiring external evaluators.

STRENGTHS AND LIMITATIONS OF SWPBS

Those considering the adoption of any approach to schoolwide discipline, as well as programs, strategies, and techniques associated with it, are wise to reflect upon that approach's strengths and limitations (see Table 2.1).

Strengths

Emphasis on Preventing Problem Behavior and Promoting "Positive" Behavior

For well over a decade now, *preventing*—rather than merely reacting to—various social, emotional, and behavioral problems has been a primary focus of nearly all mental health organizations as well as educational initiatives funded by the U.S. Department of Education (e.g., Safe and

> **SWPBS has a number of strengths. Its greatest strength is offering a variety of evidence-based behavioral techniques for preventing and correcting behavior problems.**

Healthy Schools, Character Education, and SWPBS) (Minke & Bear, 2000). SWPBS recognizes that a critical component of schoolwide discipline is the prevention of behavior problems and the promotion of appropriate behavior, which certainly includes teaching social skills. In light of the many shortcomings of the use of punishment (as discussed in Chapter

TABLE 2.1. Summary of Strengths and Limitations of the Horner and Sugai ABA Approach to SWPBS

Strengths

- Emphasis on a process.
- Emphasis on positive reinforcement as opposed to punishment.
- Goals of promoting safety and a positive school climate.
- Emphasis on evidence-based practices.
- Emphasis on collection and analysis of data.
- Behavioral interventions and supports for students who need them.
- A three-tiered approach to supports and services designed to serve all children.

Limitations

- Focus on short-term compliance, not the development of self-discipline.
- An underlying simplistic assumption that the direct teaching of rules and appropriate behavior, using principles of behaviorism, is sufficient for desired behavior.
- Limited perspective on the determinants of behavior.
- Failure to recognize the limitations of the systematic use of tangible rewards when used in a controlling manner.
- Failure to develop social cognitive and emotional competencies shown to foster prosocial behavior and inhibit antisocial behavior.
- Focus on office disciplinary referrals as a measure of effectiveness, with a lack of research demonstrating other important outcomes, including positive school climate, increased prosocial behavior, and lasting changes in behavior.
- Resistance from teachers.

1), a focus on prevention offers a much more effective—and positive—alternative to the zero-tolerance approach.

Focus on the Process of Systems Change

Consistent with research on school reform (e.g., Fullan, 2007), SWPBS clearly recognizes that successfully implementing any schoolwide program entails ongoing systems change. System change is complex, does not simply occur by decree, and rarely happens quickly. It takes time (a minimum of 3–5 years is often suggested) and is not always easy to achieve. A wide range of supports within the school system is necessary for planning, implementing, and sustaining school reform. Such supports include administrative leadership, staff commitment, ongoing staff development and training, time for staff to devote to planning and implementation, financial support, methods of communication, and perhaps most importantly team planning and decision making. Team planning and decision making involve a team of teachers, administrators, and support staff meeting frequently to plan, implement, and evaluate all phases of the program, ranging from developing goals and conducting an initial needs assessment to ensuring fidelity of implementation and evaluating data to improve the program. Largely through the Office of Special Education Programs (OSEP) Technical Assistance Center on Positive Behavioral Interventions and Supports, but also through private vendors and other agencies, thousands of schools have been provided with resources, materials, and staff training to help guide the systems changes involved in SWPBS.

Inclusion of All Students in a Three-Tiered Model of Prevention, Intervention, and Supports

The three-tier model adopted by SWPBS is certainly not new—or specific to SWPBS. It is commonly seen in mental health programs (Albee & Gullotta, 1997), and for good reasons. Not only does it emphasize the importance of prevention, especially among all students at the universal or Tier 1 level, but also perhaps more important it clearly recognizes that many students need more intensive interventions and supports. Although an estimated 15% of students at Tier 2 are deemed "at risk" and about 5% at Tier 3 have already exhibited serious and chronic behavior problems (Horner et al., 2005), research shows that in many schools, particularly urban schools, those percentages are gross underestimates of need (Wright & Dusek, 1998). Regardless of the specific percentage of students beyond Tier 1 requiring additional services and supports, an attractive feature of SWPBS is that, in emphasizing such services, it provides schools with much guidance in this area. This emphasis is consistent with its roots in special education. Providing such services and supports, including behavioral interventions, should be an important component of any schoolwide discipline program, and while it is frequently lacking in many popular models and approaches (Bear, 2005; Osher et al., 2010), it is a clear strength of SWPBS.

Emphasis on the Role of Environmental, and Alterable, Factors That Influence Student Behavior

Far too often, educators attribute the behavior problems of students to a wide range of student, home, peer, and community factors on which schools have very limited influence. Common among these factors are low ability, ADHD, poor parenting, poverty, poor role models, peer pressure, the influence of electronic media, and a student's history of problem behavior. By focusing on, or blaming, such factors, schools may inadvertently neglect factors influencing students' behavior that they *can* alter. SWPBS targets alterable factors in the school environment that commonly affect student behavior, including the clarity of expectations and rules, the quality of academic instruction, and home–school communication.

Use of Evidence-Based Behavioral Techniques

Ample research shows that positive reinforcement, punishment, and other techniques of ABA are quite effective in changing individual students' behavior, particularly in the short term (Alberto & Troutman, 2006; Landrum & Kauffman, 2006; Stage & Quiroz, 1997). Research also shows that effective classroom teachers use both behavioral and nonbehavioral techniques in preventing and correcting misbehavior among their students (Bear, 1998; Brophy, 1996). Behavioral techniques are particularly valuable in addressing the problems of students at risk of serious or chronic misbehavior or who are currently misbehaving (i.e., Tiers 2 and 3) (Kauffman & Landrum, 2008; Walker, Ramsey, & Gresham, 2004).

Positive behavioral techniques are also valuable at the schoolwide level for preventing and correcting behavior problems. While not specific to the SWPBS approach, research studies show that positive recognition of good behavior is a common characteristic of more efficacious schools (Catalano et al., 2004; Embry, 2002; Gottfredson et al., 1993, 1996). Similarly, they demonstrate that fair and consistent behavioral expectations are related to fewer behavior problems at the schoolwide level (Arum, 2003; Catalano et al., 2004; Doyle, 1986; Gottfredson et al., 1993, 1996).

Some research shows that the schoolwide use of behavioral techniques not only is effective for short-term changes in student behavior but also may lead to more lasting change. However, such research is largely limited to the Good Behavior Game (Barrish, Saunders, & Wolf, 1969; Embry, 2002; Kellam et al., 2008; Van Lier, Vuijk, & Crijnen, 2005), an interdependent group contingency program in which small groups of students within classrooms are given rewards based on good behavior, as described later in detail (Chapter 9). The extent to which the Good Behavior Game is used in SWPBS programs is unclear, however, as its use is seldom reported in the literature.

Ongoing Collection of Data

Reliable and valid data can serve multiple worthwhile purposes. For example, data from a needs assessment can indicate the areas of schoolwide discipline requiring the greatest attention as well as those areas that should be considered strengths. Similarly, evaluation data may indicate not only whether or not a given program is effective but also when and if modifications are needed. Data also are critical in persuading others (e.g., school boards and parents) that new programs are needed or that existing ones should continue to receive resources and financial support.

Limitations

Although the SWPBS approach has many notable strengths, it also has its limitations, as discussed below.

Neglect of the Role of Children's Cognitions and Emotions in Behavior and School Climate

Consistent with ABA theory and principles, environmental antecedents and consequences of behavior are seen as being the primary, if not exclusive, determinants of behavior. PBS has its roots firmly grounded in B. F. Skinner's operant behaviorism (1953), in which behavior is viewed as unidirectional, with environmental antecedents and consequences seen as the primary, if not exclusive, determinants of behavior. In this context, children's cognitions and emotions—how they think and feel—receive little, if any, attention. From its inception in January 1999 to the summer of 2009, the *Journal of Positive Interventions* published

26 articles that described SWPBS as practiced in schools, all of which reported the use of behavioral techniques, with 12 studies specifically referencing the systematic use of tokens to reinforce observable behaviors (e.g., following rules). Only 1 of those studies (i.e., Sadler, 2000) discussed children's thoughts and emotions, either in their interventions or measures of effectiveness. Generally, SWPBS programs were deemed effective if they resulted in reduced office disciplinary referrals, though no studies demonstrated a causal link between reduced ODRs and the use of positive behavioral techniques.

Peterson and Seligman (2004) have observed that "the hazards of a personless environmentalism are well-known within psychology" (p. 11). Indeed, no mainstream theory of developmental psychology views the individual as being purely passive in the process of learning and development (Dixon & Lerner, 1999). Instead, modern theories of developmental psychology clearly recognize multiple determinants of behavior and emphasize that cognitions and emotions mediate or influence, and are influenced by, one's environment (Bandura, 1986; Dodge, Coie, & Lynam, 2006; Eisenberg, 2006). In that light, undoubtedly one's environment, both immediate and distal, exerts a profound influence on student behavior, particularly in environments that are tightly controlled and regulated (such as prisons and many schools), where persons of authority, often assisted by electronic surveillance, constantly monitor and govern behavior. Yet, even in such contrived and controlling environments, an individual's thoughts and emotions influence behavior and the environment (Bandura, 1986). SWPBS neglects how thoughts and emotions of students influence both their behavior and the climate of the school.

Problems with the Maintenance and Generalization of Social Skills

Related to the SWPBS's unidirectional model of behavior and its failure to appreciate that students' thoughts and emotions often determine behavior, particularly when adults are not present, is the problem of maintaining and further generalizing social skills that are taught in SWPBS programs. That is, the social skills taught and learned through reinforcement and punishment often fail to be maintained once instruction ends. Students may also fail to generalize the new skills to settings outside of the context in which they were taught. Multiple reviews of the literature on social skills training have documented only small effect sizes for social skills training while concluding that there is little evidence that these social skills taught are either maintained or successfully generalized to other settings (Bullis, Walker, & Sprague, 2001; DuPaul & Eckert, 1994).

> "The failure of researchers to produce treatment effects that routinely generalize to other settings, times, and responses has been a sharp and essentially legitimate criticism of behavioral programming since its early application to classroom settings" (Landrum & Kauffman, 2006, p. 59).

Research also has failed to support the lecture or law-related education approach to teaching desired knowledge and behaviors (Gottfredson, 2001). This approach is similar to that of social skills training and SWPBS, in which the authorities simply tell and show students what constitutes "good behavior." The ineffectiveness of this approach is well documented in drug education programs (e.g., Drug Abuse Resistance Education [DARE]; Lynam et al., 1999). Finding that a direct approach to teaching appropriate behavior is insufficient for developing self-discipline is certainly not new in psychology and education. Some 80 years ago, in their classic studies of character that included over 10,000 students, Hartshorne and May (1928) found that directly teaching children moral knowledge, rules, or social skills did not necessarily translate into demonstrable moral behavior. Those who scored the highest on knowledge of the rules and codes of conduct were no less likely than those who scored lowest to violate such rules or codes (particularly to cheat or steal) subsequently once the external rewards, fear of punishment, and adult supervision were removed.

Underlying Assumption That All Children Require, and Benefit from, the Repeated Teaching of School Rules and Behavioral Expectations and the Systematic Use of External Rewards

Shortly upon entering elementary school, nearly all the students become familiar with the school's rules. To be sure, many fail to follow them, and very few follow them all the time, but relatively few students do not know what the rules are (just try offering one $10 to tell you the rule and to show you the appropriate behavior). Thus, repeatedly teaching school rules and reinforcing compliance are not sufficient, in and of themselves, to develop self-discipline. Programs with such an emphasis simply teach children to "be good for the sake of earning rewards and avoiding punishment," admittedly a somewhat hedonistic perspective. When the rewards and/or the fear of punishment are no longer salient, students are left with little reason to behave in the absence of their self-interest.

> **When external rewards and the fear of punishment are no longer present, students are left with little reason to behave.**

The SWPBS approach largely dismisses concerns among researchers that systematic praise and tangible rewards (particularly the latter) may have a negative long-term impact on students' intrinsic motivation. As discussed later (in Chapter 6), some research challenges the use of tokens and other tangible rewards in many SWPBS programs as the primary, if not exclusive, means of managing the behavior of students. Additional research in the area of moral reasoning shows that children who tend to focus primarily on earning rewards and avoiding punishment, rather than the impact of their behavior on others, are the ones most likely to violate school rules (Bear, Manning, & Shiomi, 2006; Manning & Bear, 2002). These findings are consistent with a wealth of research linking social and moral behavior to cognition and emotion—two aspects of development that rarely receive attention in the SWPBS approach. Cognitions and emotions, and how to develop them in the context of SWPBS, are discussed in Chapters 3 and 4.

The foregoing research findings do not mean that students should not be taught school rules, praised or rewarded for good behavior, or punished for inappropriate behavior. Instead, they suggest that such behavioral techniques are not sufficient in themselves to develop long-term self-discipline. Moreover, when not used wisely—for example, when not used in combination with techniques that focus on how students think and feel—ABA techniques that focus on external management of behavior may actually *undermine* the development of self-discipline. Fortunately, this limitation to many SWPBS programs can largely be avoided by using praise and rewards strategically.

Underlying Assumption That Because ABA Works with Individual Adults and Children with Severe Disabilities, It Must Also Work When Applied Schoolwide with All Children and Adolescents

SWPBS evolved from research demonstrating the effectiveness of ABA techniques in controlling and managing the behavior problems of adults with disabilities, particularly self-injurious behavior (e.g., head banging), aggression toward others, and pica (Dunlap, Sailor, Horner, & Sugai, 2009). Drawing largely from that research base, it is frequently stated in the PBS literature that nearly all behaviors serve one of two functions, either gaining attention or avoiding/escaping from situations or behaviors that are aversive (Crone & Horner, 2003; Day, Horner, & O'Neil, 1994). This rather simplistic understanding of the causes of human behavior is applied also to SWPBS. That is, just as special education teachers are advised to assess the functions of an individual's behavior when developing individualized education plans for students with disabilities (Day et al., 1994), so too are SWPBS schools advised to assess the functions of schoolwide behavior when they implement or modify schoolwide interventions (e.g., Bambara, 2005; Crone & Horner, 2003; Lewis, Newcomer, Trussell, & Richter, 2006; Sugai & Horner, 2009; Sugai et al., 2000). They are to determine which of those functions account for the behavior problems and to alter antecedents and consequences in the school accordingly. For example, if a large number of students were being sent to the office from several classes, the team might hypothesize that the students were misbehaving in order to avoid work and might counter the problem by further rewarding students for work completion. Although other researchers have recommended that additional functions of behavior should be recognized when conducting a functional behavioral assessment (FBA)—power/control, acceptance/affiliation, expression of self/gratification, or justice/revenge (Stoiber, 2004)—gaining attention and avoiding/escaping punishment receive primary, if not exclusive attention, in the SWPBS approach.

There are serious reasons to question the practical value of FBAs. To be sure, there is a wealth of single-subject design research that supports the usefulness of FBAs for both adults and children with serious behavior problems (Marquis et al., 2000). However, it is unclear whether FBAs can be conducted reliably in nonresearch settings; whether they lead to interventions that are any more effective than those not linked to FBAs; whether they are useful for students without disabilities, especially students beyond the early grades; whether they are useful for targeting behaviors for which antecedents and consequences are either not readily observable or are distal rather than proximal in their linkage to the behavior (e.g., substance use, many acts of aggression, stealing, cheating, lying); and finally whether they are a practical alternative in most schools, given the preceding limitations and the realization that they are not easy to conduct and often require additional personnel (Gresham et al., 2004; Landrum & Kauffman, 2006; Sasso, Conroy, Stichter, & Fox, 2001; Schill, Kratochwill, & Elliott, 1998; Scott et al., 2005). As noted by Landrum and Kauffman (2006, p. 62), "Although the idea of FBA may have legitimate conceptual roots, it has become a bandwagon on which many ride with little understanding or appreciation of its difficulty in practice."

Although the foregoing criticisms were directed primarily toward FBAs for individual students, they certainly apply to SWPBS, challenging the assertion by Sugai and Horner (2009) and others that schoolwide interventions should be grounded in FBAs. There is no research showing that FBAs can be conducted in a reliable manner at the schoolwide level or that the results improve the effectiveness of interventions.

Underlying Assumption That Teachers and Schools Are Primarily Accountable, and Thus to Blame, for the Behavior Problems of Their Students

With its emphasis on environmental antecedents and environmental consequences, an assumption inherent in the SWPBS approach is that teachers and schools—not students, families, and the wider community—are primarily responsible for student behavior. As noted by Marquis et al. (2000), "A key concept in PBS is that deficient contexts must be remediated first in order to reduce problem behavior" (p. 138). From the perspective of SWPBS, "deficient contexts" are classrooms and other school settings (e.g., cafeteria, hallways, gym) or wherever the school has authority (e.g., school bus, playground, sports events). When student behavior problems exist, such problems reflect deficit settings, which includes deficit teachers, administrators, and school staff. Student behavior is not viewed as a shared responsibility of teachers, students, and families but rather as the responsibility of those who control environmental antecedents and consequences in school.

When SWPBS is found to be ineffective, the almost automatic assumption is that the teachers and staff failed to implement interventions with fidelity. Indeed, this attribution—that the teachers, not the interventions or the programs per se, are to blame—often appears in the literature (e.g., Bohanan et al., 2006; Sugai & Horner, 2009; Sugai et al., 2008). There may be many reasons for a lack of fidelity in implementing a program—perhaps chief among them teacher resistance to, if not outright rejection of, an approach's philosophy or technique (Fullan, 2007). This observation certainly applies to SWPBS. That is, consistent with their university training and personal philosophy of school discipline, many teachers (particularly general education teachers) prefer a more student-centered perspective, or combined student-centered and teacher-centered perspective, rather than SWPBS's teacher-centered unidirectional perspective regarding school discipline. Indeed, as noted by Landrum and Kauffman (2006) in their review of the behavioral approach to classroom management, "Despite a rich history and extensive empirical underpinnings, the behavioral perspective on teaching and management is not highly regarded in the education community (see Axelrod, 1996)" (p. 47).

Landrum and Kauffman (2006) cite several reasons why educators often fail to embrace the behavioral approach, perhaps foremost among them is the lack of generalization of skills taught when behavioral techniques are used. As noted earlier, Landrum and Kauffman view this shortcoming as a legitimate criticism of the behavioral approach. Many educators are well aware that the effects of rewards and punishment are often short-term and specific to the behaviors and situations for which they are used. Although viewed by Landrum and Kauffman as a less legitimate criticism of the behavioral approach, another common reason for rejection of the approach is that many educators view behavioral techniques as forms of control, coercion, and bribery. As emphasized by Landrum and Kauffman, this criticism is valid only when behavioral techniques are *misused*. As they correctly note, behavioral techniques are "neither good nor bad" (p. 60) but are powerful tools that can be used as a means to achieve either a good or bad end. It is when the means and the end are one and the same—namely, to control or coerce students rather than to develop academic, social, and emotional competencies—that the behavioral approach is misapplied or applied in an ethically questionable manner. Unfortunately, whether the technique of choice is punishment or positive reinforcement, the behavioral approach often is used for social control. While many educators support and engage in such use, others reject it.

Empirical research also more directly challenges the SWPBS assumption that classroom and schoolwide environments determine student behavior (and thus an underlying assumption that teachers and schools are the primary source of behavior problems). The assumption that teachers and schools are the greatest determinants of student behavior is inconsistent with empirical research showing that the largest amount of variance in student behavior (Thomas, Bierman, Thompson, & Powers, 2008) and in school climate (Koth, Bradshaw, & Leaf, 2008; Vieno, Perkins, Smith, & Santinello, 2005) is explained not by differences between schools and classrooms but by differences among individual students. For example, Bierman et al. (2007) reported that 74.6% of aggressive and disruptive behavior was attributable to individual-level factors (with aggression and attention problems at home explaining most of the variance), 18.8% to classroom-level factors (e.g., teacher–student relationships, rules and expectations, classroom disruptions), and only 6.6% to school-level factors. At the practical level, these research findings are obvious to many educators, who observe that even the very best teachers and schools have students who exhibit behavior problems. It also is reflected in many students' *not* exhibiting behavior problems even when placed in poorly managed classrooms and schools. To be sure, teachers and schools still make a significant difference in student behavior, and factors in the school environment that influence student behavior should be a focus of any schoolwide discipline program. However, by focusing solely on the school environment while largely overlooking the critical importance of children's thoughts and emotions in self-discipline and of adult–student relations (other than providing support via praise and rewards), SWPBS fails to address individual and interpersonal factors that have consistently been shown to account for the greatest variance in student behavior and school climate.

ODRs Are the Primary, If Not Exclusive, Measure of Program Effectiveness

Numerous case studies of individual SWPBS schools have reported a reduction in ODRs (e.g., Bohanon et al., 2006; Ervin, Schaughency, Matthews, Goodman, & McGlinchey, 2007; Luiselli, Putnam, Handler, & Feinberg, 2002; McIntosh, Chard, Boland, & Horner, 2006; Sprague et al., 2001; Taylor-Greene et al., 1997). Indeed, reducing office disciplinary referrals, rather than improving school climate and other aspects of schoolwide discipline, is the primary, if not sole, outcome (or goal) measured in many SWPBS programs. This preoccupation with ODRs flies in the face of researchers' repeated citation of their limitations or shortcomings (Morrison, Redding, Fisher, & Peterson, 2006; Sugai et al., 2000; Tobin & Sugai, 1999; Wright & Dusek, 1998); which include:

- Inconsistencies exist across schools and over time in referral procedures (e.g., a new principal, or changes in the district's code of conduct).
- Inconsistencies exist across schools and teachers, and over time, in teachers' tolerance levels and disciplinary practices (e.g., changes due to staff turnover, staff training, time of year).
- Inconsistencies even exist within individual teachers in reasons or justifications for a referral (e.g., the same teacher might tolerate the behavior of one child but not of another or might tolerate the behavior one day and not the next).
- ODRs do not necessarily reflect the full range of social, emotional, and behavioral problems (e.g., minor classroom disruption, internalizing problems, social-cognitive deficits, etc.), and do not reflect the development of protective factors or related strategies (e.g., emotional and cognitive development). Instead, they may simply reflect changes in the use of punishment, specifically sending a child to the office.
- ODRs tend to underestimate the severity of disciplinary problems.
- A reduction in office referrals does not necessarily reflect a more positive school climate or development of self-discipline (indeed, it is just as likely to reflect the opposite—greater external control and governance by the teachers themselves).

General Lack of Research Supporting SWPBS

Although SWPBS has now been implemented in thousands of schools for over a decade, there is remarkably little empirical research supporting its effectiveness. With few exceptions, evidence of its effectiveness is limited to case studies that show the SWPBS process can be implemented with fidelity (as assessed by the SET) (Bohanon et al., 2006; McIntosh et al., 2006; Muscott, Mann, & LeBrun, 2008; Scott & Barrett, 2004) and that such implementation coincides with decreased in ODRs (Lassen, Steele, & Sailor, 2006). To date, there are no published comparative studies demonstrating that SWPBS is any more effective than other schoolwide discipline programs. Likewise, there are no longitudinal studies showing that SWPBS leads to lasting changes in any important outcome.

Particularly lacking are randomized controlled studies, deemed by most researchers as necessary for demonstrating program effectiveness. There are several exceptions, however. Using a randomized control group design, Koth et al. (2008) reported no differences in school climate between SWPBS and non-SWPBS schools after 1-year of implementation. Two randomized control group studies of elementary schools (Bradshaw, Koth, Bevans, Ilongo, & Leaf, 2008; Horner et al., 2009) reported improvements in school climate. However, in both studies school climate was evaluated by the same school staff that actually implemented the program. Moreover, improvements were found in very limited areas of school climate and/or with measures of questionable validity. Bradshaw et al. used the Organizational Health Inventory for Elementary Schools (OHI; Hoy & Feldman, 1987), a validated measure of staff reports of five dimensions of the school's organizational health. They found statistically significant differences in favor of SWPBS schools on two of the five dimensions (resource influence, which measures the principal's ability to acquire school resources and positively allocate school resources; and staff affiliation, which measures positive relations among staff) and in overall OHI scores. A marginally significant difference was found for academic emphasis, and no significant difference was found for either collegial leadership or institutional integrity. When differences were found, effect sizes were small, ranging from 0.26 to 0.34.

In their randomized wait-list control study, Horner et al. (2009) used the School Safety Survey (SSS; Sprague, Colvin, & Irvin, 1996) to measure school climate. This measure yields a risk factor score and a protective factor score. No research has been published on the validity of the measure, including its factorial validity. Nevertheless, differences between SWPBS and non-SWPBS schools and improvements in SWPBS schools (as reported by the school staff in each of the schools) were found only in risk factor scores. It is unclear, however, whether the differences in the scores reflected differences in school safety per se, as claimed by the researchers, or simply differences in risk factors related to school safety. For example, among the 13 items on the risk factor scale are "Poverty," "High student mobility," "Truancy," and "Graffiti," and "Students adjudicated by the courts." The researchers were unable to examine differences in ODR-levels because those data were either missing in too many schools or deemed by the researchers as not meeting appropriate standards. The researchers noted that the percentage of students with ODRs in SWPBS schools was slightly less than the national average. However, the same data also show that ODRs actually increased *in absolute terms* over time in SWPBS schools.

Not only is there a lack of research supporting SWPBS per se, but also reviews of the research literature should encourage educators to question the effectiveness and value of behavioral techniques in general when applied schoolwide as the primary or only means of preventing behavior problems. For example, in a meta-analysis limited to studies that employed a randomized control group design, Lösel and Beelman (2003) reported that cognitive and cognitive-behavioral programs were twice as effective as behavioral programs when one looked at studies that included a follow-up measure. Wilson, Lipsey, and Derzon (2003) reported similar findings, particularly when examining the most rigorous experimental studies (programs using randomized control groups and most likely to have been implemented with fidelity) and statistically controlling for the number of students with serious behavior problems (a correlate of program effectiveness). Under those conditions, they found that social-cognitive programs were three times more effective than behavioral programs.

Emphasis on Social Control Rather Than Self-Control or Self-Discipline

Perhaps the greatest weakness of the SWPBS approach to schoolwide discipline is that too often its primary aim is to bring about compliance to rules and expectations, as measured by reduced ODRs. The aim of schoolwide discipline—to manage or control student behavior—is the same as that of zero-tolerance programs. Only the means used to achieve that aim differ, with SWPBS employing positive instead of punitive techniques. Whether it is in the form of punishment or positive reinforcement, too often techniques of ABA are used for the purpose of social control of student behavior (Center for Mental Health in Schools, 2008; Kohn, 1996, 1999). When SWPBS programs operate—or are perceived by students and faculty to operate—in this fashion (irrespective of intent), they do little to develop self-discipline, improve school climate, or engage students in learning.

Rarely does one find in the SWPBS literature any discourse or research on how students internalize the school's societal values and norms or come to manage their own behavior when external rewards and punishment are not salient. Likewise, it often is very unclear what values and norms SWPBS advocates believe should be internalized, other than what is expected and required by adults in the school. Typically, one often finds that the schoolwide behavioral expectations and techniques used in preschool and elementary schools are the same ones used in high school. For example, responsibility and respect are taught via social skills training and token reinforcement systems. As spelled out further in Chapter 6, not only are the techniques used in SWPBS insufficient for developing self-discipline but also when used in a controlling manner they may well undermine it. SWPBS researchers either downplay or dismiss altogether research that questions the long-term positive impact of the systematic use of praise and/or tangible rewards on developing intrinsic motivation (e.g., Deci, Koestner, & Ryan, 2001). As recently observed by the Center for Mental Health in Schools (2008), "Care must be taken not to over-rely on extrinsics to entice and reward because to do so may decrease intrinsic motivation" (p. 6-9). The Center further notes that "enhancing intrinsic motivation is a fundamental *protective* factor and is the key to developing *resiliency*" (p. 6–9).

> Too often, "behavioral support" consists of a form of "social control aimed directly at reducing disruptive behavior" (Center for Mental Health in Schools, 2008, p. 6–4).

SWPBS: ADOPT? REJECT? OR INTEGRATE?

As discussed above, a major strength of ABA techniques of is that they often are effective in the management of student behavior, especially in the short term. It would be difficult to imagine classrooms and schools in which the basic principles of reinforcement and punishment were not employed. Unfortunately, however, too many schools *overemphasize* punishment to the exclusion of other methods and techniques. The SWPBS approach offers an alternative to those schools that are managing student behavior solely by using punishment, namely, using positive reinforcement instead.

Other schools, however, might have less need to manage student behavior by using external techniques of behavioral control and therefore aim as well to develop self-discipline. Such schools should not reject the use of behavioral techniques associated with SWPBS. ABA techniques are often valuable in managing and correcting student behavior. Moreover, as discussed throughout this book, when used in combination with other techniques, ABA techniques foster the long-term development of self-discipline. However, because these ABA techniques, as implemented in SWPBS programs, are insufficient to develop self-discipline, most schools should consider either (1) adopting the evidence-based SEL approach to schoolwide discipline that aims to develop self-discipline or (2) integrating the techniques of the SWPBS approach with those of the SEL approach. The latter alternative is recommended in this book.

> **There are different definitions of SWPBS. SWPBS does not have to be only behavior modification, and it shouldn't be.**

A question often emerges when the integrated/combined strategy is taken, however, namely, "Is the school now an SWPBS school?" The answer depends on what definition and perspective toward SWPBS one accepts. If one views PBS and behavior modification as the "same approach with different names" (Horner, 2000, p. 99), as seen in the SWPBS approach, then by integrating SWPBS with another approach that is not behavior modification, the resulting approach should not be referred to as SWPBS but more accurately as a combined approach. However, if one views SWPBS more broadly and as "a generic term and construct that represents a broad set of potential components" (Knoff, 2008, p. 749), then a combination of approaches to schoolwide discipline would fall under the more general umbrella of SWPBS, including the more narrowly focused and popular SWPBS approach of Horner and Sugai. Several definitions capture the more generic meaning to SWPBS. George, Harrower, and Knoster (2003) define SWPBS as

> simply . . . establishing specific guidelines and providing proactive prevention and support for all students and faculty in a given school. The goal is to nurture the emergence of a school culture that promotes positive or appropriate behavior and learning, seeks to prevent problem or inappropriate behavior, and operates through collaborative data-based decision making to build a positive school climate. (p. 171)

Similarly, Sugai and Horner (2009) emphasized "school culture" in recently defining SWPBS as "a systems approach for establishing the social culture and individualized behavior supports needed for a school to be a safe and effective learning environment for all students" (p. 309). An attractive feature these two definitions share is the emphasis on "school culture"—a major focus of the approach advocated in this volume.

SUMMARY

With its emphasis on the systematic and schoolwide use of positive reinforcement of desired behaviors, the SWPBS approach offers an attractive alternative to the frequent use of punishment seen in the zero-tolerance approach to school discipline. However, there are numerous other approaches to schoolwide discipline that emphasize the value of positive techniques, though not necessarily positive reinforcement. Key to the SWPBS approach are three features: (1) an emphasis on measurable outcomes; (2) the manner in which positive reinforcement is implemented, typically through the systematic posting of behavioral expectations throughout the school and the use of token economics; and (3) seeking to manage student behavior by controlling the external use of rewards (and punishment).

Each feature can be viewed as both a strength and a weakness. Whereas an emphasis on measurable outcomes is clearly a strength, too often the only measurable outcome is ODRs, which have several limitations. This shortcoming can be addressed, however, by using additional outcome measures, such as measures of school climate (see Chapter 11 and Appendix B). Communicating clear expectations and rules also is chiefly a strength, as research has consistently confirmed. The systematic use of reinforcement, especially token systems, may be of value in classrooms and some schools with significant behavior problems but is of questionable utility and value in most schools. As discussed in Chapters 6 and 7, praise and the occasional use of external rewards are likely to be sufficient, and often more effective, especially in the long term.

Finally, the third key feature of SWPBS—the aim of managing student behavior by controlling the external use of rewards (and punishment)—is also both a strength and a weakness. To be sure, many students do not exhibit self-discipline, and for them external rewards and punishment are often necessary and effective in managing their behavior. When used wisely, external rewards and punishment can also help foster self-discipline. Problems arise, however, when managing students' behavior, rather than developing the cognitions and feelings associated with self-discipline, becomes the school's primary aim. Fortunately, as with other shortcomings of SWPBS, this too can largely to be addressed by using ABA techniques not in a controlling manner (except when necessary) and always in combination with other techniques that focus on students' cognitions and emotions. How this can be done is the focus of the remainder of this book.

CHAPTER 3

Self-Discipline and the Social and Emotional Learning Approach to School Discipline

WHAT IS SELF-DISCIPLINE?

Used in the context of school discipline, *self-discipline* refers to students regulating their own behavior with minimal adult monitoring and use of external rewards and punishment. *Self-discipline* is often used interchangeably with the terms *responsibility, self-regulation, self-control, and autonomy. Self-discipline* refers to students deciding and choosing what actions to take and assuming responsibility for their actions. It entails knowing what's right, desiring to do what is right, and then *doing* what is right. It reflects *intrinsic* rather than extrinsic motivation. Although external rewards and the fear of punishment might certainly provide rea-

> **Self-discipline** refers to students regulating their own behavior with minimal adult monitoring and use of external rewards and punishment.

sons or motives to behave, they alone do not determine one's choice of behavior. That is, the choice to act prosocially and to inhibit antisocial behavior is made even when external rewards and punishment are not salient in a given situation. For example, the decision not to steal a purse is based not on the risk of getting caught or the promise of a reward (either money in the purse or a reward from others for not stealing) but on an understanding of the impact of stealing on others, the anticipation of feelings of guilt, and an appreciation of rules, laws, property rights, and moral principles of trust, respect, and honesty. In addition to *self-discipline*'s referring to students' behavior not being motivated by external rewards and fear of punishment, it also refers to students being able to delay gratification—to forgo immediate rewards for more important longer-term outcomes (e.g., "I don't need a token for good behavior—I can wait until my report card to be recognized for my behavior").

Unfortunately, students can be intrinsically motivated not only to behave but also to misbehave. But, just as *school discipline* is never used in the context of teaching students to misbehave, so too is *self-discipline* used in a similar manner in this book—to connote that students should learn to manage their own behavior and that such behavior should be socially and morally responsible, consistent with desired values and beliefs of society in general and hopefully of one's school. Taught both directly and indirectly throughout schooling, over time those values and beliefs become *internalized*, or adopted by students as their own (Grusec & Goodnow, 1994). As such, students strive to adhere to them and to act in a manner consistent with self-chosen social and moral values and beliefs.

As discussed in Chapter 1, developing self-discipline is one of three components of comprehensive classroom and universal-level schoolwide discipline. The other equally important, and interrelated, components are the prevention and correction of behavior problems. Developing students' self-discipline should be among every school's primary long-term aims, but it would be naïve to expect all students to demonstrate self-discipline all of the time. Very few adults do so, as may be seen in their speeding violations, littering, cheating, adultery, and countless other common violations of laws and ethical principles. Because self-discipline is a developmental phenomenon, expectations for students' self-discipline should be much less in elementary school than in high school. That is, developmentally speaking, greater adult supervision and management of student behavior should be expected with younger students (as well as with older students who continue to think and act like younger students). As children grow older, they increasingly monitor their own behavior, guided by their own values, goals, and standards that typically mirror those of significant others in their lives, including teachers. Developing self-discipline is a long-term goal. It takes time and is much more difficult to achieve than the short-term objective of complying with rules or obeying authorities.

SELF-DISCIPLINE VERSUS COMPLIANCE

To be sure, self-discipline includes compliance with rules and authority, but in developing self-discipline one's aim is to bring about what is referred to as *committed* compliance (Kochanska, 2002) or *willing* compliance (Brophy, 1996). Committed compliance is motivated by a sense of pride in one's decisions and behavior, a sense of autonomy, and respect for rules and the legitimate authority of those imposing them. This type contrasts with *situational* compliance (Kochanska, 2002) or *grudging* compliance (Brophy, 1996), which is motivated not by such appealing considerations but rather by fear of punishment or the promise of external rewards. Committed compliance should be both a short-term and long-term goal. When it is not forthcoming, however, educators must settle for situational compliance, motivated by either rewards or fear of punishment, preferably the former.

For centuries, such educators, philosophers, and researchers as Locke, Rousseau, Montessori, Dewey, Piaget, and Kohlberg have questioned whether *external* control of behavior is effective or sufficient for developing *internal* control, or self-discipline. More recently, authors of many popular models of classroom management and school discipline have emphasized the aim of developing self-discipline while questioning whether external techniques of behavior management are the best means of achieving it. Such models include those of Glasser (1965, 1969, 1986, 1998), logical consequences (Dreikurs & Grey, 1968), teacher effectiveness training (Gordon, 2003), cooperative discipline (Albert, 1996), discipline with dignity (Curwin, Mendler, & Mendler, 2008), love and logic (Fay & Funk, 1995), positive discipline (Nelsen et al., 2000), and responsive classrooms (Charney, 2002). Consistent with the views of all of the authors of those models, Glasser (1969) states that too many educators confuse conformity with responsibility and that responsibility is *"something to which we give lip service but which we do not teach in school"* (p. 22). Likewise, Curwin, Mendler, and Mendler, authors of *Discipline with Dignity* (2008), argue that there are two basic models of school discipline, the responsibility (or self-discipline) model and the obedience model, and that the latter is ineffective and insults the dignity of students.

H. Jerome Freiberg, in *Beyond Behaviorism: Changing the Classroom Management Paradigm* (1999), argues that the teacher-centered approach to school discipline, as seen in the use of behavior modification and ABA, teaches obedience and compliance but fails to develop self-discipline. He posits that a student-centered approach is needed to develop autonomy, or self-discipline. As noted by Freiberg (1999), "Self-discipline is built over time and encompasses multiple sources of experiences. It requires a learning environment that nurtures opportunities to learn from one's own experiences, including mistakes, and to reflect on these experiences" (p. 13).

Author and journalist Alfie Kohn is perhaps the most popular and harshest critic of the use of rewards and punishment to manage and control student behavior—which he refers to as the obedience model of school discipline. His books, written for the general public, are widely read by educators and parents and include *Beyond Discipline: From Compliance to Community* (Kohn, 1996) and *Punished by Rewards: The Trouble with Gold Stars, Incentive Plans, A's, Praise, and Other Bribes* (Kohn, 1999). Kohn asserts that autonomy should be the primary aim of school discipline and that an emphasis on compliance undermines autonomy. Moreover, he argues that autonomy is achieved only when students play an active role in constructing their own values—deciding which values are important, reflecting upon those values, understanding why they are important, and believing they are an important part of one's self-identity.

In sum, criticism of models of discipline that emphasize compliance and obedience is not new. Critics have included well-known researchers, philosophers, educators, and authors of books written for the general public. They argue that obedience and compliance, especially based on rewards and punishment, should never be the primary aim of education. Instead, the primary aim should be the development of cognitions and emotions that underlie autonomy and morally and socially responsible behavior, which is referred to as self-discipline in this book.

THE SEL APPROACH

The view that students' cognitions and emotions, and not just their behavior, are of critical importance in classroom and schoolwide discipline is best represented by what is referred to as the social and emotional learning approach (Collaborative for Academic, Social, and Emotional Learning [CASEL], 2005; see *www.CASEL.org*; also see Merrell & Gueldner, 2010, for a recent review of SEL). SEL refers to "the process of acquiring and effectively applying the knowledge, attitudes, and skills necessary to recognize and manage emotions; developing caring and concern for others; making responsible decisions; establishing positive relationships; and handling challenging situations capably" (Zins & Elias, 2006, p. 1).

Supporting Theory and Research

With respect to its philosophy toward education and learning, the SEL approach to classroom and schoolwide discipline is student-centered, grounded in the works of John Dewey (1908/1960) and much more in the constructivist theories of learning (Piaget, 1932/1965; Vygotsky, 1934/1987) than behavioral theory (Skinner, 1953, 1966). As such, students are viewed as active rather than passive learners, and the aim of education is believed to be not the direct transmission of knowledge and teaching of social skills, as propounded in behaviorism, but the development of self-governing and responsible citizens in a democratic society. SEL is firmly grounded in, and supported by, theory and research in many areas of psychology, but particularly the following:

- Social-cognitive theory (Bandura, 1986)
- Social information processing (Crick & Dodge, 1994)
- Social problem solving (Spivack, Platt, & Shure, 1976)
- Resilience (Doll, Zucker, & Brehm, 2004; Werner, 1982)
- Connectedness and caring (Noddings, 2002; Battistich & Ham, 1997; Battistich, Solomon, Watson, & Schaps, 1997)
- Moral development (Kohlberg, 1981)
- Prosocial development (Eisenberg, Fabes, & Spinrad, 2006)
- Emotions (Goleman, 1995; Izard, 2002; Saarni, 1999)
- Attachment (Ainsworth, 1989; Bowlby, 1982)
- Peer relations and friendship (Rubin, Bukowski, & Parker, 2006)
- Self-concept (Harter, 2006),
- Self-determination (Ryan & Deci, 2000)
- Attribution theory (Weiner, 2006)
- Social motivation (Wentzel, 2006)
- Student engagement, or school engagement (Appleton, Christenson, & Furlong, 2008; Fredricks, Blumenfeld, & Paris, 2004)
- Ecology of human development (Bronfenbrenner, 1979)
- Authoritative discipline (Baumrind, 1971, 1996)
- Primary prevention (Albee & Gullotta, 1997)

Targeted Social and Emotional Competencies

Instead of mere compliance, the primary aim of SEL is to develop individuals' qualities, strengths, assets, or competencies associated with positive mental health, which includes reducing individual, relational, and environmental risk factors associated with negative emotional, social, and academic outcomes (Durlak, Weissberg, Dymnicki, Taylor, & Schellinger, in press). In contrast to the SWPBS approach, SEL targets not only how students act but also how they think and feel. SEL also places great emphasis on relational contexts in which social and emotional competencies are best developed. As such, close and supportive teacher–student and student–student relationships are viewed as critical to developing social and emotional competencies as well as crucial aspects of school climate. Similarly, many SEL programs also emphasize school–home relationships.

Five social and emotional competencies that are critical to positive mental health are targeted in SEL programs (CASEL, 2005), namely:

- *Self awareness*, consisting of students recognizing and understanding their emotions, interests, values, strengths, and weaknesses. It incorporates both self-concept and self-confidence.
- *Social awareness*, consisting of social perspective taking, empathy, recognition and respect for individual and group differences, and the ability to seek and use family, school, and community resources.
- *Responsible decision making at school, home, and in the community*, consisting of the ability to make decisions that are socially and morally responsible—based on students' understanding and appreciation of the impact of their behavior on themselves and others, issues of justice, safety, sense of community, and caring about others.
- *Self-management of emotions and behavior*, including appropriate expression of emotions, stress and anger management, delay of gratification, impulse control, resilience, setting goals and striving to achieve them, and the ability to persevere when faced with setbacks and obstacles.
- *Relationship skills*, consisting of the ability to establish and maintain positive and cooperative relationships with others, resist peer pressures, resolve interpersonal conflicts peacefully, and seek and provide help when needed.

Those competencies are taught and developed both directly and indirectly. Directly, they are taught in curriculum lessons, either in a packaged commercial program, such as those for preventing bullying or school violence, or in the school's regular curriculum (e.g., lessons embedded in language arts or social studies). Great attention is given to the developmental appropriateness of the lessons. That is, different skills are taught at different grade levels and different strategies and techniques are used. Competencies also are directly taught in the context of class meetings, school assemblies, and disciplinary encounters. Indirectly, competencies are developed through modeling and planned activities in which students apply, practice, and hone their social and emotional skills, such as in student government, class discussions, peer mediation, service learning, clubs, and sports.

Close and Supportive Relationships, Especially between Teachers and Students

The SEL approach recognizes that, just as these five competencies promote close and supportive relationships with others, so too do close and supportive relationships with others foster the development of these competencies. Close and supportive relationships between teachers/staff and students are of particular importance in developing self-discipline, as seen in research reviewed later in this chapter. Although teacher–student relationships are a primary focus in SEL, the importance of student–student and home–school relationships is also clearly recognized and those relationships also are targeted for intervention.

> **Close and supportive relationships are critical to social and emotional learning!**

PROGRAMS INCLUDED UNDER THE SEL APPROACH

SEL includes a wide range of programs that aim to develop social and emotional competencies, including school-based preventive programs in the areas of bullying, school violence, sexual diseases, and drug, alcohol, and tobacco use (Zins & Elias, 2006). This area of emphasis includes evidence-based models of classroom management and discipline, such as Responsive Classrooms (Charney, 2002), that object to compliance as a primary aim of education and that stress the development of social and moral responsibility and positive mental health. The CASEL (2005) has reviewed 80 SEL programs, rating each as to its effectiveness and utility. Among the most evidence-based programs (i.e., those in which randomized control groups were employed) that have been shown to be effective in reducing behavior problems in school are Second Step: A Violence Prevention Curriculum (Committee for Children, 2003; Fitzgerald & Van Schoiack-Edstrom, 2006), Steps to Respect: A Bully Prevention Program (Committee for Children, 2001; see Hirschstein & Frey, 2006, for a review), Promoting Alternative Thinking Strategies (PATHS; Greenberg & Kusche, 2006), and the Caring School Community (Watson & Battistich, 2006).

Finally, SEL subsumes two other approaches to building social and emotional competencies that are currently popular in psychology and education: character education and positive psychology. Each of these two approaches is discussed below.

Character Education

The Character Education Partnership (*www.cep.org*), which is a consortium of national organizations that includes the National Association of School Psychologists and the National Education Association, defines character education as how schools help students to "understand, care about, and act upon core ethical values" (Character Education Partnership, 2004, p. 1). Character education places greater emphasis than do other SEL programs on the moral dimension of behavior, which encompasses moral values, moral action, moral emotion, moral reasoning, moral personality, and moral identity (Berkowitz & Schwartz, 2006). Thus, although character education targets each of the five SEL competencies previously listed, it specifically addresses itself to the fourth competency—decision making that is socially and morally responsible, grounded in caring about others and issues of justice. This focal point includes developing empathy, empathy-based guilt, and moral reasoning that underlie an understanding and appreciation of fairness, honesty, trust, integrity, respect, duty, safety, interpersonal relationships, and the sense of community (Berkowitz & Schwartz, 2006; Character Education Partnership, 2004). Although there are many evidence-based programs that target these competencies (Berkowitz & Bier, 2004), the Caring School Community (Watson & Battistich, 2006) stands out as being the most comprehensive research-supported program in character education and SEL (see *www.Devstu.org*).

> **SEL includes character education and positive psychology.**

Positive Psychology

SEL includes the positive psychology approach to mental health, which has gained increased attention among educators and school psychologists in recent years (Gilman, Huebner, & Furlong, 2009). Although models and programs of school discipline specific to positive psychology have not yet emerged, many programs in SEL, and especially character education programs, are consistent with the basic tenets of positive psychology (Bear, 2009). Similar to character education, positive psychology emphasizes the development of global character strengths and virtues, or personality traits that generalize across situations. However, as compared to character education and other SEL programs, greater emphasis is placed on promoting subjective self-satisfaction (i.e., happiness). With respect to schoolwide discipline, programs consistent with the basic tenets of positive psychology manifest the following four features (Bear, 2009):

1. *A primary aim is the development of character strengths and virtues of self-discipline related to mental health and emotional well-being.* Among the character strengths and virtues highlighted in positive psychology (Peterson & Seligman, 2004), the following are most important to self-discipline:

- Self-regulation—regulating one's emotions and behavior
- Social intelligence—awareness of the motives and feelings of oneself and others
- Citizenship—social responsibility, loyalty, and teamwork
- Fairness—applying principles of justice and caring in relations with others
- Authenticity—being genuine and speaking the truth
- Kindness—helping others

Each of these virtues is viewed as an aspect of one's personality that generalizes across most situations. Although situational contexts are clearly recognized as influencing student behavior, emphasis is placed on the character strengths and virtues that explain why most students act fairly consistently across different situational contexts (e.g., why across the same high school classes Madison is consistently well behaved and Katie is not).

2. *Another primary aim is to help children meet three basic human needs; namely, the need for competence, belongingness, and autonomy.* These three needs are viewed as central to self-determination and intrinsic motivation as well as to overall mental health and subjective well-being (Ryan & Deci, 2000, 2006; Ryan, Deci, Grolnick, & LaGuardia, 2006). They also are important to self-discipline in that self-discipline is readily stifled when students believe they not competent, are not accepted or loved by others, and do not have at least some measure of control over their own lives.

3. *The program develops behaviors, thoughts, and emotions reflecting certain character strengths and virtues.* Those character strengths and virtues are listed above under item 1. Consistent with the constructivist approach to human development, character strengths and virtues are seen as means of integrating an individual's thoughts, feelings, and actions. As is true with the SEL approach in general, programs consistent with the positive psychology approach place greater emphasis on strategies and techniques that develop not only desired actions but also the social and emotional mechanisms that underlie them. Teaching students *how* to decide what is right and wrong, and *why*, is viewed as being of equal, if not greater, importance than teaching students *what* to do. Thus, although students certainly learn that it is generally important to follow rules and obey those in positions of legitimate authority, they also learn that in some situations not following rules and obeying others can be a character strength or virtue (e.g., opposing unjust rules and resisting peer pressure).

4. *The program emphasizes the use of evidence-based positive techniques that prevent behavior problems.* The primary aims of positive psychology are to develop character strengths and virtues and meet the basic needs of students. In achieving these two aims, behavior problems are prevented. Just as these aims are positive ones, so too should be the

> " . . . The absence of a weakness is not in and of itself a strength" (Peterson & Seligman, 2004, p. 22).

means of achieving them. As such, rather than the frequent use of punishment and rewards to manage and correct behavior, positive psychology emphasizes the use of a variety of evidence-based strategies and techniques for developing the assets and competencies underlying self-discipline. Emphasis is placed on preventing problem behavior not only by developing self-discipline but also by creating and maintaining a positive school climate characterized by high behavioral expectations and by caring and support. Thus, although correction is used when necessary and appropriate, the emphasis is placed not on decreasing problem behavior but on developing social and emotional assets and strengths. Interventions of choice are those supported by theory and empirical research, particularly in the areas of positive emotions, positive character, and positive institutions (Seligman & Csikszentmihalyi, 2000; Seligman, Steen, Park, & Peterson, 2005).

RESEARCH SUPPORTING
THE IMPORTANCE OF SELF-DISCIPLINE AND SEL

A 2000 Gallup poll found that while the general public supports zero tolerance toward serious behavior problems, it nonetheless believes that the most important purpose of public education is "to prepare students to be responsible citizens" (Rose & Gallup, 2000). Not only does the general public support the importance of self-discipline, but so too does a wealth of research findings. Such research is derived from four main sources: (1) studies linking specific social and emotional processes, deficiencies, and competencies to the presence or absence of behavior problems; (2) studies linking social and emotional competencies, particularly self-discipline, to highly valued outcomes other than the absence of behavior problems; (3) studies supporting the important role of teacher–student relationships in developing self-discipline and improving school climate; and (4) studies demonstrating the effectiveness of programs, strategies, and techniques commonly used in SEL to develop self-discipline and other social and emotional competencies. Research in these four areas is summarized below.

Social and Emotional Processes, Deficiencies, and Competencies Linked to Self-Discipline and Behavior Problems

A large number of studies have identified various cognitive and emotional processes, deficiencies, and competencies associated with student behavior, both aggressive and prosocial, but especially the former. Many of them have been shown to serve as mediators of behavior. For example, anger has been shown to be related to aggression (Lochman, Powell, Clanton, & McElroy, 2006), with the effects of anger on other-directed aggression being indirect, mediated by such cognitive and emotional processes as whether or not the person experiencing the anger blames others and manages to regulate the anger. Educators witness examples of this nearly every day. For example, three students may experience the same teasing from others but react differently: the first one ignores the teasing and experiences no anger, another becomes angry but manages the anger well, and the third attributes hostility to the teaser, becomes angry, and then attacks the teaser verbally and physically.

Social-cognitive and emotional processes and deficiencies that have most commonly been shown to be related to problems of school discipline are listed in Table 3.1. It should be noted that many are interrelated and often work in combination. For example, on many occasions students react impulsively while failing to consider multiple alternatives and the consequences of their actions. Likewise, in a given situation the influence of each process and deficiency is often influenced by a variety of situational factors, such as the clarity of the circumstances involved, the emotional or physical closeness to others involved, peer pressure, and the saliency of adult supervision, rewards, and punishment (Crick & Dodge, 1994; Eisenberg et al., 2006). In turn, however, one's thoughts, emotions, and behavior often influence those situational factors. For example, peer pressure can influence one's decision making, but so too can one's decisions influence peers and how they act in a given situation. Likewise, just as the classroom and school climate certainly influence students' thoughts, feelings, and behavior, so too do the thoughts, feelings, and behavior of students determine classroom and school climate. The effects are reciprocal.

Given their linkage to either antisocial or prosocial behavior, the social-cognitive and emotional processes in Table 3.1 are commonly targeted in SEL programs and particularly those with the aim of developing self-discipline.

Relation of Self-Discipline and SEL to Other Important Outcomes

A growing body of research shows that the social-cognitive and emotional competencies of self-discipline, including the lack of certain deficiencies and deficits enumerated in Table 3.1, are related not only to antisocial and prosocial behavior but to additional outcomes highly valued by educators and society in general. These include (1) academic achievement, (2) positive relationships with others, (3) positive self-worth and emotional well-being, and (4) positive classroom and school climate (Bear, Manning, & Izard, 2003). Research in each of these areas is discussed below.

> **SEL promotes: (1) academic achievement, (2) positive relationships with others, (3) self-worth and emotional well-being, and (4) positive classroom and school climate.**

Academic Achievement

Numerous studies (e.g., Caprara, Barbaranelli, Pastorelli, Bandura, & Zimbardo, 2000; Duckworth & Seligman, 2005; Malecki & Elliott, 2002; Welsh, Parke, Widaman, & O'Neil, 2001) and reviews of the literature (Berkowitz & Bier, 2004; Durlak et al., in press; Zins, Weissberg, Wang, & Walberg, 2004) attest that SEL competencies, particularly self-discipline, are related to academic achievement. Among them is a study of eighth graders by Duckworth and Seligman (2005) that looked specifically at self-discipline and found that it was a stronger predictor of academic grades than IQ, school attendance, and achievement test scores. To be sure, self-discipline and academic achievement have many of the same cognitions, emotions, and behaviors in common, such as the motivation to please others and meet internalized personal standards and goals, problem solving skills, the ability to inhibit impulses and regulate emotions, feelings of pride and responsibility, perseverance, and so forth. Thus, it is readily understandable that the direction of the relationship between self-discipline and academic achievement would flow both ways, each fostering the other (Welsh et al., 2001). However, many researchers argue that the evidence is stronger supporting the positive effects of social and emotional competencies, and interventions, on academic achievement (Malecki & Elliott, 2002; Wentzel, 2006). Regardless which direction is the stronger, it is clear that schools can foster self-discipline by providing excellent academic instruction and they also can improve academic achievement by developing social and emotional competencies, especially self-discipline.

TABLE 3.1. Common Social Cognitive and Emotional Processes, Deficiencies, and Deficits Related to Antisocial Behavior

	Examples of why and when the process, deficiency, or deficit is a problem related to discipline
Anger	
Arsenio, Gold, & Adams (2004); Camodeca & Goossens (2005); Deming & Lochman (2008); Geunyoung, Walden, Harris, Karrass, & Catron (2007); Hubbard, Dodge, Cillessen, Coie, & Schwartz (2001); de Castro, Merk, Koops, Veerman, & Bosch (2005); see Lochman et al. (2006) for a review of anger and aggression	• Easily frustrated and moved to anger. • Experiences anger more often and intensely. • Fails to regulate emotions, especially anger and frustration.
Empathy	
See Eisenberg (2006); Eisenberg et al. (2006); Hoffman (2000); Jolliffe & Farrington (2004); Lovett & Sheffield (2007) for reviews	• Doesn't feel the same emotion experienced by others appropriate to the given situation (e.g., chuckles when someone gets hurt, ignores someone who is crying, doesn't care about feelings of others). • Expresses little concern about others.
Guilt and shame	
Ahmed (2006); Menesini & Camodeca (2008); see Eisenberg et al. (2006); Frick & White (2008); Hoffman (2000); Tangney et al. (2007) for reviews	• Fails to experience a sense of responsibility for his or her own behavior (lack of guilt). • Does not feel any less about him- or herself after harming another (lack of shame). • Lacks feelings of remorse over wrongdoings, is cold and callous (lack of shame and guilt). • Lacks sense of pride in moral behavior, or integrity. Moral behavior is not central to self-concept and self-esteem.
Moral reasoning and motivation	
Arsenio & Lemerise (2004); Bear & Rys (1994); Blair, Monson, & Frederickson (2001); Covington (2000); Crick & Ladd (1990); Guerra, Huesmann, & Hanish (1995); Kuther (2000); Laible, Eye, & Carlo (2008); Malti, Gasser, & Buchmann (2009); Manning & Bear (2002); O'Brennnen, Bradshaw, & Sawyer (2009); Palmer & Hollin (2001); Quiggle, Garber, Panak, & Dodge (1992); Sijtsema, Veenstra, Lindenberg, & Salmivalli (2009); Stams et al. (2006); Weiner (2006)	• Moral reasoning is self-centered, based on and motivated by seeking rewards, avoiding punishment, and retribution rather than the needs and perspectives of others, a sense of responsibility or integrity, social approval, caring, or issues of fairness, justice, and respect. • Believes that antisocial behavior is easy, acceptable, justified, and effective in achieving positive, self-serving outcomes and rewards (including tangible rewards, peer approval, and feelings of power and control).

(cont.)

TABLE 3.1. *(cont.)*

	Examples of why and when the process, deficiency, or deficit is a problem related to discipline

Moral reasoning and motivation *(cont.)*

- Goals in a given situation are consistent with the above reasoning and beliefs—self-centered and focused on the present rather than the future (e.g., seeks immediate rewards and is unable to delay gratification)

Awareness of, and sensitivity to, the emotions of others and to social and moral problems

Cohen & Strayer (1996); Hoglund, Lalonde, & Leadbeater (2008); Hubbard, Dodge, Cillessen, Coie, & Schwartz (2001); Schultz, Izard, & Ackerman (2000)

- Fails to recognize when others are angry, frustrated, sad, etc. (e.g., continues inappropriate behavior when teacher shows that he or she's becoming frustrated and angry).
- Fails to consider the perspective of others, such as how they might perceive a given situation.
- Fails to perceive that there is a social or moral problem in a given situation (e.g., isn't aware of impact of behavior on others, that there is a rule governing the behavior or situation).
- Reads social cues incorrectly or makes errors interpreting the situation.

Cognitive scripts reflecting personal beliefs, attitudes, and values that support antisocial behavior

Burks, Laird, Dodge, Pettit, & Bates (1999); Crozier et al. (2008); Huesmann (1988); Werner & Nixon (2005); Zelli, Dodge, Lochman, & Laird (1999)

- Like a script in a film, cognitive scripts guide antisocial behavior, such as "Hit others when threatened" or "Don't let others push you around." (Cognitive scripts also can guide prosocial behavior, however: "Be kind to others," Follow the Golden Rule.")

Hostile attributional bias

Camodeca & Goosens (2005); Crozier et al. (2008); Lansford et al. (2006); see de Castro, Veerman, Koops, Bosch, & Monshouwer (2002), for review

- Overly attributes the behavior of others to their hostile intentions while overlooking mitigating circumstances (e.g., when bumped in the hallway, quickly assumes that the other person meant to do it).

Impulsivity

Barkley et al. (2002); Deming & Lochman (2008); Lösel, Bliesener, & Bender (2007)

- Fails to inhibit antisocial behavior, responding automatically to a situation without reflecting or problem solving (e.g., grabs desired object from peer, tells teacher to "shut up").

(cont.)

TABLE 3.1. *(cont.)*

	Examples of why and when the process, deficiency, or deficit is a problem related to discipline
Generating alternative solutions and evaluating their consequences	
Crozier et al. (2008); Fontaine, Yang, Dodge, Bates, & Pettit (2009); Guerra (1989); Guerra & Slaby (1989); Lansford et al. (2006); Lösel et al. (2007); Mikami, Lee, Hinshaw, & Mullin (2008)	• Generates fewer solutions to social problems than prosocial peers. • Generates solutions of lesser quality (more aggressive, atypical, and socially maladaptive). • Fails to reflect upon consequences of behavior and alternatives considered.
Mechanisms of moral disengagement (also referred to as cognitive distortions)	
Bandura (2002); Bandura, Caprara, Barbaranelli, Pastorelli, & Regalia (2001); Gina (2006); Weiner (2006)	• Avoids negative feelings by deflecting and not accepting responsibility. • Blames others, uses excuses and mechanisms to avoid responsibility and protect him- or herself (e.g., "He deserved it," "I was just joking," "Others did it too," "He made me do it," "He started it first").
Perceptions of self-efficacy	
Bandura (1997); Erdley & Asher (1999); Quiggle et al. (1992)	• Self-efficacy, or self-confidence in performing a behavior, is lacking with respect to desirable behaviors. • Self-efficacy is not lacking with respect to undesirable behaviors (e.g., one is confident that he or she can win a fight, not get caught stealing, etc.).

Positive Relationships

Both students and teachers prefer students who demonstrate self-discipline. For example, students who inhibit aggression and antisocial behavior and exhibit prosocial behavior tend to be more accepted and popular among their peers, whereas those who frequently fight, lie, steal, bully, and exhibit other aggressive and antisocial behaviors tend to be rejected (Rubin et al., 2006). Note that it is the frequency and severity of such behaviors—when they significantly deviate from the norm—that are most detrimental to peer acceptance and close friendships. Occasional and minor acts of misbehavior are unlikely to lead to peer rejection. Indeed, students are more likely to reject the "teacher's pet" than someone who occasionally exhibits minor misbehavior or even more serious acts of aggression but for what are perceived to be good reasons, such as fighting when provoked, fighting to protect a friend, or being aggressive in sports (Bear & Rys, 1994; Wentzel, 1994).

Teachers also prefer students who demonstrate self-discipline—those who inhibit aggression and antisocial behavior and exhibit prosocial behavior—and who thus require little supervision (Birch & Ladd, 1998). Not only are teachers more fond of students with these qualities, but they also tend to provide them with more social support (Hughes, Cavell, & Willson, 2001).

Positive Self-Worth and Emotional Well-Being

Research shows that children and adolescents perceive behavioral conduct, or moral behavior, to be an important aspect of self-concept and to be critical to overall perceptions of self-worth (Harter, 1999, 2006). Behavioral conduct is one of five major domains of self-concept consistently found among children and adolescents (Harter, 1999, 2006). The other domains are academics, social acceptance, physical appearance, and athletics. Self-perceptions of competence or adequacy in those domains largely determine overall self-perceptions of self-worth, or self-esteem. Positive self-perceptions, especially in those domains of perceived importance, are associated with greater overall happiness and general emotional well-being (Harter, 1999). Self-perceptions of behavioral conduct are of particular importance because most students highly value competence in this domain. Whereas students might discount the importance of other domains (e.g., athletics, social acceptance), it is very difficult for them to discount the importance of their behavior and still maintain high positive self-worth (Clever, Bear, & Juvonen, 1992). Indeed, for many individuals a "moral identity" is critical to their overall sense of self and happiness (Hardy & Carlo, 2005; Hart, Atkins, & Donnelly, 2006).

Positive Classroom and Schoolwide Climate

In developing self-discipline, schools reduce behavior problems, foster academic achievement, improve relationships between students, teachers, and staff, and enhance self-perceptions of overall self-worth and happiness. In turn, schools foster a positive school climate. That is, each of these obejectives is recognized as either an important aspect of school climate or as a factor that influences or is influenced by school climate. For example, ample research shows that students feel a stronger sense of belonging and view their schools more favorably when respectful, caring, and supportive relationships exist among themselves and between teachers/staff and students (Osterman, 2000). Students tend to reciprocate by demonstrating caring, respect, and support toward others and creating fewer behavior problems (Battistich, Schaps, Watson, Solomon, & Lewis, 2000). Likewise, researchers have viewed academic achievement and behavior problems as components of school climate as well as both determinants and outcomes of school climate (Anderson, 1982; Cohen et al., 2009). From the perspective of positive psychology, self-worth and subjective happiness can be viewed similarly—as factors that influence school climate in a reciprocal fashion: just as positive students help create a positive school climate, so too do positive school climates, characterized by few behavior problems, high academic achievement, and supportive relationships among teachers and teachers, foster student self-worth and happiness.

Research Supporting the Importance of Caring and Supportive Relationships

Research supports the importance of teacher–student, student–student, and school–home relationships in SEL programs and in developing self-discipline. Support is strongest, however, for teacher–student relationships. This correlation is consistent with the degree of emphasis placed on those categories of relationships in most SEL programs.

Teacher–Student Relationships

Ample research in the areas of classroom management, school discipline, and school climate strongly supports the importance of teachers' demonstrating caring, warmth, respect, and emotional support (e.g., Battistich et al., 1997; Birch & Ladd, 1998; Hamre & Pianta, 2006; Osterman, 2000; Marzano, 2003; Pianta, 1999). Those qualities have been shown to be associated with the following outcomes:

- Greater school completion (Croninger & Lee, 2001; Reschly & Christenson, 2006)
- Greater on-task behavior (Battistich et al., 1997; Battistich & Hom, 1997)
- Less cheating (Murdock, Hale, & Weber, 2001)
- Greater academic achievement (Fredricks et al., 2004; Gregory & Weinstein, 2004; Hamre & Pianta, 2001)
- Greater peer acceptance (Hughes et al., 2001)
- Greater motivation to act responsibly and prosocially (Wentzel, 1996, 2006)
- Less oppositional and antisocial behavior (Bru, Murberg, & Stephens, 2001; Bru, Stephens, & Torsheim, 2002; Meehan, Hughes, & Cavell, 2003; Murdock, 1999; Ryan & Patrick, 2001)
- Less bullying and victimization (Gregory et al., in press)
- Less use of weapons (Henrich, Brookmeyer, & Shahar, 2005)
- Fewer conflicts with teachers, irrespective of degree of problem behavior (Hamre & Pianta, 2001; Hamre, Pianta, Downer, & Mashburn, 2008).

Students are more likely to internalize their teachers' (and school's) values, as evidenced in the above behaviors, when teachers are perceived to be caring, warm, fair, respectful, and supportive (Wentzel, 1997, 2006). Research shows that caring, warm, respectful, and emotionally supportive relationships, although important to all students, are particularly important for those at greatest risk for the foregoing negative outcomes, especially school disengagement and problem behaviors (Balfanz, Herzog, & MacIver, 2007; Hamre et al., 2008; Juvonen, 2007; Wentzel & Wigfield, 2007), and those lacking support from other sources, such as parents, peers, and close friends (Harter, 1999; Pianta, 1999). In light of these studies, some researchers (e.g., Hughes et al., 2001) argue that schools should focus more on enhancing teacher–student relationships than interventions that focus on the direct teaching of social skills. This argument is supported by research showing not only that supportive teacher–student relationships are associated with a number of positive student outcomes but also that improvements in those outcomes are mediated by improvements in teacher–student relationships and the school environment (Solomon, Battistich, Watson, Schaps, & Lewis, 2000).

Student–Student Relationships

Just as teacher–student relationships have been shown to be related to various important outcomes, so too have student–student, or peer, relationships. However, less research has been conducted in this area, especially the role of student–student relationships in developing self-discipline. As noted earlier, self-perceptions of social acceptance are a critical aspect of overall self-worth and emotional well-being. This observation applies to having one or more close friends as well as not being accepted and socially rejected by one's overall peer group (Waas, 2006). Without a close friend, students experience loneliness and are at risk of depression (Parker & Asher, 1993). Students who are socially rejected are at increased risk for disruptive behavior, poor achievement, disliking of school, and the avoidance and noncompletion of school (Buhs & Ladd, 2001; Buhs, Ladd, & Herald, 2006; French & Conrad, 2001; Welsh, 2000). Outcomes are less unfavorable for those who are neglected but not rejected (Waas, 2006). Overall, however, the lack of social support is related to behavior problems, with social support from classmates moderating victimization and distress (Davidson & Demaray, 2007) and predicting externalizing and adaptive behaviors (Rueger, Malecki, & Demaray, 2008). Classroom norms also play an important role in aggression and behavior: Students are more likely to be disruptive and aggressive in those classrooms in which peers are disruptive and aggressive (Stearns, Dodge, & Nicholson, 2008; van Lier et al., 2005).

Home–School Relationships

Obviously, families exert a strong influence on the academic, social, and emotional development of children (Parke & Buriel, 2006). Thus, as recognized in SEL (Elias et al., 1997), as well as in nearly all school reform efforts (e.g., Comer, Haynes, Joyner, & Ben-Avie, 1996), it makes sense to include families in interventions for developing self-discipline and for preventing and correcting misbehavior. Such inclusion might range from active participation of parents in planning, implementing, and evaluating schoolwide programs to home-school communication and collaboration at the individual-student level (Christenson & Sheridan, 2001).

Research Demonstrating the Effectiveness of SEL Programs

Empirical research demonstrating the effectiveness of SEL in improving various positive outcomes originates from two sources: (1) studies of the effectiveness of SEL programs and (2) studies of the effectiveness of social cognitive techniques used in SEL programs. Several reviews of the literature have demonstrated the effectiveness of universal programs that target social cognitive, emotional, and ecological factors. These include general reviews of school-based programs for promoting mental health and preventing school violence, aggression, and conduct problems (Durlak & Wells, 1997; Greenberg, Domitrovich, & Bumbarger, 2001; Hahn et al., 2007; Lösel & Beelman, 2003; Wilson, Gottfredson, & Najaka, 2001; Wilson & Lipsey, 2007) as well as more focused reviews of programs identified as SEL (Collaborative for Academic, Social, and Emotional Learning, 2005; Durlak et al., in press; Zins et al., 2004), character education (Berkowitz & Bier, 2004), positive youth development (Catalano et al., 2004; Durlak et al., 2007), and classroom management and school discipline (Freiberg & Lapointe, 2006).

In a recent comprehensive meta-analysis of 207 studies that implemented SEL programs, Durlak et al. (in press) found significant gains in academic achievement, SEL skills (e.g., student and teacher reports of interpersonal problem solving, identifying emotions from social cues, conflict resolution strategies, emotion regulation, coping strategies), student attitudes toward self and others (e.g., self-esteem, self-concept, self-efficacy, attitudes toward school and teachers, beliefs about violence, helping others, social justice, and drug use), and positive social behaviors (e.g., daily skills of getting along with others, cooperating with and respecting others). They also found significant decreases in behavior problems (e.g., classroom disruption, noncompliance, aggression, bullying, school suspensions, and delinquent acts) and emotional distress (e.g., depression, anxiety, stress or social withdrawal). Compared to students in control groups, improvements translated into an impressive 23% increase in percentile rank in SEL skills, an 11% increase in academic performance, and a 9–10% increase in the other measured outcomes. Significant improvements continued to be found 6 months or more after the programs ended. Another important finding, with significant implications for schoolwide discipline, was that programs implemented at the schoolwide level were no more effective than those implemented only at the classroom level. On two measured outcomes, SEL skills and positive social behavior, schoolwide programs were less effective. Other meta-analyses of prevention programs also reported no increased value to schoolwide programs as compared to classroom-level programs (Corcoran & Pillai, 2007; Lipsey & Wilson, 2007).

> **Compared to students not in SEL programs, on average those in SEL programs show 23% greater improvement in SEL skills, 11% in academic performance, and about 10% in other measured outcomes.**

Durlak et al. (in press) also found that a major determinant of program effectiveness was (1) fidelity, or integrity, of program implementation—a finding replicated in several other reviews (see Chapter 11)—and (2) the extent to which SEL programs followed four recommended practices. Those four practices, identified by the acronym SAFE, consisted of *sequenced* activities that were planned in a step-by-step manner; *active* forms of learning, such as role plays, discussions, and rehearsal with feedback; a *focus* on developing social and emotional skills and providing sufficient time to teach and practice those skills; and the targeting of *explicit* and specific social and emotional skills.

Studies of Techniques Used in SEL

Several comprehensive reviews of the literature for preventing behavior problems among children and youth suggest that programs are more effective when they combine social cognitive and behavioral techniques than when they use behavioral techniques alone. For example, Lösel and Beelman (2003) reported that at the end of intervention phases programs that emphasized behavioral, cognitive, or cognitive-behavioral techniques were equally effective. However, when a follow-up phase was included, programs using cognitive and cognitive-behavioral techniques were found to be twice as effective as programs using behavioral techniques alone. Thus, the effects of behavioral techniques tended to be more short-term and less lasting. Wilson et al. (2003) also reported larger effects for social cognitive programs than for behavioral programs.

As reported by Osher et al. (2010), perhaps the best comparison of the two approaches comes from a recent meta-analysis by Wilson and Lipsey (2007). In that review there was a focused comparison of various types of universal school-based programs for preventing aggressive and disruptive behavior. Both quasi-experimental and randomized control experimental studies were used. No significant differences in effect sizes were found between programs that emphasized cognitive or emotional techniques, behavioral techniques, or social skills training. The researchers found that the average universal prevention program reduced the percentage of students exhibiting behavior problems from 15 to 20%.

SUMMARY

Developing self-discipline is one of three components of comprehensive classroom and schoolwide discipline. Since the onset of public education, schools have recognized the importance of developing social, emotional, and moral competencies that will enable students to function as responsible self-governing citizens when no longer under the supervision of adults. In this chapter I argued that the best approach to developing self-discipline is that of social and emotional learning, which includes character education and positive psychology.

Support for SEL, especially its focus on self-discipline versus compliance, comes from multiple theories and lines of research. Studies have identified a variety of specific social and emotional processes, deficiencies, and competencies associated with either the presence or absence of behavior problems. Those areas are targeted for intervention in SEL. Research also has linked SEL competencies, particularly self-discipline, to valued outcomes other than simply the absence of behavior problems. Those outcomes included academic achievement, positive relationships with others, positive self-worth and emotional well-being, and positive classroom and schoolwide climate. Research strongly supports not only SEL's emphasis on social and emotional competencies but also its emphasis on the ecological contexts in which those competencies are developed, and especially the context of caring and supportive teacher–student relationships. Finally, research supports the effectiveness of SEL programs and the social-cognitive techniques that characterize the approach.

In sum, self-discipline should be the primary long-term aim of classroom and school-wide discipline, and SEL is the best approach for achieving it. As noted in Chapter 1, however, whereas techniques for developing self-discipline are a major strength of the SEL approach, techniques for correcting behavior problems is a relative weakness of SEL and a strength of the SWPBS approach (*prevention* of behavior problems being a strength of both approaches). Thus, for comprehensive classroom and schoolwide discipline, SWPBS programs should be integrated with the SEL approach. Similarly, in classrooms and schools with students with behavior problems who are not responsive to the SEL approach, techniques commonly found in SWPBS programs should be used in combination with SEL not only to correct problem behavior but also to help develop self-discipline.

CHAPTER 4

Strategies for
Developing Self-Discipline
(and a Positive School Climate)

In the first three chapters, I argued that managing student behavior and developing self-discipline are equally important aims of education but that too often schools focus on the short-term aim of managing or controlling student behavior and on preventing and correcting behavior problems. In doing so, they neglect the long-term aim of developing self-discipline. I argued that, while this situation exists among schools with a zero tolerance approach to discipline, it also applies to many schools with an SWPBS approach. Chapter 3 presented an alternative approach—the SEL approach. Although the SEL approach is not specific to school discipline, it includes various models and programs for classroom management and schoolwide discipline. In each of them, the primary aim is to develop social and emotional competencies either directly or indirectly related to self-discipline.

The purpose of this chapter is to review the evidence-based strategies and techniques found in SEL programs that are designed to develop the social cognitions and emotions underlying self-discipline. Particular attention is focused on the SEL strategies and techniques that are infused throughout the curriculum and the everyday life of the school, but which are not treated in later chapters on prevention and correction. As discussed in Chapter 1, some strategies and techniques for comprehensive discipline serve multiple aims. For example, praise and rewards, when used wisely, can be effective in preventing and correcting misbehavior and also in developing self-discipline. Indeed, it is for this reason that the strategic use of praise and rewards is presented in two separate chapters (Chapters 6 and 7). Likewise, as discussed in Chapter 5, structure (including high expectations as well as clear rules and their enforcement) and supportive relationships play key roles in prevention. Structure and supportive relationships are critical to the effectiveness of nearly all strategies, whether used for prevention, correction, or developing self-discipline. How one responds to behavior problems also has a strong impact on self-discipline, and thus the vari-

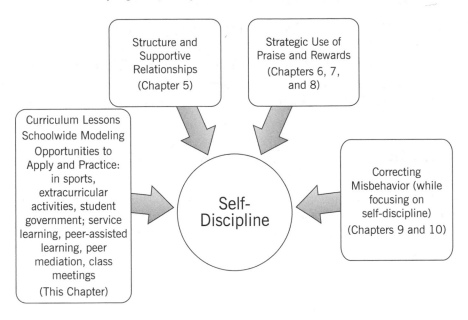

FIGURE 4.1. Strategies for developing self-discipline and a positive school climate.

ous strategies for developing self-discipline during disciplinary encounters are presented in both Chapters 9 and 10. Figure 4.1 illustrates the multiple strategies that help develop self-discipline while showing which ones are the focal point of this and subsequent chapters.

WHAT SHOULD BE DEVELOPED?

As previously noted, SEL targets five areas of social and emotional competence: self-awareness, social awareness, responsible decision making, self-management of emotions and behavior, and relationship skills. Self-discipline requires skills in each of these areas, but particularly the ability to make and act upon responsible decisions. This capability includes self-managing emotions and behavior throughout the process of making decisions and when carrying out what one decides. Indeed, as defined in this book, self-discipline *is* socially and morally responsible decision making and behavior. It is only when students fail to make socially and morally responsible decisions, and act accordingly, that external discipline is needed. To be sure, the other areas of SEL also are important to self-discipline. In making and acting upon socially and morally responsible decisions, students need to be aware of their own emotions, thoughts, and other aspects of self; be aware of the emotions and thoughts of others; and possess good relationship skills. However, skills in those three areas do not define self-discipline. Students can be well aware of self and others, have excellent relationship skills, and manage their emotions and behavior well but nonetheless think, feel, and act in socially and morally *irresponsible* ways. Indeed, skills in those areas can actually enhance such irresponsible behavior, as seen in the actions of cold and callous criminals who are well aware of their emotions and how others think and feel, who are skilled at manipulating others, and who can skillfully plan and execute the most hideous crimes. Thus, whereas all five areas of SEL should certainly be included in SEL programs for school discipline, and to a certain degree they are addressed in strategies presented in this chapter, the focus of this chapter is more specifically on strategies and techniques for helping students make, and act upon, decisions that are socially and morally responsible.

FOUR STEPS TO DEVELOPING SELF-DISCIPLINE

Table 3.1 in Chapter 3 presented various social cognitive and emotional processes that mediate problem behavior (or the absence thereof). A useful framework to help guide educators in targeting those processes, while focusing specifically on self-discipline, is to think of responsible decision making and behavior as consisting of four basic components (Bear, 2005, 2006; Bear et al., 2003; Rest, 1983):

1. Perceiving that a social or moral problem exists
2. Determining what one *ought* to do
3. Deciding among alternatives
4. Doing what one decides to do

Within each of these four components, biases, deficits, and deficiencies in social cognitive processes often explain why some children and adolescents (and adults) exhibit aggressive and antisocial behavior often, as well as why others do so occasionally. Although the four components are presented separately for heuristic purposes, all are interrelated. Processes within each component influence other processes within the same component, but also other processes in the other components. This interaction often occurs in a simultaneous and reciprocal fashion. Thus, although it helps to teach the components as a step-by-step problem-solving process, it should be understood that decision making does not always occur in such a sequential fashion (Dodge et al., 2006). Likewise, not all components apply in a given situation. Typically, a combination of processes and skills across more than one component are used. Indeed, it is a combination of social cognitive and emotional processes and skills that best predicts behavior (Lansford et al., 2006).

The above four components are translated below into four steps that should guide educators in the goal of developing self-discipline.

Step 1: Develop Student Sensitivity to Social and Moral Problems

Before students can begin to think about a problem situation, much less act or inhibit impulses to act, they need to recognize that a given situation calls for the processing of information and perhaps an action on their part. Recognition, awareness, and sensitivity to social and emotional cues in problem situations are often lacking among aggressive and antisocial children and youth (see Table 3.1 in Chapter 3 for references; see Bear et al.,

2003, and Dodge et al., 2006, for reviews). When asked about a problem situation, they might know the socially desired response, but when presented with those situations in real life they are often unaware or insensitive to the need to respond, or they respond impulsively without much thought.

Step 2: Determine What One Ought to Do

Upon recognizing that a situation calls for some type of action (including thinking) or non-action (including inhibiting impulses and regulating emotions), the next step to socially and morally responsible behavior is to decide what *is* the right thing to do. Often, this step simply consists in students automatically retrieving well-rehearsed cognitive scripts stored in memory that have been reinforced in the past (see Table 3.1 in Chapter 3 for references; see Bear et al., 2003, and Dodge et al., 2006, for reviews). Those scripts can support either responsible behavior (e.g., "Respect others," "Follow school rules," "Be kind to others") or aggressive and antisocial behavior (e.g., "Don't let others tell you what to do," "Be tough," "Don't snitch on others"). When the latter occurs, greater emphasis should be placed on teaching students to stop and think about alternative choices before deciding upon the first action or solution that comes to mind. In many other situations, however, students stop and think but come up with few good alternatives and choose the least likely to be productive. This scenario is seen in aggressive and antisocial students tending to generate alternatives that lack in both quantity and quality (see Table 3.1 in Chapter 3 for references; see Bear et al., 2003, and Dodge et al., 2006, for reviews).

The greatest difference in the quality of alternative solutions generated by aggressive and antisocial students, compared to those who are more prosocial in their behavior, is in the moral reasoning used to support the alternatives chosen. Aggressive and antisocial students tend to focus on personal, hedonistic consequences—gaining external rewards and avoiding punishment—and retribution or revenge. In contrast, other students focus more on the impact of their behavior on others, empathy, caring, anticipation of feelings of guilt or shame, and issues of fairness or justice (see Table 3.1 in Chapter 3 for references; see Bear et al., 2003, and Dodge et al., 2006, for reviews). As noted in earlier chapters, a major implication of this finding is that schools that emphasize earning rewards and avoiding punishment may actually be developing the type of reasoning most commonly found among those students who *are* the most aggressive and antisocial (Bear et al., 2006; Manning & Bear, 2002), including bullies

> **Schools that emphasize earning rewards and avoiding punishment may actually be developing the type of reasoning most commonly found among those students who are the most aggressive and antisocial.**

(Menesini & Camodeca, 2008; Minesini et al., 2003). Thus, rather than preventing future behavior problems, especially in the absence of adult monitoring, those schools may well be contributing to it.

In addition to focusing on the quality of solutions, at this step one also should encourage students to accept responsibility for their own behavior. Determining the right thing to do often hinges on attributions of responsibility. If students believe that they are not responsible for their actions (or lack thereof), it is unlikely they will reflect carefully upon what they *should* do. Students (and adults) often avoid assuming responsibility by using various *mechanisms of disengagement*, or cognitive distortions (see Table 3.1 in Chapter 3 for references; see Bear et al., 2003, and Dodge et al., 2006, for reviews). Those mechanisms are commonly seen in excuses, denials, and attempts to blame others. When students use them, it is important to tactfully challenge them; otherwise, they are likely to be negatively reinforced (i.e., students avoid getting into trouble for their actions). Chapter 10 presents techniques for confronting mechanisms of disengagement when correcting misbehavior.

Step 3: Decide among Alternatives

Far too often, students know multiple alternative solutions and can clearly explain why some are good ones and others are not, but nevertheless they decide upon a poor solution (which might be not acting at all). This may occur for a variety of reasons: they might decide that, although a chosen solution is the right thing to do, it would be either ineffective, too difficult, or not worth the effort. They might decide that it is not their responsibility to do anything (i.e., mechanisms of moral disengagement, discussed above, come into play at this point). Peer pressure or other environmental and situational factors might be exerting a strong influence on behavior in the given situation. Emotion regulation or impulse control might be a problem, or their competing values and goals ("I don't like getting into trouble, but it was worth it"). A self-serving bias also helps explain why many individuals fail to act in a manner consistent with their social and moral reasoning. That is, most tend to look out for themselves before, or instead of, looking out for others (Eisenberg et al., 2006). These factors, often working in combination, largely account for differences in behavior between students with and without significant behavior problems. They also often explain why even the best-behaving students sometimes misbehave (see Table 3.1 in Chapter 3 for references; see Bear et al., 2003, and Dodge et al., 2006, for reviews). Thus, it is important that they be targeted at this step.

Step 4: Do What One Decides to Do

Many of the same factors under Component 3 ("Deciding among alternatives") that explain why students (and adults!) decide not to do what they think they *should do* also help explain why they often decide to do what they should *but still do not do it*. In addition to the factors above, there are four others that often come into play at this step: (1) social skills, (2) coping and resilience skills, (3) perceptions of self-efficacy, and (4) moral emotions.

Social Skills

Although this term is sometimes used broadly to encompass social information processing or decision-making skills, it is used here in a more narrow sense to refer to students having the necessary skills to execute what they decide and plan to do. If those skills are not already in the student's repertoire, then they must be taught directly. Beyond the early grades, the lack of social skills

per se is seldom an issue for most students. That is, few students have social skill deficits. Instead, they are more likely to have performance or fluency deficits, as seen in the failure to exhibit social skills that they already possess (Gresham, 2002). Such failure can be attributed to any number of reasons discussed above that come into play after a decision has been made (e.g., competing values, peer pressure), but also to the factors below.

Coping Skills and Resilience

Many social skills are difficult to practice when one is faced with stressors, obstacles, and hardships. Despite the best social problem-solving, decision-making, and social skills, not all stressors, obstacles, and hardships can be avoided or overcome—and, even when they can, success is not assured. Thus, to solve social problems effectively and act responsibly, students often require not only these various social, emotional, and behavioral skills but also the ability to cope with adversity. They need to cope with situations in which they have little control and to bounce back after experiencing failure or hardships. For example, the best social problem-solving skills, as well as efforts by others, are not always sufficient for protecting students from being victims of ongoing bullying outside of the school setting. Likewise, both within and outside the school environment, nearly all students experience day-to-day stressors, such as being teased or rejected by peers or a sibling, not doing as well on a test as hoped, or being grounded by parents. Indeed, students report that the most common sources of stress in their lives are not those that many educators might guess (e.g., violence, abuse, divorce, poverty) but "minor" day-to-day stressors, especially those involving relationships with others (peers, parents, siblings, teachers) (Spirito, Stark, Grace, & Stamoulis, 1991). When students fail to cope with or bounce back from these stressors, performance or fluency deficits in social skills, as well as in all other areas of social and emotional competence, are likely to emerge.

Perceived Self-Efficacy

Perceived self-efficacy refers to people's belief about their capability to achieve what they actually intend to achieve or to otherwise influence events that affect their lives (Bandura, 1997). Beliefs about self-efficacy clearly influence students' decision making, but they also have a strong impact on their motivation to act in accordance with their moral reasoning and decision making. High perceptions of self-efficacy motivate individuals to engage or persist in prosocial acts (Colby & Damon, 1999). Unfortunately, students who exhibit frequent antisocial behavior also hold high perceptions of self-efficacy, believing that they are quite capable of engaging in transgressions toward others (e.g., "I am very good at fighting and am confident that I can win this fight") (Arsenio & Lemerise, 2001). Often, however, those students are lacking perceptions of self-efficacy about their ability to act prosocially (Goldstein, Harootunian, & Conoley, 1994).

Moral Emotions

Although emotions exert an influence at each of the four steps, certain emotions provide the spark, or motivation, often needed for individuals to follow through with their intentions and decisions. Although anger motivates aggression (see Table 3.1 in Chapter 3 for references; see Bear et al., 2003, and Dodge et al., 2006, for reviews), it can also account for prosocial behavior. For example, out of anger a student might come to the assistance of another student being victimized by a bully. Self-regulation of anger also certainly plays a role in the absence of aggression. Three other emotions, however, are viewed as the "moral emotions" that most often influence and motivate prosocial behavior (see Eisenberg et al., 2006; Hoffman, 2000; Tangney et al., 2007): empathy (and sympathy), guilt, and shame (see Table 3.1 in Chapter 3 for references; see Bear et al., 2003, and Dodge et al., 2006, for reviews). Sharing the perspective of others (empathy), and especially caring or feeling sorry about them (sympathy), often motivates helping others. Guilt, including empathy-based guilt, also motivates prosocial behavior (e.g., "I would have felt badly for not helping"). Likewise, the *anticipation* of experiencing guilt frequently motivates students to *refrain* from actions that might harm others, either physically or psychologically, and to otherwise act consistently with their values and moral reasoning. Finally, shame serves similar functions as guilt. Although guilt and shame are closely related, the primary difference is that with guilt negative feelings are directed to a specific action ("I feel badly for doing that") whereas with shame they are global ("I am a bad person for doing that"). Anticipated guilt as well as pride (though not an emotion per se) are often linked to responsible behavioral choices in the classroom (Ford, Wentzel, Wood, Stevens, & Sisfield, 1989). Inducing empathy-based guilt and pride, which is often done when reminding students of the importance of socially and morally responsible behavior, is much more effective in developing self-discipline and social conformity than the common techniques of correcting misbehavior by inducing fear or shame (Izard, 1991).

STRATEGIES FOR DEVELOPING SELF-DISCIPLINE

The purpose of presenting the strategies below, as well as throughout this book, is not to present educators with a menu from which they are to select. Rather, *all* of the strategies presented should be implemented throughout the school if one's aim is to develop self-discipline *and* foster a positive school climate. This is not only because many of the strategies are interdependent (e.g., the strategic use of praise helps build strong teacher–student relationships) but also because their effects should be cumulative and no strategy is designed to replace the other. Six strategies for developing self-discipline are presented below. Although they are very important in developing self-discipline (as noted earlier), the first three strategies receive only brief attention here because they are covered thoroughly in other chapters.

Strategy 1: Use Praise and Rewards Strategically and Wisely, with the Aim of Developing Self-Discipline

Praise and rewards can be very effective in helping to develop self-discipline, but only when used strategically and wisely. When not used in that manner, they have the potential of causing more harm than good. As discussed in depth in Chapter 6, in recent years the use of praise and rewards has been the center of much controversy. The criticism has been strongest against the use of tangible rewards, with many researchers asserting that rewards harm intrinsic motivation. Other researchers, however, argue that this rarely happens in the classroom. Although few researchers advise against the use of praise, many argue that it is often used ineffectively. These issues are discussed in Chapter 6, and specific recommendations for the strategic use of praise and rewards are presented in Chapter 7. For now, it is important to remember that praise and rewards, when used strategically and wisely, are useful in developing self-discipline.

Strategy 2: Build and Maintain a Positive Teacher–Student Relationship Characterized by a Balance of Structure and Support

As discussed in Chapter 5, positive teacher–student relationships play a critical role in preventing behavior problems, and (as noted in Chapter 9) they are equally important when correcting behavior problems. In both chapters it is shown that effective teachers and schools are authoritative rather than authoritarian or permissive in their approaches to discipline. As such, they exhibit a balanced combination of structure, or *demandingness*, and support, or *responsiveness*. Specific techniques for structure and support are provided in those two chapters. Two additional techniques for providing student support are presented below: *dialoguing* and *scaffolding*. Although they certainly apply to both prevention and correction, and especially the latter, they are presented here because they should be used in each of the strategies below for developing social and moral problem solving and decision making.

> **Dialoguing and scaffolding are effective ways to provide students with the structure and support needed for developing self-discipline.**

Guidance and Support with Dialoguing

As pointedly noted by Myrna Shure (2001), "Punishing, threatening, suggesting, or even explaining to children what they should and should not do are monologues. The adult is doing all the talking for the child" (p. 278). Instead of a monologue, Shure recommends a dialogue. In dialoguing, teachers provide support by posing guiding questions designed to help students apply and practice social problem-solving skills. Those skills include ones that should have been taught previously in curriculum lessons and in schoolwide activities designed to develop self-discipline. Form 4.1 (at the end of the chapter) presents questions that teachers might use during dialoguing to guide students through the four steps to responsible decision making and behavior. Although adaptations would need to be made for lower grades, they should prove valuable in multiple contexts in which self-discipline is the focal point, including discussions of curriculum lessons, class meetings, and disciplinary encounters.

Scaffolding

A good metaphor for conceptualizing the amount of support and guidance a student needs to successfully achieve a given task, including during dialoguing, is that of scaffolding, which is a support system used when constructing a building (Brown & Palincsar, 1989; Stone, 1998). Following this metaphor, some buildings require more scaffolding than others. When construction is completed, the scaffolding is removed and the building stands on its own. As in constructing buildings, just enough support, or scaffolding, as necessary should be used in teaching students to solve social and moral problems on their own. As such, the amount of scaffolding should be systematically reduced, and ultimately removed, as students improve their social and moral problem-solving skills and assume greater responsibility in applying them. Because one's aim is to develop self-discipline, what is being scaffolded is not solving the specific problem, but instead it is developing social problem-solving skills that students can apply across multiple problem situations. When needed, scaffolding helps students achieve tasks that they would not ordinarily achieve on their own. Whereas students with undeveloped or poor problem-solving skills require a lot of scaffolding (e.g., direct instruction and modeling), more skilled students require much less (e.g., reminders, Socratic questioning).

Strategy 3: Implement Curriculum Activities That Directly Teach Social, Emotional, and Behavioral Competencies

To one extent or another, every school has a curriculum that teaches social and emotional competencies, although many schools are unaware of their curriculum. That is, in all schools at least a "hidden" curriculum exists. In many schools, however, the curriculum is more visible and is one of two types or a combination thereof: (1) a packaged curriculum, consisting primarily of lessons taught in one or more classes or in a separate course, and preferably with strategies included for promoting generalization of those skills to other settings; and (2) curriculum lessons that are integrated into the general curriculum (but not "hidden") and deliberately taught to promote self-discipline.

Packaged Programs

Although some schools and individuals develop their own SEL programs, most programs are commercially produced. There are many SEL programs supported by research that attests to their effectiveness in showing improvement on at least one desired outcome using quasi-experimental research designs. However, very few have undergone the rigor of empirical research using random assignment and a control group while showing decreased behavior problems. Exceptions include Second Step: A Violence Prevention Curriculum (Committee for Children, 2003; see Fitzgerald & Van Schoiack-Edstrom, 2006, for a review), Steps to Respect: A Bully Prevention Program (Committee for Children, 2001; see Hirschstein & Frey, 2006, for a review), Promoting Alternative Thinking Strategies (PATHS; Kusche & Greenberg, 2000; see Greenberg & Kusche, 2006, for a review), and the Caring School Community (see Watson & Battistich, 2006, for review). Before adopting any packaged program, school officials are strongly advised to consult reviews of programs being considered and to evaluate the program itself (see Collaborative for Academic, Social and Emotional Learning, 2005, for a review of 80 such programs, and Merrell & Gueldner, 2010, for recent reviews of selected SEL programs). Form 4.2 (at the end of the chapter) presents a checklist designed to help review programs.

Among empirically validated programs, Second Step: A Violence Prevention Curriculum (Committee for Children, 2003; see *www.cfchildren.org*) contains units that cover each of the four components of socially and morally responsible behavior. Using discussion, direct teaching, and role playing, the program teaches students to follow five steps in dealing with interpersonal problems through social and moral problem-solving skills. They are:

1. Ask first: What is the problem?
2. Next ask: What are some solutions?
3. For each solution, ask: Is it safe? How might people feel? Is it fair? Will it work?
4. Choose a solution and implement it.
5. Determine whether the solution is working and, if not, what to do next.

An attractive feature of Step 3 is that it emphasizes issues of fairness and the effects of the student's behavior on others, including aspects of moral reasoning and empathy.

The Strong Kids programs (Strong Start, PreK–3; Strong Kids, 3–8; Strong Teens, 9–12; see *strongkids.uoregon.edu*) is another commercially packaged SEL curriculum that is well grounded in social and emotional theory and research and covers the four components of responsible decision making and behavior presented in this chapter. An attractive feature of these programs is that they include lessons on coping and resilience. Only a few small-scale studies have been conducted to date on the effectiveness of these new programs, but results have been promising. For example, in a recent quasi-experimental design study of Strong Start, significant improvements were found among second graders in peer ratings of prosocial behavior and teacher ratings of internalizing behaviors (Caldarella, Christensen, Kramer, & Kronmiller, 2009). No significant decrease was found in behavior problems, however.

Integrating Lessons into the General Curriculum

Packaged programs have many advantages, especially the convenience of having lessons already prepared and field-tested materials for presenting them. However, they also have their disadvantages. Among the disadvantages are the sometimes prohibitive costs of materials and training as well as potential resistance from teachers when asked to add another thing to their already busy and demanding day (Fullan, 2007). When resistance occurs, programs are often not implemented as designed (i.e., with fidelity). Fidelity of implementation has consistently been shown to be related to the effectiveness of prevention and promotion programs, and lack of fidelity is frequently cited as a common problem among both researchers and those implementing packaged programs (Catalano et al., 2004; Durlak & Dupre, 2008).

As an alternative to adopting a packaged program, school officials should consider examining their "hidden" curriculum closely and making it more visible by deliberately and systematically integrating SEL lessons into the existing general curriculum, such as in literacy, health, and social studies. For example, skills related to all four of the previously cited steps to developing self-discipline could be taught in literature that addresses social and moral issues (e.g., *Pinocchio, Lord of the Flies, Diary of Anne Frank, To Kill a Mockingbird*) as well as in covering such topics in social studies such as slavery, the Holocaust, civil rights, and constitutional rights. Similar social and moral issues could be addressed when discussing the daily media. Moral and social issues also could be addressed in creative writing assignments, journal writing, poetry, debates, video and theatrical productions, art, music, and research surveys and interviews. For generalization and additional teaching skills development, SEL-related concepts could be infused throughout all other instructional practices, including class meetings and disciplinary encounters (as discussed later). This approach is taken by the Caring School Community and supported by multiple studies that have measured and assessed a variety of academic, social, and emotional outcomes (Watson & Battistich, 2006).

> **By integrating lessons into the general curriculum, schools avoid many of the limitations of packaged curriculum programs for SEL.**

When adopting an integrated approach, the methods of instruction should be considered to be as important as the curriculum content. Those teaching the lessons need to use a variety of evidence-based instructional strategies for promoting social problem solving and decision making, such as those found in Second Step and PATHS (e.g., modeling, role playing, active discussion, rehearsal, positive reinforcement). They also need to be given sufficient time to develop the integrated lesson plans while ensuring that they target the cognitive and emotional processes shown to be most closely associated with antisocial and prosocial behavior (see Table 3.1 in Chapter 3). Likewise, careful steps must be taken to assure that all processes are taught in a sequenced, developmentally appropriate fashion (for an excellent list of sequenced SEL standards to guide SEL curriculum development, see *www.isbe.state.il.us/ils/social_emotional/standards.htm*).

Strategy 4: Provide Multiple Models of Social and Moral Problem Solving, Moral and Regulated Emotions, and Responsible Behavior

It is through observational, or incidental, learning rather than the systematic use of techniques of operant learning (e.g., shaping a behavior by reinforcing specific steps or successive approximations) that most social learning occurs (Bandura, 1986). Modeling promotes learning by (1) informing students of appropriate ways of thinking and acting, (2) motivating them to think and act the same, (3) fostering values and standards that underlie the behaviors observed, and (4) often triggering the same emotional reactions they observe that are associated with prosocial behavior, such as empathy, sorrow, and pride (Bandura, 1986).

Before entering school, most children have already observed countless acts of antisocial behavior, either at home, in the community, or in multiple forms of media expression (e.g., movies, television, video games, storybooks). Fortunately, children and adolescents also observe countless acts of prosocial behavior. Thus, it makes sense for schools not only to try to curtail observations of aggression but to capitalize on observational learning by taking deliberate actions to ensure that models of desired social, emotional, and behavioral competencies are provided throughout the school and its curricula. The first place to begin should be with the adult models in the school. As discussed in Chapter 5 on prevention, adult modeling of desired behavior is an important strategy for both preventing behavior problems and developing self-discipline. There are many other ways, however, in which positive models can be provided. Form 4.3 (at the end of the chapter) is a sample checklist for school officials to use in providing a variety of effective models of desired behaviors.

> **Other than sleeping, children and adolescents spend more time (an average of about 8 hours per day) exposed to multiple forms of media than in any other activity, with the average student observing over 200,000 acts of violence on television prior to the age of 18 (American Academy of Pediatrics, 2001).**

Modeling also should be used more directly when social, emotional, and behavioral skills are lacking or when they need to be reviewed. This is a common method used in most evidence-based SEL programs, including Second Step and PATHS. When used in this manner, the targeted skill is first explained; its importance and relation to positive outcomes are discussed; the skill is then modeled by the adult or students; students rehearse the skill in role-play situations and receive feedback on their performance from classmates and the teacher; and the class members then discuss where, when, and how the skill might be used in real-life situations. Efforts are made to provide for practice and reinforcement of the skills outside of the training sessions.

Strategy 5: Provide Multiple Opportunities for Students to Apply and Practice Social, Emotional, and Moral Competencies of Self-Discipline

Knowledge is of little value if it is not applied in practice, and this observation is especially true of self-discipline. It is not sufficient that students know what to do and how to do it; they also need to apply and practice these skills in the classroom, school, and elsewhere. Five evidence-based opportunities for students to apply and practice the social and emotional competencies of self-discipline are reviewed below: (1) sports and extracurricular activities (including student government), (2) service learning, (3) peer-assisted learning, (4) peer mediation, and (5) class meetings.

Sports and Extracurricular Activities (Including Student Government)

Extracurricular activities include student government, clubs (e.g., business and vocational clubs, religious clubs, game clubs, service clubs, academic clubs, foreign language clubs), and fine arts (music, band, chorus, drama, art club). Participation in sports and extracurricular activities can promote social and emotional learning in numerous ways (Fredricks & Eccles, 2008):

- Increasing opportunities for positive interactions with both peers and school adults
- Promoting leadership skills
- Exposing students to positive role models
- Increasing engagement in school
- Fostering a sense of school community
- Enhancing self-concept and self-confidence (as a result of successful experiences)
- Engaging students in democratic decision making (especially student government at the classroom and schoolwide levels)

Of course, for these benefits to be realized, the learning opportunities must be meaningful ones, offering genuine opportunities for social and moral decision making. For example, student government must involve much more than just fund-raising.

Participation in sports and extracurricular activities in general has been shown to be associated with a number of positive academic and social-emotional outcomes. Academically these may include higher grades, test scores, and educational aspirations as well as greater school engagement and valuing of the school (Fredricks & Eccles, 2006a, 2008). Socially and emotionally, favorable outcomes include higher self-esteem and resiliency and lower depression (Fredricks & Eccles, 2006b, 2008; Mahoney, Schweder, & Stattin, 2002); having more friends who are prosocial (Fredricks & Eccles, 2008) and who hold high academic aspirations (Barber, Eccles, & Stone, 2001); and exhibiting fewer behavior problems (Fredricks & Eccles, 2008; Mahoney & Cairns, 1997; Youniss, Yates, & Su, 1997). The greatest impact that participation in sports and extracurricular activities has on reducing behavior problems is generally found among high-risk adolescents (Mahoney, 2000; Mahoney & Cairns, 1997).

Research findings are not always consistent across studies, however, given that multiple factors mediate or influence the value and effectiveness of sports and extracurricular activities. Such factors might include the qualities of the coach or instructor, the number of activities the student is involved in, whether the student's participation is voluntary or required, the intensity of involvement, the student's motivation in the activities, the age of the student, and the types of peers in the group. Upon reviewing the literature on sports and character development, Reeve and Weiss (2006) concluded, "The bottom line is that sport has the potential to build character and the types of experiences afforded children in the competitive environment" (p. 489). They provide excellent recommendations for maximizing positive outcomes for students engaged in sports. Although their recommendations are specific to sports, most also certainly apply to other extracurricular activities. These recommendations are summarized in Form 4.4 (at the end of the chapter).

Service Learning

The Corporation for National and Community Service (n.d., see their website for excellent resources on service learning: *www.servicelearning.org*) defines service learning as a "teaching and learning strategy that integrates meaningful community service with instruction and reflection to enrich the learning experience, teach civic responsibility, and strengthen communities." Typically the strategy is integrated with an academic course such that students participate in a service activity while watching films, researching, reading articles, writing essays, and discussing related topics. They also reflect upon those academic activities and more importantly their service experience, such as by writing about them in a journal. For example, students might work at a soup kitchen while studying poverty and societal change (Yates & Youniss, 2001).

Although relatively few studies have been conducted on the effects of service learning, the ones that have been conducted suggest multiple positive effects, including reduced negative behaviors (i.e., fewer arrests, fewer pregnancies, less alcohol consumption, fewer behavior problems and suspensions in school) and increased positive behaviors, including academic achievement and behaviors reflecting social, emotional, and moral development and competence (i.e., greater empathy, dependability, trustworthiness, greater self-efficacy in helping others, greater civic engagement after graduating from high school; see Hart, Matsuba, & Atkins, 2008, for a recent review). Interestingly, there is little research supporting the following common features of service learning programs (Hart et al., 2008): (1) that service learning is more effective when integrating service activities with curriculum activities, as opposed to providing service learning without such integration; (2) that students benefit more when they volunteer to participate, as opposed to being required to participate; and (3) that structured reflection is necessary for students to benefit (interestingly, writing about their experience was found to be much more effective than verbal discussion).

Based upon a review of service learning programs and research, the Corporation for National and Community Service recommends that K–12 service learning programs should have the following qualities or features to order to be effective (RMC Research Corporation, 2009):

- Sufficient duration and intensity
- Intentional use of service learning as an instructional strategy to meet the program's goals
- Active engagement of students in meaningful and personally relevant service and learning activities
- Providing students, with guidance from adults, with a strong voice in planning, implementing, and evaluating their service learning experiences

- Promoting understanding of diversity and mutual respect
- Arranging collaborative and mutually beneficial partnerships that address community needs
- Encouraging or requiring meaningful and ongoing reflection about the service learning experiences, especially about how they relate to one's self-concept (or moral identity) and one's relationship to society

Peer-Assisted Learning

Peer-assisted learning (PAL) refers to small-group or dyadic learning activities in which academic instruction or problem solving is led and shared by students (Ginsburg-Block, Rohrbeck, Fantuzzo, & Lavigne, 2006). The most popular models of PAL are cooperative learning (Johnson & Johnson, 1999), classwide peer tutoring (Greenwood, Maheady, & Delquadri, 2002), and reciprocal peer tutoring (Fantuzzo & Ginsburg-Block, 1998). Compared to traditional instruction, PAL has consistently been shown to have a greater positive impact on academic, social, and emotional outcomes, including academic achievement, less behavior problems, greater class cohesion and peer acceptance (including greater acceptance of minority students and students with disabilities), and increased social perspective taking and self-esteem (see Ginsburg-Block, Rohrbeck, Fantuzzo, & Lavigne, 2006, and Natasi & Clements, 1991, for reviews). PAL has been shown to be particularly effective with students in grades 1–3; when same-gender groupings are used; when interdependent group reward contingencies are included; and with urban, minority, and low-income students who are at greatest risk of negative academic and social and emotional outcomes (Ginsburg-Block, Rohrbeck, & Fantuzzo, 2006; Ginsburg-Block, Rohrbeck, Fantuzzo, & Lavigne, 2006).

The advantages of PAL over traditional methods of instruction have primarily been attributed to (1) instruction being student-centered, which fosters motivation and enhanced self-concept, and (2) peer interactions that foster motivation. However, it also has been suggested that in many situations PAL provides increased clarity of instruction and greater cognitive challenge (Ginsburg-Block, Rohrbeck, Fantuzzo, & Lavigne 2006). With respect to fostering social, emotional, and moral development, the greater cognitive challenge includes understanding and respecting the perspective of others and learning how to resolve disagreements and controversy before being able to reach group agreement and attain a common goal (Mitchell, Johnson, & Johnson, 2002).

In all of the studies included in the reviews of PAL cited above, peer assistance was provided in the area of academic instruction but not in the area of social and emotional learning. It is impressive then that, despite not being the target of those PAL programs, the programs were nevertheless shown to be associated with a number of positive social and emotional outcomes. One SEL program that includes both academic *and* social and emotional learning as targets of PAL is the Caring School Community (Watson & Battistich, 2006). The program includes *Buddies*, a component in which older elementary school students tutor and coach younger students in both academics and prosocial behavior (see *www.devstu.org/csc* for a description and activity books).

Peer Mediation

Several SEL programs that focus on school discipline are designed to equip students with the skills of peer mediation and conflict resolution, for them to routinely apply to assist other students in resolving and managing peer conflicts. Peer mediators assist others throughout the school, including in classrooms, hallways, and on the playgrounds. Peer mediation programs can increase negotiation and mediation knowledge and skills; reduce peer conflicts, suspensions, expulsions, and disciplinary actions; and improve overall school climate (Burrell, Zirbel, & Allen, 2003; Johnson & Johnson, 2006). The peer mediation program with the most extensive research is the Teaching Students to Be Peacemakers Program (Johnson & Johnson, 2005).

Class Meetings

Although empirical research is lacking as to the effectiveness of class meetings per se, several evidence-based multicomponent programs for elementary schools use class meetings as a context in which students learn and practice social problem-solving skills and in which prosocial values are highlighted. In those programs, class meetings also serve the purpose of promoting close teacher–student and student–student relationships as well as a positive classroom climate and sense of community. Two popular evidence-based programs that make frequent use of class meetings are Responsive Classroom (Brock, Nishida, Chiong, Grimm, & Rimm-Kaufman, 2008; Charney, 2002; see *www.responsiveclassroom.org*) and the Caring School Community (Watson & Battistich, 2006; see *www.devstu.org/csc*; see both programs' websites for books and support materials for conducting class meetings). Although found most often in elementary school, class meetings also have been used in high schools to foster social and moral reasoning (Power, Higgins, & Kohlberg, 1989).

Class meetings can be used for group problem solving of a wide range of social and moral issues pertaining to the classroom and school community. ClassMaps (Doll et al., 2004, 2009) is an excellent tool to use in classrooms to identify areas of concern and stimulate interventions. In using ClassMaps, students share and graph class results of the Class-Maps survey, review and analyze their scores, identify the classes' strengths and weaknesses, and develop, implement, and monitor a plan that addresses areas of shared concern. Although designed primarily for elementary classrooms, with adaptations the tool can be used in solving schoolwide problems even beyond elementary school.

> **Class meetings should not be only for elementary students, but for students of all grades. However, the content, process, frequency, and duration of class meetings would differ greatly from the lower to upper grades.**

Finally, class meetings can be used to discuss classroom and schoolwide issues more specific to matters of discipline, including preventing and correcting behavior problems and developing self-discipline. When used for this purpose, however, discussion of individual students should be avoided or done with extreme care. There should be minimal risk of students' feeling anxious, upset, embarrassed, or ostracized. The following recommendations are suggested for conducting class meetings, but especially when addressing behavior problems (adapted from Bear, 2005):

- Ensure that the classroom atmosphere is nonthreatening and characterized by mutual respect and trust. Students should be allowed to freely voice their opinions and challenge others, but only in a respectful manner.
- Arrange chairs in a circle or semicircle so that all students can see one another.
- If feasible and where appropriate (depending on time considerations and the issue under discussion), arrange for small-group as well as whole-class discussions. Smaller groups (e.g., four to eight participants) provide greater opportunities for all students to share their views.
- Encourage peer discussion. Participation of all students should be encouraged, and no students (nor even the teacher) should be allowed to monopolize the discussion.
- Do not use the meeting as the time to lecture students about their inappropriate behavior.
- Make sure that the teacher acts as a *problem-solving facilitator* who models good listening and thinking skills and a *moral advocate* who advocates for the moral principles of fairness, justice, caring, and the rights and welfare of others (DiBiase, Gibbs, & Potter, 2005; Power et al., 1989).
- As a moral advocate, do not hesitate to tactfully confront or challenge excuses, distortions, denials, blaming others, and poor solutions (see DiBiase et al., 2005, for specific techniques).
- Use dialoguing and scaffolding to guide discussion (see guiding questions in Form 4.1).
- If the behavior of specific individuals is discussed in the meeting, those involved should agree in advance to its inclusion.
- Focus on solutions and how to prevent reoccurrences of the behavior.
- Avoid blaming and proposing punitive consequences for the misbehavior. Make sure that the meeting does not become a "kangaroo court" in which students are tried for their misbehavior.
- Use praise strategically and wisely to encourage and reinforce good reasoning, listening and discussion skills, social problem solving, and the development of self-discipline (see Chapters 6 and 7).

Strategy 6: Use Disciplinary Encounters to Help Develop Self-Discipline

This strategy is the focus of Chapters 9 and 10 on correcting behavior problems but is listed here to emphasize that imposing punishment should not be one's primary goal when correcting behavior problems. As noted in Chapter 1, punishment is often required in the school's code of conduct. When used wisely and in combination with other strategies and techniques, it also can be helpful in developing self-discipline. However, when correcting behavior problems, one's primary aim should be to help students develop the social and emotional competencies of self-discipline, such that they, rather than adults, manage their behavior and do so in a manner that is socially and morally responsible. As explained and shown in Chapters 9 and 10, disciplinary encounters provide an excellent context for helping to develop self-discipline.

SUMMARY

In this chapter, four components to self-discipline were presented that organize and integrate a wealth of research on the social-cognitive and emotional processes that underlie or influence socially and morally responsible behavior, or self-discipline. Derived from those four components, four steps were given to guide educators on how students should think, feel, and act when faced with social and moral problems: (1) develop student sensitivity to social and moral problems, (2) determine what one *ought* to do, (3) decide among alternatives, and (4) do what one decides to do. Six strategies were presented to develop social and emotional processes within each of those steps, three of which were a primary focus of this chapter.

The first strategy emphasized is to implement curriculum activities that directly teach social, emotional, and behavioral competencies. Two ways in which this is commonly done is to either adopt a packaged curriculum or integrate lessons throughout the existing curriculum. Examples of evidence-based packages were presented, and the advantages of the integrated approach were noted. The second strategy is to provide multiple models of social and moral problem solving, moral and regulated emotions, and responsible behavior. The importance of modeling was discussed, and specific techniques were given for using modeling schoolwide and for enhancing its effectiveness. The third general strategy discussed in this chapter is to provide multiple opportunities for students to apply and practice the social, emotional, and moral competencies of self-discipline. Five more specific strategies for achieving this general strategy were discussed: (1) sports and extracurricular activities (including student government, (2) service learning, (3) peer-assisted learning, (4) peer mediation, and (5) class meetings. Recommendations for implementing those strategies also were given.

The strategies in this chapter were presented, with their common aim being the development of self-discipline. In helping develop self-discipline, these strategies also achieve two other important, and interrelated, goals of most schools, namely, preventing behavior problems and improving the school's climate.

Questions Teachers Should Ask Students, and Students Should Ask Themselves, during Social Problem Solving

To Help Develop Student Sensitivity to Social and Moral Problems

- What is the problem in this situation? How do you know, or suspect, that there is a problem?
- Is there a rule that is being broken? Is someone likely to get hurt or have his or her feelings hurt? Is there the potential for harm to a relationship or friendship?
- What might be the emotions or feelings of everyone in the situation? What might have happened earlier? What might happen next?
- What happened the last time in situations you remember like this one?
- In sum, what exactly is the problem (or potential problem) and why is it important?

To Help Determine What One Ought to Do

- What should you do? What is the *right* thing to do?
- How do you determine the right thing to do—or what one *ought* to do? How do others determine the same? What makes a choice right or wrong, moral, responsible, or ethical?
- How about the perspectives and feelings of others who are not immediately involved in the situation? What are the goals and intentions of those involved? How do they matter and why?
- What is the fairest or most just thing to do? Is fair the same as right? Is it fair to hit someone who hits you first? Is it the right thing to do?
- Will everyone involved think it is fair and right?
- What actions might show respect of the rights and welfare of others? The lack thereof?
- What might be the consequences if you did what you ought to do? If you didn't?
- What action(s) would be most caring or prosocial?
- What might others—especially those you respect or admire the most—think you should do? Your family? Other relatives? Your teacher? Classmates? Coach? Religious leader? Other role models?
- What might judges decide? How would they make their decisions?
- Does your choice respect the rights of others? Will it harm them either physically or emotionally?
- What choice would be consistent with the Golden Rule of treating others as you would like them to treat you?
- What are your personal beliefs and values that help guide you in this situation?

Questions to Help Students Decide among Alternatives and Choose What They Ought to Do

- What did you do the last time there was a problem like this one? Did it solve the problem or make the matter worse? Should you do the same thing, or do you need to think more about this situation?
- What are all of the alternative solutions to the problem?
- Which solutions are consistent with what you ought to do? Which ones are not?
- Is there more than one way to achieve your goals—to do what you think you ought to do?
- Which solutions are most likely to "work"?
- How does one determine what is likely to work or to be most effective? What criteria are most important?
- What would you like to happen? What are your goals? Are they realistic? If more than one, which are the most and least important goals to you and others?
- Are your goals consistent with what you ought to do?
- How do you choose among competing goals and values?

(cont.)

- What do you do when what you *want* to do is not the same as what you *ought* to do?
- How might "what works" not be the same as what one ought to do?
- Which alternatives are most consistent with what you ought to do *and* are likely to work? What is the first choice? Second choice? Third choice? Which are your last choices? Are there any alternatives that you would never choose?
- Are there any other problems that your chosen solution might actually create?

Questions to Help Students Do What They Actually Decided to Do

- Do you need a plan to do what you decided to do? If so, what might it look like?
- Can you do it? Do you have the skills to do what you ought to do and decided to do? Do you have the self-confidence?
- What might help motivate you to do what you ought to do—what thoughts and feelings might help?
- Who might help you, and in what ways?
- If your first choice doesn't work, what will you try next that is consistent with what you ought to do? Do you have the skills and self-confidence for other choices to work?
- What obstacles might get in the way of your doing what you ought to do and intend to do?
- What might you do to avoid or overcome those obstacles? What will you do if you face them?
- How might you resist negative peer pressure?
- Might your feelings or emotions be a problem? For example, will you need to control your anger or make sure you don't say or do something impulsively?
- How will you know if your first choice, or any other choice, "works"? Will you feel better?
- Will others feel better? How might others react? Will there still be a problem?
- Do you need assistance? If so, who might help you? How would you seek their assistance?

Checklist to Help Schools Officials Select among Alternative Programs for Developing Self-Discipline

_____ The program's goals are consistent with those highly valued by the school staff, parents, and community.

_____ Research shows that implementation of the program leads to important social-cognitive (e.g., problem-solving skills), emotional (e.g., empathy, anger regulation), or behavioral (increased prosocial behavior, reduced antisocial behavioral) outcomes that school officials hope to achieve, especially those reflecting self-discipline.

_____ The program is likely to be accepted by teachers or others implementing it. Its demands on their time and training are reasonable, and the program's philosophy and recommended techniques are consistent with those who will be implementing the program.

_____ Measures are provided, or readily available, to evaluate the program's effectiveness. Where needed, the publisher provides outcome measures that are not readily available elsewhere, such as those that align with the specific goals of the program (e.g., pre–post evaluation tools for assessing the social-cognitive skills targeted in the program).

_____ Measures are provided, or readily available, to assess whether the program is being implemented as intended (i.e., with fidelity). For example, observational or self-report checklists are provided.

_____ In addition to curriculum lessons, the program provides support materials designed to promote generalization of skills outside of the environment in which the lessons are taught. For example, specific recommendations or activities are given to foster generalization in other locations in the school and outside of school, supporting materials are provided for parents, homework lessons are provided, etc.

_____ Professional development training opportunities, as needed, are provided, including training both before implementation begins and during it.

_____ The program is affordable to the school. Sufficient funds are available to purchase whatever materials in sufficient quantities are needed and to provide any necessary training.

_____ Other schools that have implemented the program have been contacted and asked about their evaluation of the program, including the practicality and fidelity of its implementation, its acceptability and prospective impact, and any potential obstacles to its implementation.

Checklist for Using Modeling to Help Develop Self-Discipline

____ Adults in the school provide positive role models for self-discipline. Adults throughout the school exhibit the same qualities they expect of their students, such as respect (e.g., they treat students with the same respect that they expect from them), responsibility (e.g., they come to class on time, return graded papers promptly).

____ Deliberate efforts are made in classrooms to provide and highlight multiple models of self-discipline, using a variety of methods, such as:

    ____ Multiple forms of media (literature, films, websites, documentaries, newspaper articles)

    ____ Curriculum units that profile positive role models

    ____ Lessons throughout nearly all curriculum areas (social studies, literacy, science, etc.)

    ____ Publicly recognizing the prosocial behaviors of students (e.g., verbal recognition through postings on bulletin boards, such as a Star Student of the Week, news clippings; articles in a class newsletter; students sharing with the class their achievements and achievements of others)

Deliberate efforts are made schoolwide to provide and highlight multiple models of self-discipline, using a variety of methods, such as:

    ____ Schoolwide assemblies

    ____ Morning announcements

    ____ A theme of the month, in which individuals are highlighted who represent that theme (e.g., courage, perseverance, honesty, trust, caring, respect, tolerance)

____ Efforts are made to curtail student exposure to negative role models and increase exposure to positive role models outside of school, using such methods as:

    ____ Curriculum lessons that teach students about the effects of the media, especially exposure to violence, on behavior

    ____ Newsletters to parents

    ____ Class discussions

    ____ Informing students of prosocial books, movies, and video games that are read or viewed by their own school role models (e.g., the biographies of desired role models read by their school role models)

____ Not only desired behaviors but also desired thoughts and emotions are modeled, such as social problem-solving skills (models think out loud or explain their thinking) but also positive emotions and regulation of negative emotions. Including:

    ____ Empathy

    ____ Sorrow

(cont.)

Checklist for Using Modeling to Help Develop Self-Discipline
(page 2 of 2)

_____ Pride

_____ Self-regulation of frustration and anger

_____ Feelings of responsibility

_____ Most of the models are characterized by the following features that enhance the effectiveness of modeling:

     _____ The models are well liked by the students or possess interpersonal qualities that students are attracted to, such as friendliness, caring, and a sense of humor.

     _____ The models are viewed by students as being competent in the skills modeled.

     _____ The models possess qualities desired by the students (athletic, musical, artistic skills; financial success, popularity, etc.)

     _____ Diversity is seen in the role models provided. For example, they vary in age, gender, race, socioeconomic status, careers, and cultural backgrounds.

     _____ Both specific skills (e.g., self-talk to calm oneself down) and more general dispositions (e.g., kindness, responsibility) are highlighted in the models.

     _____ All school staff members recognize and reinforce students publicly who model the desired social and emotional skills, and they do so strategically and wisely.

     _____ Models exhibit a wide range of skills or solutions to problems, not just one way to solve a problem.

     _____ Solutions to real-life problems are modeled. When hypothetical situations are used, they are realistic and linked to real-life situations.

     _____ When undesired behaviors are modeled, desired replacement behaviors are also modeled and receive greater attention.

     _____ In general, all adults model those qualities that the school hopes to see in students, both in the present and in the future when they are adults, such as respect for others, responsibility, kindness, caring, cooperation, honesty, trustworthiness, self-confidence, and self- discipline.

Recommendations for Maximizing the Social and Emotional Benefits of Sports and Extracurricular Activities

1. *Provide an optimal level of challenge.* Although expectations should be high, they also must be realistic. The level of challenge should foster motivation and learning while avoiding stress and anxiety.

2. *Make the experiences enjoyable.* Learning can and should be fun, and this is particularly important for nonrequired activities. Otherwise, burnout and dropping out are likely to occur.

3. *Create a motivational climate that encourages mastery.* Effort and improvement are highly valued and recognized.

4. *Maximize social support.* This includes support and positive guidance not only from the coach or instructor but also from parents and peers. The amount of praise should always exceed the amount of constructive criticism; in sports, this requirement might include keeping spectators at a distance.

5. *Make sure the coach or instructor is a role model.* The coach or instructor should model those social, emotional, and moral qualities that the school and community desire in their children and youth, including respect, honesty, fairness, and taking a stand against acts of injustice.

6. *Deemphasize winning.* This is especially important at younger ages. Skill development and fun should be the priorities.

7. *Ensure that instructors and coaches are appropriately trained.* Although most coaches and instructors of extracurricular activities are certified, not all are necessarily trained in the sport or activity they are coaching or teaching; such training should be required for all coaches and instructors of school-sponsored sports and activities.

8. *Where feasible, make special adaptations to requirements or rules to increase student involvement and the likelihood of success.* Such adaptations are not generally allowed in competitive events, but they should be made at the instructional and recreational levels.

9. *Provide opportunities commensurate with the student's age and skill level.* For example, emphasize recreational-level sports and activities in elementary school, and in the higher grades continue to offer recreational level sports and activities while also providing competitive opportunities at higher skill levels.

10. *Help the student—and, where appropriate, his or her parents—to decide whether he or she should participate in the sport or extracurricular activity.* The sport or activity should match the interest, and in many cases the skills, of the student. Often students and their parents need customized guidance as to which sports and activities are best for them, both in and outside of school.

CHAPTER 5

Preventing Behavior Problems

As discussed in the preceding two chapters, both the SEL approach and the SWPBS approach have been shown to be effective in preventing behavior problems. This is true at the classroom and schoolwide levels, although evidence supporting SWPBS at the schoolwide level is limited largely to reducing disciplinary office referrals and suspensions. One might argue that the zero tolerance approach also is effective in preventing behavior problems. Indeed, surveillance cameras, student identification badges, metal detectors, locker searches, school resource officers, and extensive and harsh codes of conduct are generally instituted for the purpose of deterring or preventing behavior problems. But, as argued in Chapter 1, their effectiveness is short-term and situational in that these techniques work only so long as they are salient, and they are likely to create a climate that is not conducive to developing self-discipline, learning, or positive mental health (American Psychological Association Zero Tolerance Task Force, 2008). Thus, the effectiveness of prevention programs should not be judged solely by the extent to which they reduce behavior problems, as typically indicated by reduced ODRs, suspensions, behavior ratings of students, or other indicators of safety. Although reduced problem behaviors and increased safety *are* important outcomes, schools should make sure that achieving them is never done at the expense of maintaining a positive school climate or developing students' self-discipline.

Strategies and techniques presented in this chapter are those designed to prevent behavior problems while simultaneously promoting positive classroom and schoolwide climates conducive to social, emotional, academic, and moral development. Few, if any, of the strategies and techniques presented are new to schools. They can be found in most textbooks on classroom management and school discipline (e.g., Bear, 2005; Charles, 2008a, 2008b; Evertson & Emmer, 2008; Evertson, Emmer, & Worsham, 2006; Good & Brophy, 2007; Jones & Jones, 2010; Martella, Nelson, & Machand-Martella, 2003; Weinstein & Mignano, 2007). Indeed, many of them appeared in books written for American educators over 100 years ago (e.g., Bagley, 1908; Raub, 1882). They also are commonly cited as recommended evidence-based practices in reviews of the literature on classroom management and school discipline (e.g., Charles, 2008b; Epstein, Atkins, Cullinan, Kutash, & Weaver, 2008; Evertson & Weinstein, 2006; Marzano, 2003). Finally, they are found in most SEL and SWPBS programs, although some receive greater emphasis in one approach than in the other. For example, the role of caring and supportive teacher–student relationships in preventing behavior problems receives greater emphasis in SEL than in SWPBS programs. On the other hand, behavioral antecedents, especially clarity of expectations and rules and the systematic use of praise and rewards for desired behavior, receive greater emphasis in SWPBS.

WHAT WORKS
IN THE PREVENTION OF BEHAVIOR PROBLEMS?

Two different lines of research provide answers to the question of what works best in preventing behavior problems. The first has been guided largely by research in child development, educational psychology, and school psychology on differences in discipline between effective and ineffective parents, teachers, and schools. This line of inquiry includes differences in the beliefs, perceptions, and goals of students, teachers, and parents; relationships among children and their parents and teachers; and differences in strategies and techniques used by parents and teachers. The outcome measures have largely been those related to social and emotional adjustment, including behavior problems. The second line of research has been guided more by research in special education and school psychology on the effectiveness of specific behavioral techniques in bringing about improvements in student behavior. Whereas the first line of research is consistent with the SEL approach to discipline, and its valuing of the importance of how educators think, feel, and act, the second line is more consistent with the SWPBS approach and its emphasis on specific observable actions taken by educators to change observable student behavior.

Both lines of research provide educators with valuable guidance for preventing behavior problems as well as for developing self-discipline and correcting misbehavior. The first provides guidance on the best general approach to prevention—namely, an authoritative approach. This approach is especially useful when one's goals are developing self-discipline and positive school climate, but it is also valuable for the more immediate goal of short-term compliance. Educators who adhere to the authoritative approach are both demanding and responsive. They communicate high behavioral expectations while simultaneously demonstrating their responsiveness to the social and emotional needs of students. The second line of research has provided educators with more specific techniques designed primarily to achieve short-term compliance via prevention and correction. Too often these educators are authoritaritian—that is, demanding but not necessarily responsive to the social and emotional needs of students.

This chapter first presents the authoritative approach to classroom and schoolwide discipline and the research supporting it. Next, more specific preventative strategies and techniques for effective classroom and schoolwide discipline are presented. Those strategies and techniques draw from and integrate research on the authoritative approach to discipline with comparable research on the effective use of behavioral techniques.

THE AUTHORITATIVE APPROACH TO CLASSROOM AND SCHOOLWIDE DISCIPLINE

Roughly 40 years ago Diana Baumrind (1968, 1971) identified three general types of child-rearing: *authoritative, authoritarian,* and *permissive.* She found that the most effective parents are authoritative in their approach to childrearing and discipline. They demonstrate two coexisting qualities, or high scores on two empirically supported dimensions of childrearing, *responsiveness* and *demandingness* (Baumrind, 1996), which are described below. Authoritative parents are high on both dimensions, authoritarian parents are high on demandingness but lacking in responsiveness, and permissive parents are high in responsiveness but lack in demandingness.

> **Both effective parenting and effective classroom management consist of a blend of responsiveness and demandingness.**

Responsiveness

Responsiveness is seen in how adults respond to the social, emotional, cognitive, and physical needs of students. Responsive adults prefer to guide rather than direct or control students. They prefer to influence student behavior through modeling, persuasion, and reasoning rather than using punishment or exercising their authority. They understand that a caring and supportive relationship is critical not only in meeting students' needs but also in developing self-discipline and preventing behavior problems. Thus, they demonstrate positive affect, as seen in warmth, understanding, respect, acceptance, enjoyment in working with students, and concern for and interest in the lives of all students. Responsive adults listen and communicate openly and clearly. When appropriate, they include students as active participants in classroom and schoolwide decision making. They model and reinforce desired behavior—but also desired thinking and emotions. In addressing the need for autonomy, they emphasize the development of social problem solving, moral decision making, and acceptance of responsibility for one's behavior.

Demandingness

In being responsive, authoritative adults demonstrate caring and support, but they are not pushovers when it comes to preventing and responding to misbehavior, rather, they demand appropriate behavior. In demonstrating demandingness, they hold high expectations but make every effort to help students meet them. They closely monitor and supervise student behavior, set clear and fair rules, and are firm, consistent, and fair in their enforcement of the rules and their consequences. Although they understand that student misbehavior is normal, they do not tolerate actions that are harmful or that interfere with learning.

Although they prefer to guide rather than direct, they do not hesitate to *use* discipline (e.g., time out, removal of privileges) when students fail to exhibit self-discipline or to act responsibly. However, when authoritative adults find it necessary to use punishment, they prefer mild over harsh forms of punishment and use it in combination with persuasion and reasoning and in a context of a caring and supportive relationship.

Supporting Research

Research strongly supports responsiveness and demandingness, but especially the two in combination. Compared to children and adolescents raised by authoritarian or permissive parents, those raised by authoritative parents (i.e., ones characterized by responsiveness and demandingness) tend to rank higher on measures of moral maturity, social competence, self-esteem, and academic achievement as well as exhibit fewer behavior problems (Baumrind, 1996; Kurdek & Fine, 1994; Lamborn, Mounts, Steinberg, & Dornbusch, 1991; Steinberg, 1996; Steinberg, Elmen, & Mounts, 1989). Such positive outcomes are largely attributed to responsiveness, which promotes autonomy, and demandingness, which encourages compliance (Baumrind, 1996)—two important parts of self-discipline.

Responsiveness and demandingness help to develop self-discipline in several ways. Responsiveness does so by modeling and teaching social and emotional competencies, especially empathy and social and moral responsibility, and by creating caring and supportive relationships, which are also conducive to its development. As noted in Chapter 3 on SEL and self-discipline, students are more inclined to adopt and internalize the values and standards of adults when communicated in the context of a caring and supportive adult–student relationship (Wentzel, 1997, 2004). Demandingness promotes self-discipline by requiring students to actually demonstrate those social and emotional competences that are associated with self-discipline, such as impulse control, anger regulation, delay of gratification, and prosocial behavior. It also promotes self-discipline by creating a structured and safe environment in which desired behaviors are practiced and reinforced while undesired behaviors are discouraged.

Research on both classroom and schoolwide discipline also strongly supports the key importance of responsiveness and demandingness. As reviewed in Chapter 3, research shows that positive teacher–student relationships, in which teachers demonstrate responsiveness, are related to favorable academic, social, and emotional outcomes. Students also are more inclined to seek help and assistance from teachers ranked high in terms of responsiveness (Unnever & Cornell, 2004). Research at the schoolwide level shows that positive adult–student relationships in school are a critical aspect of school climate, that is, students like and prefer teachers and schools characterized by responsiveness (e.g., Battistich et al., 1997; Birch & Ladd, 1998; Hamre & Pianta, 2006; Osterman, 2000; Pianta, 1999). The correlation is especially strong when responsiveness is combined with demandingness, such that the adults are neither overly permissive nor controlling (Wubbels, Brekelmans, van Tartwijk, & Admiral, 1999).

With respect to demandingness, research shows that clear expectations, the fairness of rules, and the fair enforcement of rules and consequences are related to fewer behavior problems—ranging from minor classroom disruptions to more serious bullying as well as aggression and delinquent behavior—and to greater student engagement and academic achievement (Arum, 2003; Benner, Graham, & Mistry, 2008; Brand, Felner, Shim, Seitsinger, & Dumas, 2003; Catalano et al., 2004; Doyle, 1986; Gottfredson et al., 1993, 2005; Mayer & Leone, 1999; Welsh, 2000). When demandingness is either lacking or is unfair and too harsh, behavioral and academic outcomes are likely to be far less positive. Whereas overly permissive teachers and schools create behavior problems and a disorderly environment, overly demanding ones create poor adult–teacher relationships that often result in students disliking their teachers (and school) and challenging their authority (Gregory et al., in press; Mayer & Leone, 1999).

Classroom and schoolwide research supports the importance of both responsiveness and demandingness in discipline—but especially their combination—and thus the authoritative approach. A healthy balance of responsiveness and demandingness has been found to be a key characteristic of effective discipline at both the classroom level (Brophy, 1996; Brophy & McCaslin, 1992; Gregory & Weinstein, 2004, 2008; Wentzel, 2002) and more recently at the schoolwide level (Gregory et al., in press). For example, in a comprehensive study of 96 classroom teachers, Brophy and McCaslin (1992) identified beliefs and practices that differentiated the most effective from the least effective teachers with respect to classroom discipline. Effectiveness was determined based on a combination of measures, including classroom observations, teacher interviews, and ratings of teachers by administrators. The researchers concluded that the authoritative approach to discipline best differentiated effective from ineffective teachers. The most effective teachers preferred to guide rather than demand appropriate behavior and emphasized social problem solving, decision making, and responsibility for one's own behavior. They understood that although correction was necessary at times, including the use of punishment, the most effective form of correction was not punishment alone but a combination of positive and mildly punitive techniques that reduced problem behavior and helped develop self-discipline. Thus, even in correcting students' misbehavior, they demonstrated both responsiveness and demandingness.

Similar support for the authoritative approach comes from research at the schoolwide level. In a recent study that included 290 high schools, Gregory et al. (in press) found that the safest schools, as evidenced by less bullying and victimization, were those perceived by students and teachers to be ranked high on both structure (demandingness) and support (responsiveness). These researchers concluded that "discipline practices should not be polarized into a 'get tough' versus 'give support' debate because both structure and support contribute to school safety for adolescents" (p. x).

PREVENTIVE STRATEGIES AND TECHNIQUES FOR EFFECTIVE CLASSROOM AND SCHOOLWIDE DISCIPLINE

The remainder of this chapter presents 10 evidence-based strategies for effective classroom and schoolwide discipline, and multiple techniques for implementing those strategies. Each strategy is consistent with the authoritative approach to classroom and schoolwide discipline.

The strategies are derived from research on authoritative discipline in educational psychology, developmental psychology, and school psychology, including research discussed above. The strategies and techniques also come from research in special education that has focused more specifically on the antecedents of behavior and effectiveness in preventing behavior problems (Kern & Clements, 2007). Few, if any, of the strategies and techniques are important only in prevention. Most also help develop self-discipline and should be included in individual or group programs focusing more on correction, or one's response to misbehavior after it has already occurred. For example, Strategy 1, "Demonstrate caring and support for all students," certainly applies to all three components of comprehensive school discipline, whereas Strategy 7, "Frequently monitor student behavior and respond quickly to early signs of misbehavior," is critical to both prevention and correction. Similarly, the use of praise is of utmost value in prevention but also in developing self-discipline and correcting misbehavior; thus, this strategy is presented in greater detail in Chapters 6, 7, and 8.

Strategy 1: Demonstrate Caring and Support for All Students

As reviewed in Chapter 3 on the SEL approach, there is a wealth of evidence that schools can prevent behavior problems by building and maintaining caring and supportive teacher–student relationships. Obviously, the more adults in a school who demonstrate caring and support, the better, but it is especially important that each student believe that there is at least one adult in the school who is caring and supportive of him or her (Osterman, 2000). Table 5.1 lists techniques that teachers and other school personnel use to demonstrate caring and support. The techniques are ones commonly cited in the research literature, drawn from classroom observations, teacher interviews, and teacher reports, but also ones that educators have shared with me in my courses and workshops on classroom management and school discipline.

Strategy 2: Promote Positive and Prevent Negative Peer Interactions

Relationships between students, or peer relationships, are often as critical to academic, social, and emotional development as are teacher–student relationships. This is clearly seen in the detrimental impact of bullying, peer rejection, and loneliness on both social and emotional adjustment and learning (Rubin et al., 2006; Waas, 2006). Peer relationships can be a problem in and of themselves, but they also are a frequent source of other behavior problems for which students are often corrected. Moreover, peer relationships are a widely recognized component of classroom and school climate, and frequently the component that students suggest is in need of the greatest improvement (Bear, Smith, Blank, & Chen, under review). It is for these reasons that effective teachers strive to establish a sense of community characterized by positive

> **Developing social and emotional competencies related to peer relations, and creating school norms and a culture of caring and supportive relations, are primary goals of most SEL programs.**

TABLE 5.1 Techniques to Demonstrate Caring and Support

- Increase time available for teachers and staff to interact positively with students, either individually or in small groups. For example, reduce teacher–student ratios; promote clubs, sports, and extracurricular activities supervised by adults; offer mentoring; and divide the school into separate units (e.g., ninth-grade academy).

- Limit classroom interruptions (e.g., unnecessary announcements, transitions), as they disrupt learning, reduce time for quality teacher–student interactions, and increase the potential for negative teacher–student interactions by often requiring greater compliance (e.g., "Listen to the announcement," "Stay in your seats while I talk to someone in the hall").

- Demonstrate knowledge of and a sincere interest in the lives of students, including knowing their interests, hobbies, concerns, wishes, strengths, and weaknesses. For example, gain such knowledge about students by conducting oral or written interviews with them (i.e., through individual oral interviews or written surveys), especially early in the school year. Interview or talk to their parents, peers, and previous teachers to obtain similar information. Have peers interview one another and report their findings to their teacher. In language arts, ask students to write their autobiography (with photos) or maintain a journal that the teacher reads and comments on. Information obtained from those sources would then be used to help teachers convey caring, understanding, and interest.

- Where feasible, adjust the curriculum, based on individuals' interests and the needs of students. For example, encourage students to read books and complete projects of their own choice.

- Hold class meetings in which students are encouraged to express and share their concerns. Although some programs recommend daily classroom meetings of approximately 30 minutes in elementary school, meetings do not have be every day or to last that long.

- To the extent practical and feasible, greet students as they enter the classroom and school building in the morning and leave in the afternoon.

- When the opportunity arises, and where appropriate, advocate for students. For example, defend their actions toward peers ("I can understand why you said that to him and will speak to him about it myself") or ask parents or administrators to be more lenient when a student is in trouble.

- Arrange to place suggestion boxes in classrooms and at a central location in the building, in which students can provide comments and suggestions (while remaining anonymous if so desired). Teachers can respond to suggestions at a class meeting or to the individual student when applicable.

- Post photos and news clippings of students or otherwise share with others the achievements and accomplishments of students. (e.g., class and schoolwide morning announcements, website newsletters). This would include photos and news stories originated by school staff members as well as stories or articles in local newspapers.

- Acknowledge all birthdays (e.g., with a card and/or announcement).

- Demonstrate humor. As is true with caring, warmth, trust, and respect, humor promotes positive relations. It also makes learning more enjoyable and fun.

- Attend out-of-school events of students (e.g., games in sports, music performances, fund-raising events, club activities).

- Actively participate *with* students in school and community activities such as service learning, games, and club activities.

- Use a variety of ways to recognize and reinforce desired behaviors, such as praise, personal notes or letters to students, positive messages to the parents (see Strategy 10).

- Make yourself maximally available for brief, regular interactions with individual students, especially those needing additional attention.

- Emphasize the positive aspects of students during parent–teacher conferences and in other communications with parents (see Strategy 9). Not only does this approach enhance teacher–parent relations, but its effects are likely to carry over to teacher–student relations.

- Provide adequate support services, especially to students during times of difficulty, most particularly including mentoring (for a review of programs, see Jekielek, Kristin, Moore, & Hair, 2002; for an evidence-based program and practical techniques, see (*ici.umn.edu/checkandconnect*).

teacher–student *and* student–student relationships (Osterman, 2000). Likewise, developing social and emotional competencies related to peer relationships and creating school norms and a culture of caring and supportive relationships are primary goals of most SEL programs, especially those for preventing bullying (for reviews of the literature and research, see Batsche & Porter, 2006; Espelage & Swearer, 2004; Merrell, Gueldner, Ross, & Isava, 2008).

Student-centered techniques for developing social and emotional competencies pertaining to peer relationships and self-discipline, such as empathy, conflict resolution, social problem solving, communication skills, and resisting peer pressure are presented in the next chapter. Table 5.2 lists additional techniques that effective teachers and schools use to promote positive and prevent negative peer relationships.

Strategy 3: Create a Physical Environment That Is Safe and Conducive to Teaching and Learning

While the first two strategies deal with the social and emotional environment, particularly relationships, this strategy focuses more specifically on the physical environment. Crowded, uncomfortable (e.g., poor cooling or heating), and physically unattractive environments contribute to aggression and violence (Berkowitz, 1989a, 1989b). Likewise, behavior problems are much more frequent when students are in close physical proximity to one another (especially when supervision is lacking), such as in hallways, cafeterias, playgrounds, and on school buses (Astor, Benbenishty, Marachi, & Meyer, 2006). The seating arrangements, the

---

TABLE 5.2. Techniques to Promote Positive and Prevent Negative Peer Relationships

- Emphasize cooperative rather than competitive activities, such as peer-assisted learning, clubs, team sports, chorus, band, service learning, and within class or across grade-level "buddy" systems.

- Throughout the curriculum and everyday life of the school, including in-class discussions, lessons, disciplinary encounters, and assemblies, emphasize the importance of a sense of community and the qualities that characterize it, such as respect, trust, caring, and shared responsibility.

- Take a strong stance against all forms of bullying—including verbal, physical, and relational (e.g., excluding others)—and lack of respect for diversity and different perspectives. Expect and encourage students to do the same.

- Encourage students to seek assistance from adults for friends and peers needing help, especially during times of stress, including teaching and encouraging students to recognize warning signs of potentially serious acts of school violence among their peers, such as a threat or harassment, to share their concerns with adults in schools, and to seek their assistance.

- Provide a wide range of school-sponsored clubs, sports, and other extracurricular activities, and encourage every student to participate in at least one or in other adult-supervised clubs and group activities outside of school, such as the YMCA, YWCA, 4-H Club, Scouts, church groups, sports teams, Boys Club, Girls Club, and the like.

location of the teacher, the organization of materials, supplies, and equipment, and the general attractiveness of the classroom are all widely recognized as important components in classroom management (e.g., Weinstein & Mignano, 2007). The same phenomenon applies to the school environment outside of classrooms, including not only physical appearance but also the flow of student traffic, proper scheduling, and adequate lighting, heating, and cooling (Hunley, 2008). Unfortunately, poor existing structures, inadequate resources, and overcrowding often limit what many teachers and schools can do to improve their physical environments. However, there are still things they can do, as elaborated in Table 5.3. Where appropriate and feasible, students (and parents) should be active participants in decisions pertaining to each of these recommendations, as well as in their implementation, as such

TABLE 5.3. Techniques to Help Create a Physical Environment That Is Safe and Conducive to Teaching and Learning

- Enhance the physical attractiveness of classrooms, hallways, and other areas of the building and school grounds, which entails attractively painted walls, colorful and interesting posters and bulletin boards, attractive trees and plants, and comfortable furniture.

- Arrange chairs, desks, tables, supplies, equipment, and materials in a well-organized and efficient manner.

- Arrange chairs and desks to reduce congestion, enhance student engagement, minimize distractions, and maximize teacher monitoring and movement around the class (especially quick movement toward students when assistance or close physical proximity is needed). While arranging desks in rows tends to be most conducive to students' attending to teacher-led lessons and individual seatwork, it is recommended that students work at tables for cooperative learning activities and that chairs be placed in a circle or horseshoe shape for discussions.

- Arrange materials, supplies, and equipment (including pencil sharpeners and staplers) such that students can use them without disrupting the class or taking time away from learning (e.g., locate some near the teacher's desk and/or spread them out around the room to avoid congestion).

- At gym and recess, arrange equipment such that it can be quickly and easily accessed and used by students. Remove, lock, or cover up materials, supplies, and equipment when students should not be using them.

- Allow students to sit where they prefer, but make it clear that this privilege can be withdrawn when self-discipline is not exhibited. This instruction would apply to seating in classrooms, the cafeteria, at assemblies, and on the bus. When students' behavior disrupts learning or teaching or is harmful to others (e.g., teasing, bullying), this privilege should be removed and the student(s) moved to where close adult monitoring and supervision can occur.

- Assure that the school campus has appropriate lighting, locks, two-way communications systems, alarm systems, and additional safety equipment as appropriate and needed, including fences, metal detectors, and surveillance cameras.

- Arrange schedules and direct traffic-flow patterns to minimize congestion (and potential conflicts between different age groups) during class transitions, lunch periods, recess periods, and in loading and unloading buses.

involvement enhances shared responsibility and ownership as well as a sense of community.

Strategy 4: Establish Social, Emotional, and Academic Expectations That Are Clear, High, Reasonable, and Responsive to Developmental, Cultural, and Individual Differences

As discussed earlier in this chapter, authoritative teachers and school officials make it clear that they expect students to demonstrate self-discipline, as demonstrated in students' following school rules, regulating their emotions and behavior, and otherwise acting in a responsible and respectful manner toward adults and peers. They also expect students to work hard and achieve high academic standards. Their expectations are both reasonable and responsive to developmental, cultural, and individual differences in learning. For example, the expectations in high school are not be the same as in elementary school, and many children with disabilities should not be expected to achieve the same academically as those without disabilities. Nevertheless, high expectations apply to all students—they are expected to reach their highest potential in all areas of learning and development. In addition, classroom and schoolwide expectations should be:

- Communicated clearly in policies and practice (e.g., in the school's code of conduct and mission statement through specified procedures and routines). The SWPBS approach recommends that behavioral expectations be posted throughout the school building and grounds.
- Emphasized during the early days of each school year and revisited as often as needed throughout the year.
- Taught directly and indirectly (e.g., via modeling; see Strategy 4, Chapter 4, on the use of modeling, pp. 66–67). Students should be reinforced by teachers, staff members, peers, and parents seeking to comply with all rules.
- Backed up by a system of supports for students who frequently fail to comply.
- Few in number (four to six) and positively worded. Common ones pertain to responsibility ("Be responsible"), respect ("Respect others"), effort ("Do your best"), and obeying authority or rules ("Follow directions"). A long list of expectations and rules is not always needed. In a private school for children at which I work as a school psychologist, only one behavioral expectation is posted throughout the building (and emphasized throughout the school curriculum), namely, "Be kind." Most of the students are children with learning disabilities or attention-deficit/hyperactivity disorder, but they quickly learn that being kind incorporates a variety of socially and morally responsible behaviors.

Strategy 5: Establish Predictable Procedures and Routines

A procedure defines the appropriate course of action one is to take to carry out a particular activity or function (Weinstein, 2006). A procedure becomes a routine after it has been repeated over and over and is performed habitually, requiring little if any adult supervision. Like rules, procedures and routines are used to help guide student behavior and maintain orderly classrooms and schools. They differ from rules, however, in that procedures and routines are typically not written and not used to control student behavior, especially with punitive consequences.

Evertson et al. (2006) recommend that teachers establish six types of procedures and routines in their classrooms. Four of them are specific to the classrooms: (1) those for room use, such as the use of the pencil sharpener and other equipment, materials, and supplies; (2) those for guiding individual work and teacher-led activities, such as for obtaining assistance from the teacher or peers, turning in classwork and homework, and engaging in appropriate activities upon completing assignments early; (3) those for small-group instruction, such as those that facilitate entering and leaving the group and clarify what is expected of group members; and (4) those for cooperative learning group activities, such as how to work together and how individual accountability will be demonstrated.

Two additional types of procedures and routines apply classwide and schoolwide: (1) those for class transitions into and out of the classroom and other areas of the school such as the cafeteria, library, auditorium, and hallways; and (2) those that are general, such as for distributing materials, requesting help from the teacher or others in school, taking attendance, morning announcements, fire and other safety drills, use of lockers, and for individual students to go to the bathroom, water fountain, the office, library, and elsewhere.

As is true of general behavioral expectations, procedures and routines should be taught, discussed, modeled, practiced and reinforced early in the school year, and retaught as often as needed throughout the school year. Sometimes it is also helpful to use *foreshadowing* for procedures and routines, especially when behavior problems are likely to occur, such as during transitions. In foreshadowing, students are reminded what will happen soon and how they should respond (e.g., "The bell will ring in 5 minutes, so please finish up and get ready"). Additional ways to reduce behavior problems during transitions is to minimize the number of transitions, reduce the size of groups involved in a transition (e.g., let one group go first, followed by another), turn transitions into a game in which teams are challenged to complete the transition in a given amount of time or without disruptions (recognize them with privileges or praise), and to assign a "buddy," or partner, to assist students at risk for behavior problems.

Strategy 6: Establish Fair Rules and Consequences

As is true with behavioral expectations, procedures, and routines, rules serve to help manage student behavior but generally more directly and explicitly than the former. While behavioral expectations tend to be general ("Respect others"), rules often are more specific ("Be in class when the bell rings"); However, it is not uncommon to find behavioral expectations and general classroom rules backed up by more specific and often unwritten rules. Rules are generally codified in writing (e.g., a code of conduct), not only to regulate behavior but also often to exercise adult authority. Rules also differ from behavioral expectations in that they are almost always linked to punitive consequences for their violation.

Whether or not students perceive classroom and school rules to be clear and fair has been shown to be a determinant of student behavior, school climate, and school safety (Arum, 2003; Benner et al., 2008; Brand et al., 2003; Gottfredson et al., 1993; Gottfredson, Payne, & Gottfredson, 2005; Mayer & Leone, 1999; Welsh, 2000, 2003). Perhaps the most convincing evidence of the importance of fairness of rules comes from Arum's (2003) comprehensive national study of over 30,000 students. Like other researchers, Arum found fairness to be associated with multiple positive outcomes, but he also demonstrated further support for the authoritative approach to school

> **When students perceive rules to be fair—neither too lenient nor overly harsh—they are most willing to obey them.**

discipline by showing a curvilinear relationship between fairness and strictness. That is, strictness was found to be related to student perceptions of fairness, but only up to a certain point. In schools where students perceived rules as too lenient, they generally perceived them as unfair, but they also perceived them as unfair when they thought the rules were too strict. Students perceived rules to be most fair when they were neither too lenient nor overly harsh, and *it was in those schools that students reported the greatest willingness to obey rules.* Students also demonstrated higher grades in schools in which they perceived rules to be fair. Interestingly, the impact of perceptions of fairness on academic achievement was shown to be strongest among African American students: their grades were worse in schools in which rules were perceived by students as either too lenient or overly strict.

Arum's (2003) findings and those of others (e.g., Mayer & Leone, 1999) confirm that an authoritarian zero tolerance approach to school discipline, characterized by overly strict rules and consequences intended to induce fear, is generally ineffective. It is likely to increase misbehavior and disengagement from school and to foster further strictness and harshness by school administrators and staff ("If one day of suspension isn't enough to stop this, let's make it three days"). However, Arum's findings also show that a *fair* and *reasonable* degree of strictness, or demandingness, is critical to effective school discipline. One key to the effectiveness of moderately strict rules is that they are perceived by students as being imposed by adults with *legitimate* moral authority—by adults who are respected and viewed as fair and supportive, not overly controlling (Arum, 2003). As recently noted by Gregory and Weinstein (2008), this view is consistent with research in social psychology on procedural justice showing that adults are more likely to obey police and judges whom they trust and believe to be fair (Tyler, 2006; Tyler & Degocy, 1995). Trust and perceptions of fairness are especially important for compliance during adolescence, when students are seeking greater autonomy and have a greater understanding of fairness and respect.

Researchers and authors of textbooks on classroom management and school discipline (e.g., Canter & Canter, 2001; Curwin, Mendler, & Mendler, 2008; Dreikurs & Grey, 1968; Duke, 2002; Evertson et al., 2006; Jones & Jones, 2010; Weinstein, 2006) generally concur about what characterizes effective rules. Those characteristics are summarized below. Although they apply to rules at both the classroom and school levels, emphasis is placed on classroom rules because school rules are usually determined at the district level, with individual schools having little leeway in determining their own rules:

1. *Effective rules are clear to students, their parents, and teachers/staff.* Everyone clearly understands what each rule means, which entails not only the use of language that is clear to all readers of the rules (e.g., written in the language used in the home and at the student's reading level) but also giving specific examples of where and when each rule applies. Rules should state clearly and positively the behaviors that students are to exhibit (e.g., "Raise your hand to speak") rather than not exhibit ("Don't call out"). Examples, however, should certainly include both expected and prohibited behaviors.

Rules should be presented both orally and in writing (where developmentally appropriate for students) to all parties at the very beginning of the school year (e.g., in staff meetings, open house for parents, and during the earliest days of school for students). Parents should sign that they have reviewed classroom and school rules with their children and understand them (with a record kept for future reference). Where age appropriate, students should sign that they understand the rules. Teachers might also ask students to take a test of their knowledge and understanding of the rules.

Classroom rules should be clearly posted in the classroom. If schoolwide behavioral expectations are used in the school, they too should be posted and discussed together with the classroom rules (e.g., how specific classroom rules convey the behavioral expectations of responsibility and respect). To avoid too many rules and expectations, however, the classroom rules might be the same as the schoolwide expectations (with more specific examples and details given about how each general behavioral expectation translates into a more specific written or unwritten rule).

2. *Effective rules are fair and reasonable.* Whereas schoolwide school rules are typically developed by a committee that includes teachers, administrators, support staff, and parents (and at times students in upper grades), classroom rules are typically developed by the classroom teacher (with or without student involvement, as discussed later in this section). In determining what is *fair* and *reasonable*, the perceptions of all parties involved in applying and following the rules, including those of the students, should be considered. As noted previously, students—and especially adolescents—are likely to protest, ignore, or resist those rules they perceive as overly harsh, trivial, or otherwise unfair and unreasonable.

Duke (2002) and Gathercoal (2001) argue that it is easier to defend the fairness of rules when they are grounded in constitutional rights, such as safety, property rights, respect for the rights and needs of others, and personal and social responsibility. To help ensure that classroom rules are not unreasonable or unnecessary, Weinstein (2006) recommends that teachers ask themselves: (1) Is there a compelling reason for the rule? (2) Will the rule enhance classroom climate and learning? and (3) Can a clear rationale for the rule be given to students, parents, and administrators?

3. *Effective rules are taught, and behaviors consistent with the rules are reinforced.* Often teaching the rules should entail more than just reviewing, explaining, and discussing the rules. Particularly in the lower grades and with students at risk of behavior problems, it also should include modeling the desired behaviors and having students demonstrate and

rehearse them. At all grades students should be recognized and reinforced for following the rules (see Chapters 6 and 7 on the use of praise and rewards).

4. *Effective rules are backed up by fair, reasonable, and judicious consequences for their violation.* It is important that rules be fair and reasonable if students are expected to follow them in a committed rather than grudging fashion, and this requirement also applies to the consequences exacted in enforcing them. As discussed further in Chapter 9 on correcting misbehavior, with respect to being fair and reasonable, consistency is important but not as important as being judicious—considering all the circumstances of a given situation of a rule violation, such as the student's intentions and previous history, before invoking the consequences. School officials should serve not just as knee-jerk enforcers but also as judges capable of determining one's guilt or innocence based on fair consequences. Normally this approach means considering consequences, on a case-by-case basis and making sure that the consequences "fit the crime."

5. *Effective rules are limited to no more than four or five general ones at the classroom level.* Generally, it is recommended that classroom rules be no more than four to five in number (Gable, Hester, Rock, & Hughes, 2009). It is difficult for students to remember, and for teachers to manage, more than that. A long list also runs the risk of the teacher being more authoritarian than authoritative, thereby creating a negative classroom climate. Again, in many cases the classroom rules might be the same as, or similar to, schoolwide expectations such as:

- Be responsible (or show self-discipline).
- Respect the rights and views of others.
- Be prepared and do your best.
- Be kind toward others.
- Solve social conflicts peacefully.

Should Students Help Develop the Rules?

Although most researchers and writers agree on most other aspects of rules, many disagree on the answer to the question of whether students should help to develop them. There also is a lack of research to guide one in answering it properly (Duke, 2002). Some argue that teachers and students should develop rules collaboratively because the active involvement of students increases their understanding and appreciation of the rules and thus their commitment to following them (e.g., Charney, 2002; Curwin et al., 2008; Epstein et al., 2008; Jones & Jones, 2010; Kerr & Nelson, 2009). Others argue that teachers should simply develop the rules themselves and discuss them with their students while giving a clear rationale for each one, welcoming and respecting student comments (e.g., Duke, 2002; Evertson et al., 2006). The latter approach is often the most efficient, recognizing that students rarely have as much choice as school officials about matters pertaining to rules, especially schoolwide rules.

Strategy 7: Monitor Student Behavior Frequently and Respond Quickly to Early Signs of Misbehavior

With respect to preventing behavior problems at both the classroom and schoolwide levels, the most effective school officials function much like air traffic controllers. They constantly monitor the movement of a large number of planes (read students) while sharing responsibility with the pilots (students) for the outcomes of their decisions, including the planes' movements in the skies and on the runways (in the classroom and school).

Effective teachers are a lot like air traffic controllers!

They are constantly alert as to the status of each plane and well aware which ones require more guidance than others (e.g., those lacking skills and those flying in challenging environments, and *especially* those both lacking skills *and* flying in challenging environments). They understand that greater guidance is needed at certain times than at others, such as during landings (i.e., when students enter the classroom or begin assignments) and takeoffs (when students finish assignments or get ready to transition) and in congested areas (hallways, the playground, the cafeteria). They anticipate which planes (students) might be in trouble and respond immediately to avoid possible crashes (crises)—which includes providing as much guidance and support as needed, and doing so without delay.

Like good air traffic controllers, effective educators demonstrate two qualities that have consistently been shown to prevent behavior problems: *withitness* and *overlapping* (Doyle, 1986; Kounin, 1970; Kounin & Gump, 1974). In demonstrating withitness (i.e., classroom awareness), effective teachers (and school officials) closely monitor student behavior and respond immediately to early signs of misbehavior, such as when a student first appears to be disengaged from learning, gets out of his or her seat, or becomes upset, angry, or frustrated. This hyperawareness often prevents a full-fledged behavior problem from taking form and the misbehavior from becoming contagious and spreading throughout the class. Withitness helps prevent disruptions in learning, possible harm to others, and the need to use intrusive and time-consuming forms of correction. Withitness may be observed when teachers closely scan and move about the classroom, using eye contact, physical proximity, verbal prompts, reminders, and praise—but also warnings—at the earliest signs of potential or actual misbehavior. In demonstrating overlapping (i.e., attending to multiple things at the same time), effective teachers use such techniques as the foregoing—but seamlessly. For example, they simultaneously prevent potential misbehavior by two students on opposite sides of the room by standing near one and giving the evil eye to the other—all while continuing to teach a lesson. Frequent monitoring of and early response to potential misbehavior are always important, but they are especially important for (1) those students who lack self-discipline and (2) during times and in places that are most conducive to misbehavior.

In monitoring student behavior, effective educators demonstrate withitness and overlapping in their use of the following techniques:

• They frequently circulate throughout the classroom and building while questioning, assisting, and providing feedback and praise. They recognize that this is more important during independent seat work and group work than during teacher-directed activities (Weinstein, 2006).

• They make students aware that they are being monitored, whether through physical proximity, visual contact, or verbal reminders, instruction, or feedback.

• They ensure that their students remain well aware of what they should be doing, periodically reminding them, as needed (e.g., "Everyone should be working on page 59 of your math book right now," or "Mustafa, you should be on your way to class, or you're going to be tardy"). This requires that the teachers themselves be aware what each student should be doing.

• They provide increased monitoring, supervision, and support during times and in places that behavior problems are most likely to occur, especially in congested areas and at times when students think they are not being observed by adults. In classrooms, this period would include the beginning and end of assignments and transitions and during difficult assignments and cooperative learning activities. At the schoolwide level, this period would include the beginning and end of the school day (especially toward the beginning of the school year), during transitions, and in such hot spots as hallways, the playground or student parking lot, bus loading area, bathrooms, stairwells, and the cafeteria.

• They devote the bulk of their attention to specific students at the greatest risk of behavior problems owing either to their previous history, the particular difficulty of a given task (i.e., one likely to be more challenging or frustrating than usual), or other special circumstances (e.g., a given student enters the classroom upset).

• At the schoolwide level, they maximize the amount of monitoring provided, as needed, by requiring most teachers and staff members to be in the hallways or outside of their classroom doors during transition periods. In schools where misbehavior is rife, this heightened monitoring effort might include the use of school resource officers and surveillance cameras.

• They are alert to and respond immediately to signs of behavior problems. In the classroom such signs might include talking without permission, getting out of one's seat, not following directions or working on assigned tasks, not completing an activity successfully, or putting one's head down on the desk. At the schoolwide level indications might include students not being where they are supposed to be, shoving or name calling, and gathering to observe a potential fight.

• At the classroom level, they try to catch and correct errors on assignments early, before the task becomes increasingly frustrating. When providing feedback, they do so quietly, trying not to disturb others who are working productively.

• They solicit help from students in monitoring the behavior and academic progress of their peers, where appropriate. In the classroom, this help might include providing assistance to others on assignments. At the schoolwide level, it would include immediately reporting to adults any threats of violence.

• They encourage self-monitoring of behavior while emphasizing the importance of self-discipline and social responsibility. They encourage students to seek assistance from peers and adults whenever it is needed, including not only academic assistance on classroom assignments but also assistance when faced with such social and emotional stressors as bullying, peer rejection, problems at home, and the like.

Strategy 8: Provide Academic Instruction and Activities That Engage and Motivate Learning

Comparatively few behavior problems occur in classrooms where teachers provide instruction and learning activities that truly motivate students and actively engage them in learning (Brophy, 2004; Morrone & Pintrich, 2006; Osterman, 2000; Stipek, 2002). Effective teachers and school officials understand that they can prevent many behavior problems from developing by undertaking to accomplish the following practical goals (Bear, 2005):

1. *Provide momentum and smoothness.* These are two more characteristics of effective teachers (in addition to withitness and overlapping) observed nearly four decades ago by Kounin (Kounin, 1970; Kounin & Gump, 1974) that researchers have consistently found to be important in preventing misbehavior (Doyle, 1986). *Momentum* refers to the pacing of instruction: ideally, once students enter the classroom, the lesson begins promptly, is presented at a brisk pace, and elicits a high rate of student responses. *Smoothness* refers to the even flow of instruction, in which any misbehavior and/or interruptions are handled with but minimal impact on instructional effectiveness.

Both momentum and smoothness are qualities seen not only during instruction but also during transitions. Transitions occur quickly and seamlessly, thereby avoiding behavior problems. Little time is wasted. Methods used for transitions and to avoid wasted time include:

- Enforcing the implicit "rule" that students need permission to be engaged in nonlearning activities during those times that student engagement is expected of them. That is, not only are they not allowed to misbehave but also they are not allowed to do "nothing" upon finishing an assignment early or at other times when the rest of the class is engaged. For example, after finishing one task, students are instructed and expected to immediately turn their attention to multiple other tasks, whether reading a book, working on homework, working on the computer, completing activities at work centers, or completing work on a folder of enrichment or fun educational activities kept either in their desks or elsewhere in the room.
- Using *foreshadowing*—informing or cuing students what is coming next (e.g., what the next assignment will be and what materials will be needed).
- Ensuring that lesson plans and materials are prepared and organized in advance.
- Reminding students of behavioral expectations and rules.
- Using praise strategically, such as praising students for desired behavior (e.g., "I see that Michael is getting ready for the next class. Thanks for reminding me, Michael").

2. *Provide class instruction and materials that motivate student engagement in learning.* Instruction and materials should never be boring or unchallenging, nor too difficult or frustrating—they should be just right! They should clearly demonstrate interest and enthusiasm in the subject matter, communicating to students why it is important. Do not repeat the same activities over and over, whether lectures, direct instruction, or worksheets. Instead, to spark motivation, engage learning and higher-order thinking, and prevent behavior problems, use novelty and variety as often as possible and seek to match instructional content and materials with the interests of students whenever possible, including the use of discussions, cooperative learning, peer-assisted learning, computer-assisted learning, and instructional gaming. Give particular attention to cooperative learning, because it motivates not only academic learning but also prosocial behavior (Johnson & Johnson, 1999).

3. *Provide students with opportunities to participate in instructional decisions.* For example, allow students to choose topics of study and the means by which they can demonstrate mastery. Obviously, such choices should be reasonable ones and generally limited to those offered by the teacher. To foster motivation one might allow students to choose topics for further investigation in social studies, how they will research them (e.g., interviews, surveys, computer searches, library searches), and how they will demonstrate their knowledge (e.g., written report, poem, song, video, play). Additional opportunities to participate in instructional decisions might include student goal setting, self-monitoring, teacher–student conferencing, and class meetings.

4. *Adapt the instruction, curriculum, and materials to individual needs and cultural differences.* This suggestion includes differentiating instructions and making adaptations to meet the needs of students with learning disabilities, attention deficit/hyperactivity disorder, and other disabilities, as well as those who are gifted and talented. It also means being responsive to racial, cultural, and ethnic diversity.

5. *Communicate high academic expectations.* As is true with behavioral expectations, effective teachers hold academic expectations that are high (yet realistic) and convey that they are optimistic that all students will achieve them.

6. *Communicate that teachers and students should be accountable for academic success.* To be sure, teachers are the ones held most accountable for student learning, but students (and parents) also should share in accountability. Together, teachers and students can set academic goals and monitor progress toward meeting them. The accountability for meeting or not meeting those goals and standards is then rightfully shared.

7. *Ensure that high rates of success occur, especially when new concepts are first introduced.* The experience of failure stifles motivation, particularly when repeated or occurring early in a task. Effective teachers assign tasks with a high probability for early and continued success. To maintain momentum and student engagement in learning, more difficult and challenging material is gradually introduced and interspersed with material already mastered. Students understand the directions and how to complete the assigned tasks. While student engagement and on-task behavior are important, it is also important that the time expended on an assignment to be spent productively (Weinstein, 2007).

8. *Give frequent feedback—and especially praise—to foster academic learning.* Effective teachers provide frequent feedback: they praise correct academic responses (and effort) and use constructive criticism when expectations are not met and when effort and achievement are lacking. Positive reinforcement, especially praise, is much more common (and welcome) than constructive criticism.

Strategy 9: Establish and Maintain Close Communication with Each Student's Parents and Work Hard to Garner Their Support

There are two major reasons why this recommended strategy is important. First, parents have the ethical, and often legal, right to be well informed about their children's behavior—academic, social, and emotional, and both positive and negative (Jones & Jones, 2010). Second, parents, together with school officials and peers, exert a powerful influence on their children's academic, social, emotional, and moral development (Parke & Buriel, 2006). Parental support helps schools and school officials to achieve their academic, social, emotional, and moral goals or objectives, while the lack of that support can make achieving them very difficult. Parents can be the source of considerable reinforcement or, alternatively, much stress. Thus, close communications and collaboration with parents are important not only in fostering student learning and preventing behavior problems but also in promoting a positive school climate.

Teachers and school officials should initiate positive communications with parents early in the school year and continue them throughout the year. Too often, school officials make the mistake of allowing this first contact with parents to be a negative one, the most obvious example being when parents are first contacted about their child's behavior or academic problems. However, even in the absence of such problems, the initial contact with parents is not always very positive. For example, the first contact often consists of mailing parents the school's code of conduct and a list of what they are expected to purchase and do. Although those items are important, they should be secondary to the message that parents are valued participants in the process of educating their children, that their support is needed and their active involvement and collaboration are appreciated. Parents should be informed of the best methods of communicating with the school and their child's teacher and provided with specific ways in which they can become actively involved (e.g., visit the school; join the PTA; volunteer to help in various ways, such as on committees, with field trips, in the classroom). Likewise, they should be informed, how their child's classroom teacher and school officials will communicate with them. A letter should come from both the school and the child's teacher (or a group letter from teachers in middle school and high school).

> Parents not only have the right to be informed about their children's behavior, but informing parents also is often simply a wise practice for helping develop student self-discipline.

Positive communications should continue throughout the school year. For example, positive notes (in a homework notebook or separately), e-mails, or phone calls should be sent periodically to the homes of all students. Additional methods of positive communications include class and school newsletters, parent conferences, announcements on class and school web pages, articles in local newspapers, and parent–teacher meetings.

Strategy 10: Use Praise and Rewards in a Wise and Strategic Manner

Praise and rewards—especially praise—should be used in implementing each of the foregoing strategies, but used in a manner that improves behavior while minimizing the risk of diminishing intrinsic motivation. This last strategy is perhaps the most important one for preventing behavior problems. Because praise and rewards can be very effective not only in motivating academic learning and bringing about compliance but also perhaps more importantly in developing and motivating self-discipline, they are covered in detail in Chapters 6, 7, and 8.

SUMMARY

The preceding chapter focused on student-centered strategies designed primarily to develop discipline but which also certainly serve to help prevent behavior problems. Strategies in the current chapter are more teacher-centered, focused not on the long-term development of social and emotional competencies within students but on the actions of teachers and other school staff that greatly influence the behavior of students while they are in school. These actions commonly fall under the general category of classroom management, with the primary goal being the prevention of behavior problems.

The best approach to classroom management and school discipline is an authoritative approach—an approach that gives equal attention to two important qualities, demandingness and responsiveness. Research shows that, in contrast to the authoritarian approach (which is high in demandingness but low in responsiveness) and the permissive approach (which is high in responsiveness but low in demandingness), the authoritative approach leads to a number of positive academic, social, and emotional student outcomes. The authoritative approach to discipline is the one used in SEL. Authoritative educators combine both teacher-centered and student-centered strategies. In doing so, they both prevent behavior problems in the short term and develop self-discipline in the long term. While in Chapter 4 I presented 6 strategies, mostly student-centered ones, that are used by authoritative educators and in SEL programs to develop self-discipline, in this chapter I presented 10 strategies used by authoritative teachers that are more teacher-centered and specific to preventing behavior problems.

CHAPTER 6

Praise and Rewards
Use with Caution?

Just as students have been spanked, reprimanded, and suspended for their behavior over the centuries, so too have they been praised and rewarded for good behavior. As noted by O'Leary and Drabman (1971), as early as the 12th century it was reported that children were awarded with nuts, figs, and honey in the teaching of the Torah (Birnbaum, 1962), and in the early 16th century Erasmus argued that, instead of the cane, teachers should use cherries and cakes to help their pupils learn Latin and Greek (Skinner, 1966). Based largely on the early research of John Watson (1913), Edward Thorndike (1920), and B. F. Skinner (1953, 1966) on the use of positive reinforcement and punishment, those techniques received widespread application in classrooms in the 1960s and 1970s. Today, praise and rewards are the techniques that often come to mind when one thinks of "positive" techniques for classroom management and schoolwide discipline. Indeed, they are the foundation of Canter and Canter's popular model *Assertive Discipline* (Canter & Canter, 2001) and of the SWPBS approach to schoolwide discipline.

To be sure, praise and rewards can be powerful techniques for behavior change. However, often they are not. Like any other educational technique, they can be used effectively or ineffectively. Likewise, they can be used for either worthwhile or for dubious purposes, such as to help develop self-discipline or simply to control student behavior. This chapter focuses on critical issues pertaining to the use of praise and rewards, giving good reasons for their use but also reasons why school officials should be cautious when using them. Particular attention is given to an issue of considerable controversy in recent years—the potential harmful impact of praise and rewards on intrinsic motivation. This chapter serves as a foundation for the succeeding two chapters. In Chapters 7 and 8, specific strategies and techniques are presented for the strategic and wise use of praise and rewards to increase desired behaviors while also developing self-discipline.

DISTINGUISHING AMONG
POSITIVE REINFORCEMENT, REWARDS, AND PRAISE

Praise and rewards serve multiple functions, as discussed below, but educators typically use them to teach or strengthen student behaviors while following principles of positive reinforcement. They are viewed as effectively serving this function when the targeted behaviors increase in strength or frequency following their use. Only when they are used successfully in this manner should they be referred to as *positive reinforcers*, or techniques of positive reinforcement. Because praise and rewards do not necessarily reinforce behavior (and can actually serve as punishers) they will not be referred to in this chapter as *positive reinforcers*, but simply as *praise* and *rewards*. This distinction allows one to address the critical question "Under what conditions do praise and rewards *function* as positive reinforcers?"

In addition to distinguishing rewards from reinforcers, it is important to differentiate praise from rewards. Praise *can* be used to reward and reinforce behavior. However, research shows that teachers do not always use praise for this purpose, but for multiple other purposes. Another reason to differentiate praise from rewards is that research, as discussed in this chapter, indicates that teachers should be much less concerned about any potential negative impacts from the use of praise than from the use of rewards.

Praise is one type of reward called *social* rewards. Social rewards in the classroom include praise, but they also include attention from the teacher, peers, parents, siblings, and others. Praise and attention have several major advantages over other classroom techniques used to reward or reinforce behavior: They are relatively easy to use, occur naturally, and students are less likely to get tired of them (i.e., they are less likely to be "satiatins") (Kazdin, 1981). Thus, teachers are much more prone to use praise and attention than other rewards. Also, unlike many other rewards, praise has the advantage of being appropriate for students of all ages and abilities.

In addition to social rewards, teachers use four other types of rewards, although more so in lower grades than higher grades:

Privileges, such as assisting the teacher, preferred parking for high school students, "hat day," and listening to music during classwork.

Preferred activities, such as extra recess, free time, watching a video, listening to music, and playing a game.

Tangibles, such as stickers, toys, certificates, and candy.

Tokens, such as coupons, tickets, chips, or points that can be exchanged for tangibles, preferred activities, or privileges.

Although praise can be expressed in writing and nonverbally such as in a gesture or physical response (e.g., applause, smile, or hug), it is typically expressed verbally. Praise is similar to *feedback*, but whereas feedback can be neutral, negative, or positive, praise is intended to be positive—conveying an evaluation of approval or satisfaction of another person's behavior, performance, product, or attribute (Kanouse, Gumpert, & Canavan-Gumpert, 1981). For example, mere feedback would be "You were correct" or "You followed the rule about raising your hand," whereas praise would be "Great job!" or "Thanks for raising your hand."

THE CONTROVERSY OVER THE USE OF PRAISE AND REWARDS

Despite their common use in classrooms and schools, praise and rewards have always been the subjects of controversy and criticism, including by authors of popular models of school discipline (e.g., Dreikurs & Grey, 1968; Kohn, 1999; Nelson et al., 2000) and leading theorists and researchers in psychology and education (Brophy, 1981; Kohlberg, 1981; Piaget, 1932/1965; Deci, Koestner, & Ryan, 1999, 2001). For example, both Dreikurs (Dreikurs & Grey, 1968) and authors of more recent models of his popular approach to discipline (e.g., Nelsen et al., 2000) have claimed that praise and rewards discourage self-discipline and self-esteem; foster dependency on adults; convey authority, power, and a lack of trust and respect; are a form of bribery; and often contribute to a sense of failure. The last consequence is believed to occur when students expect to receive praise or rewards but do not. Driekurs

> **An important question is: Under what circumstances, if any, might praise and rewards not only be ineffective in changing behavior, but be harmful to intrinsic motivation and moral reasoning?**

advised teachers to avoid punishment, rewards, and even praise, and to rely instead on "encouragement" and "consequences." Likewise, Alfie Kohn, a journalist and author of several popular books, including *Punished by Rewards: The Trouble with Gold Stars, Incentive Plans, A's, Praise, and Other Bribes* (1999), has repeatedly warned parents and educators of the dangers of praise and rewards.

Recent criticism of praise and rewards, and especially tangible and token rewards, has been directed primarily to their use in managing and controlling behavior via principles of reinforcement and the potential harm such use might have on intrinsic motivation—a core ingredient of self-discipline. At issue are two primary concerns. First, an overemphasis on rewards might encourage students to be extrinsically motivated and self-centered by learning to exhibit behavior only if that behavior is rewarded by others. As such, students' behavior becomes determined by the saliency and power of rewards in their environment. This is the same criticism as that leveled at the use of punishment, as discussed in Chapter 1: when neither the allure of rewards nor fear of punishment is salient, there is little motivation for students to follow school rules, respect others, and/or engage in other socially and morally responsible behaviors. The second major concern about the overuse of rewards concerns those students who are intrinsically motivated (as evidenced by their exhibiting the desired behaviors when no external rewards are apparent). It is argued that for those students rewards might actually harm or undermine their intrinsic motivation, especially when used to control or manage their behavior (or even given that appearance). Such concerns over the use of praise and rewards (but especially tangible rewards) to control and manage student behavior are not new. Montessori (1912/1974), Piaget (1932/1965), and Kohlberg (1984) are among prominent psychologists in the past who viewed rewards as manipulative and potentially harmful to intrinsic motivation and human development.

GOOD REASONS TO USE PRAISE (AND REWARDS), OTHER THAN TO MANAGE OR REINFORCE STUDENT BEHAVIOR

Before discussing limitations to the use of rewards and the debate over their potential harm to intrinsic motivation, it is important to emphasize that teachers and schools use praise and rewards, and particularly praise, for reasons other than managing students by reinforcing desired behavior. There are many other good reasons for using praise as well as rewards, as discussed below.

Based on his own research and that of others, Brophy (1981) found that teachers' use of praise seldom functions as reinforcement of specific behavior, and thus it often is not used for that intended purpose. In a more recent review of the literature, Beaman and Wheldall (2000) reached the same conclusion: Teachers seldom use praise contingently as positive reinforcement. Instead, teachers are much more inclined to use praise more globally (e.g., "The class is doing a good job," "You're doing fine, Katelyn"), and for reasons other than behavior management (Brophy, 1981). When used in this manner, praise serves the worthwhile function of helping to build, strengthen, and maintain positive teacher–student relationships. As was discussed in Chapters 3 and 4, demonstrating caring and support, which includes the frequent use of positive feedback, praise, and rewards, is a common characteristic of teachers whom students like the most, and it also is a critical feature of positive school climate.

Brophy (1981) and others have identified the following five ways in which praise and rewards function to help create positive classroom and schoolwide climates. Let us discuss each in turn.

> **There are many good reasons to use praise and rewards other than to manage student behavior.**

1. *Praise and rewards provide positive feedback and guidance, highlighting behaviors, thoughts, and emotions that are desired, important, and normative.* In praising and rewarding how students act, think, and feel, educators communicate important behavioral expectations that are commonly valued in our society and that are important to overall success and happiness. These expectations include learning such values and virtues as responsibility, respect, caring, and trustworthiness. To be effective in the process of socialization, praise and rewards do not necessarily have to function as reinforcers of targeted behaviors. Instead, they can effectively help serve in socialization by providing feedback as to how students are performing. Indeed, teachers' use of informational feedback (e.g., "This is the mistake you made, and here is how to fix it") is commonly found to have a stronger influence on improving academic achievement in the classroom than either praise or rewards. This is because praise and rewards often contain little informational value (Hattie & Timperley, 2007). Praise and rewards also serve in socialization by highlighting the importance of values and virtues, especially when they are normative. Although exceptions certainly abound, behaving in a manner that is consistent with the norm is a powerful motivator of student behavior (Bugental & Grusec, 2006).

2. *The use of praise and rewards helps to avoid or reduce the use of criticism and other punitive techniques.* Both praise and criticism are used routinely by both effective

and ineffective teachers to inform students of the correctness of their behavior. However, the more effective classroom managers tend to use praise more frequently than criticism and punishment (Brophy & McCaslin, 1992). They recognize that doing so not only helps maintain a positive teacher–student relationship and classroom climate but also helps avoid the *use* of criticism and punishment—it's difficult to criticize and punish when you're busy praising and rewarding.

3. *Praise and rewards serve as spontaneous expressions of surprise, caring, and appreciation.* A surprise announcement such as "You have been great this week, so I'm giving 10 minutes extra recess today!" or "No homework!" is likely to make most students happy and to view the teacher announcing the reward more favorably. As noted by Brophy (1981, p. 17), "Ironically, this kind of praise, which is given spontaneously rather than as part of a systematic effort to reinforce, probably is the most reinforcing in its effects on students."

4. *Praise and rewards can help to repair damage done to the teacher–student relationship after criticism or punishment has been used.* This function is seen when a teacher attempts to restore the teacher–student relationship that has been harmed as a result of criticizing or punishing a student. It also applies when a teacher predicts inappropriate behavior (e.g., "I think you're going to get into trouble if I leave you alone in the classroom") but that behavior never happens.

5. *Praise and rewards can serve as vicarious reinforcement.* Many behaviors are learned simply by observing others. Individuals are much more likely to imitate those behaviors if the person being observed is praised or rewarded (Bandura, 1986). In the classroom, this aspect is seen when a teacher calls the class's attention to the good behavior of a student and praises that student. For example, in the presence of peers, several of whom are out of their seats when they should not be, a teacher loudly states, "Thank you, Thomas, for being in your seat!" This function is especially useful during transitions (e.g., "Michael gets to be first in line"), the intention being to motivate the behavior of others more than that of the student singled out for praise. Teachers must be very careful when using praise and rewards in this manner, however, especially with students beyond elementary school. Too often teachers praise students in the class who are not the ones classmates desire to be like. Not only does this strategy fail to motivate classmates who are observing, but it also might fail to motivate the student singled out. As noted by Brophy (1981, p. 17), "Unless the student singled out for such 'praise' is very immature and teacher dependent, they are likely to feel manipulated or punished rather than rewarded by it."

The extent to which teachers use praise and rewards for the foregoing reasons, as well as for the purpose of reinforcing and managing student behavior, is largely determined by their educational philosophy, training, personality, and style of teaching. For example, most special education teachers are trained in applied behavior analysis, whereas general education teachers are more likely to have been trained in programs with a constructivist student-centered philosophy (Brownell, Ross, Colón, & McCallum, 2005). As such, one should expect general education teachers to be less inclined than special education teachers to use praise and rewards in a planned, contingent, and systematic fashion to manage student behavior.

It is not only teacher preferences, however, that determine how often and in what manner praise and rewards are used. Students also greatly influence a teacher's use of praise and rewards, and it is not just by behaving. For example, Brophy (1981) found that some students condition their teachers to praise them by actively seeking the praise and responding favorably to it. This phenomenon is commonly seen among students who strongly desire teacher approval and attention, such as students who frequently ask teachers to check their work and those who are always raising their hands, eagerly waiting to give the right answers. Students who strongly value teacher attention and thus exhibit appropriate behavior to gain such attention are often the ones who elicit the most praise.

PRACTICAL LIMITATIONS TO PRAISE AND REWARDS

Although praise and rewards serve each of the important functions already cited, their most common intended function with respect to classroom management and school discipline is positive reinforcement. That is, praise and rewards are dispensed with the aim of reinforcing or strengthening desired behaviors. Unquestionably, a wealth of research shows that praise and rewards function as powerful techniques of positive reinforcement for reducing a variety of behavior problems (Alberto & Troutman, 2006), particularly at the individual student and classroom levels, with research demonstrating that praise, social awards, privileges, preferred activities, tangibles, and tokens can be effective in managing student behavior (Landrum & Kauffman, 2006; O'Leary & O'Leary, 1977). As noted in Chapter 2 on SWPBS, substantially less research has been conducted on the effectiveness of the systematic use of praise and rewards at the schoolwide level.

As reviewed in Chapter 5 on authoritative discipline, research also shows that at the individual student and classroom levels effective teachers use praise and rewards in combination with other techniques. They use them to prevent and correct behavior problems but also to develop self-discipline. Interestingly, such research suggests that the most effective teachers are not overly effusive in their use of praise and rewards but, rather, use them more strategically. For example, expert tutors use praise much less often than the least effective tutors (Lepper & Woolverton, 2002).

> As with the use of punishment, educators should be aware of the limitations to the use of praise and rewards.

In sum, effective educators use praise and rewards, although not as often as advocates of SWPBS and applied behavioral analyses recommend (e.g., Maag, 2001; Sugai & Horner, 2009). Brophy (1981) concluded that the (in his view) relatively infrequent use of praise and rewards largely reflected the fact that the effectiveness and feasibility of their use to improve student behavior "has been seriously oversold." Furthermore, he noted, "Reinforcement of specific behaviors in an ongoing class situation simply is not feasible, even with praise as the reinforcer (assuming its effectiveness). At most, the teacher can concentrate on a few specific behaviors for the class as a whole, or on a larger number of specific behaviors for a few individuals" (p. 21).

Brophy (1981) cited limitations inherent in the use of praise that reduce its effectiveness and feasibility, most of which were repeated by Hattie and Timperley (2007) in their review of the literature on feedback. Most of those limitations and others, as listed below, apply not only to praise but also to tangible rewards.

1. *Individuals differ in their preferences and responses to praise and rewards.* What is reinforcing to some students is not reinforcing to others. Individual students vary in the rewards they prefer and in their responses to praise and rewards (Alberto & Troutman, 2006; McLaughlin, 1975). For example, not all children like candy or at least not the same kind, not all enjoy extra recess or free time (although most do), and not all are pleased when praised by teachers (especially some adolescents when praised in front of their peers). When the rewards are not what students like, it is very doubtful that they will reinforce the behavior rewarded. It is not uncommon to find that the rewards chosen by teachers do not match the preferences of their students (Daly, Jacob, King, & Cheramie, 1984; Fantuzzo & Rohrbeck, 1991).

2. *Teachers and schools often do not have access to, or control over, the rewards that are the most powerful reinforcers of behavior.* This situation is seldom a problem in the early grades, where most young children cherish their teacher's attention and are easily motivated by tangible rewards (e.g., stickers), preferred activities (e.g., recess), and privileges (e.g., helping the teacher). Likewise, it is less of a problem in restrictive settings, such as alternative schools for students with serious behavior problems, where educators are able to manipulate the strongest reinforcers in those settings (e.g., tokens or points to leave). However, by the time students enter middle school, those rewards typically lose their reinforcing value. Autonomy and peer attention replace teacher attention in value, recess is no longer an option, and prized tangibles cost much more (e.g., iPods, cars, clothing). Rewards with potential reinforcement value still exist that teachers might manipulate, such as a homework pass, free time, and tokens that serve as raffle tickets for an iPod (which is likely to be of interest only to those who do not already own one). However, they are fewer in number and are often more difficult to provide. Whereas finding rewards that are positive reinforcers is a challenge at the individual student and classroom levels, it is a particularly daunting task at the schoolwide level, and especially beyond elementary school.

To avoid this limitation, some SWPBS schools use privileges instead of tangible rewards. However, one should be aware that there is a risk of harming rather than improving student perceptions of fairness, and thus the effectiveness of privileges, by requiring students to earn them when they were previously not contingent upon their behavior (e.g., a field trip, school dance).

3. *Public praise and rewards are not appropriate at all ages.* Unquestionably, the use of praise and rewards to reinforce and manage behavior is very effective with young children and those individuals with disabilities who are functioning cognitively as young children. Developmentally, young children are much more externally oriented, motivated by rewards rather than concern about the impact of their behavior on others, respect for rules and order, and issues of fairness and justice (Stipek, 2002). Likewise, young children

are much more likely than preadolescents and adolescents to value teacher authority and adult attention. With increasing age, students become more concerned with the approval of their peers and have a greater desire for autonomy (Lepper, Corpus, & Iyengar, 2005). This changeover largely explains why many adolescents do not like to be praised publicly, preferring either private praise or none at all (Burnett, 2002; Elwell & Tiberio, 1994). To adolescents, public praise and being given a token for good behavior in front of their peers may actually be embarrassing and thus serve as punishment rather than positive reinforcement. As discussed later in this chapter, the embarrassment can be especially acute when the behavior that is publicly recognized is relatively easy to enact and not behavior viewed as truly deserving public recognition (e.g., walking in the hall, being quiet and compliant).

An awareness of the developmental inappropriateness of lavishing public praise on adolescents or giving them tokens and rewards may largely explain why middle school and high school teachers are consistently found to use praise and rewards less often than preschool and elementary teachers. That is, rather than simply resisting change or the use of ABA techniques, they understand that for developmental reasons adolescents differ from preschoolers in their response to tangible rewards and public praise.

Another important developmental difference in the effectiveness of rewards is that after about the third grade students become more sensitive to *how* praise and rewards are administered (Henderlong & Lepper, 2002). That is, they are much more likely to be aware of situations in which those administering praise and rewards are not sincere and are using the rewards to manipulate their behavior. Before the third grade, however, this reaction pattern is seldom an issue.

4. *Praise—and especially rewards—can be satiating.* Rewards lose their effectiveness when students have "had enough." An excellent example is the teacher who disseminates large amounts of candy and other edibles lavishly throughout the day for good behavior—the kids eventually get full, if not sick. More common and realistic examples can also be found in many schools. For example, satiation is likely to occur when younger students are rewarded every day with stickers, a special badge, or with lunch with their teacher. It also is likely to occur among older students when repeatedly rewarded with the same privilege of listening to songs while working (especially the same ones). Although a major advantage of praise over other rewards is that satiation is less likely to occur (Kazdin, 1981), satiation also can occur with praise. For example, saying "Great!" over and over quickly loses its effectiveness.

5. *To maximize their usefulness in teaching new behaviors, praise and rewards must be given immediately and contingently.* When teaching a new behavior, or one that is seldom exhibited, teachers are advised to reinforce that behavior immediately, continuously, and contingently (Alberto & Troutman, 2006). This requirement is difficult to implement in a class of 25–30 students or more, and it is especially challenging to apply it schoolwide. As noted earlier, Brophy (1981) found that teachers seldom reinforce specific behaviors, instead preferring to reinforce behaviors more globally. This requirement is one reason why they do so.

6. *The skilled and systematic use of praise and rewards to reinforce and manage student behavior requires considerable training.* Assuming that the control and modification of students' behavior is one's aim (and that this can be achieved in spite of all the limitations listed here), to achieve this aim teachers need training in applied behavior analysis. The lack of training in ABA (rather than these other various reasons) is frequently cited by behaviorists as the primary reason why behavioral programs fail—that is, because poorly trained teachers do not know how to use positive reinforcement correctly (Maag, 2001).

7. *The effects of praise and rewards often do not generalize outside of the setting in which they are systematically applied* (Kazdin, 1981; Landrum & Kauffman, 2006). Ideally, once students have learned a new behavior via principles of reinforcement, then that behavior will become habitual and its occurrence will be reinforced, at least intermittently (or occasionally) by natural reinforcers in the environment. Such intermittent reinforcement should maintain the behavior and foster its generalization to multiple settings. A good example is in the early grades, when students are taught, praised, and called on when they raise their hands to ask or answer questions. For many students this behavior becomes a habit, reinforced not by the teacher continuously praising students for raising their hands but simply by the more naturally occurring reinforcers of being called on by the teacher, receiving praise or attention from the teacher, and the personal satisfaction of knowing the correct answer. The students have learned to raise their hands, and this behavior is seen across classroom settings and with other teachers. As such, there is evidence that maintenance and generalization occurred.

Unfortunately, not all desired behaviors become habitual, nor do they automatically transfer and generalize to other settings. This observation is true more for some students than for others. Likewise, it often is seen in certain behaviors more so than in others (e.g., being reinforced in social skills training for resisting peer pressure and managing one's anger). As such, improvements in behavior brought about with the deliberate and systematic use of praise and rewards often are short-lived, occurring only when the reinforcement is salient in the student's environment. Recall from Chapter 1 that this limitation also applies to the systematic use of punishment: when external rewards (or punishment) are withdrawn or are no longer present, behavior often reverts back to its previous state.

8. *To be effective, praise and rewards must be sincere and credible.* This effect may largely be determined by the actual sincerity of the person delivering the praise or reward, but it is the students' *perceptions* of sincerity (irrespective of the teacher's intentions) that are most important. The risk of praise or a reward being perceived as insincere—and thus dismissed—is greatest under the following conditions (Henderlong & Lepper, 2002):

- The praise is overly general and effusive ("You are the greatest!" or "You are the most respectful kid in this class!").
- It is inconsistent with the student's actual behavior or personal beliefs about him- or herself (e.g., the student's behavior actually has not been "the greatest" or "most respectful").

- The student recognizes that there is little reason to believe that the teacher, or evaluator, is being honest and sincere (e.g., nearly everyone is given a token, including those who often misbehave, because the teacher has been directed to give out lots of tokens).
- The praise is contradicted by other verbal or nonverbal behavior (e.g., the facial expression or tone of the teacher does not convey satisfaction).
- The actual relationship between the teacher and student is a poor one.

Under such conditions as these, in which praise and rewards are perceived by students to be insincere, there is increased risk that they will be perceived as controlling and manipulative. As a result, they are likely to be ineffective and potentially harmful to the teacher–student relationship and school climate. As noted earlier, this is most likely to happen after the third grade, when students become more sensitive to a lack of sincerity.

9. *Under certain conditions praise—and especially tangible rewards—may undermine the development of self-discipline.* Of all the limitations cited, this one is most directly relevant to developing self-discipline. At issue is not when praise and rewards are likely to be ineffective in reinforcing behavior, but rather when they might be harmful to intrinsic motivation and teach students that the primary reason to act in a socially and morally responsible manner is to earn external rewards. Because this issue is at the core of an ongoing controversy over the use of praise and rewards to manage or control student behavior, this limitation is discussed below in greater detail.

DO PRAISE AND REWARDS UNDERMINE INTRINSIC MOTIVATION, AND, IF SO, *WHEN* DO THEY?

During the past several decades researchers and educators have debated the potentially harmful effects of praise and rewards on intrinsic motivation. The debate received heightened interest with the publication of Alfie Kohn's popular book *Punished by Rewards: The Trouble with Gold Stars, Incentive Plans, A's, Praise, and Other Bribes* (1998) and a series of literature reviews and commentaries on the negative effects of praise and rewards in several highly respected journals. In one of these reviews, Deci et al. (1999), prominent researchers in educational psychology, concluded, "Although rewards can control people's behavior—indeed, that is presumably why they are so widely advocated—the primary negative effect of rewards is that they tend to forestall self-regulation." Similar messages were presented in popular magazines for teachers. For example, the cover story of the October 2007 issue of *Instructor* magazine was titled "Are Kids Over Praised?", and an article in *American Educator* written by Dr. Carol Dweck (1999) of Stanford University was titled "Caution: Praise Can Be Dangerous."

Researchers have posed the question: What might be the effects of lavishly praising or rewarding children for completing puzzles, drawing pictures, or sharing with others when they already enjoy performing those activities in the absence of any apparent rewards? Might giving stickers to students who enjoy sharing with others not only be effective in increasing that behavior but actually discourage it in certain students? How might students who are frequently praised and rewarded for good behavior respond under conditions of few rewards (e.g., after moving from one classroom to another, or upon transitioning from an elementary school that uses praise and rewards often to a middle school in which praise is less frequent and rewards are rare)? In the absence of praise and rewards, will those students persevere in the their good behavior when faced with challenges?

A related issue, but one that has received much less attention in the literature, is the impact of the systematic overuse of praise and rewards on the development of self-discipline. More specifically, are the praise and rewards currently used in most SWPBS programs harmful to the development of self-discipline? If not harmful, are they *sufficient* for developing self-discipline? That is, do they teach students why certain behaviors are important *irrespective* of external rewards? How can rewards be made useful to promoting self-discipline when they are no longer so salient?

Before discussing the debate and such questions, it is important to clarify what the debate over the use of praise and rewards is *not* about, at least not among most researchers (Bear, 2005, 2008):

What the Debate Is Not About

1. *The debate is not over the advantages and limitations of praise and rewards (which were previously listed and discussed).* That is, most researchers are not debating whether or not teachers *should* praise and reward students. No researchers are unalterably opposed to the use of praise and rewards (although some might call them different things, such as encouragement or positive consequences). Instead, the debate is about *how* and *how often* praise—and especially tangible rewards—should be used.

2. *The debate is not over the effectiveness of praise and rewards in controlling student behavior and in helping to bring about short-term compliance.* As noted earlier, research convincingly demonstrates that praise and rewards are often quite effective in controlling and managing student behavior. Not only does their use often increase appropriate behavior, but it also decreases inappropriate behavior. Positive reinforcement is particularly effective

> It is important to know what the debate is *not* over: the use of praise and rewards to manage student behavior when self-discipline is not evident.

in bringing about compliance when combined with punishment (Landrum & Kauffman, 2006). Whereas many researchers and experts in school discipline question whether short-term compliance should be the primary aim of school discipline, few question that there are times when compliance is important and that praise and rewards (and punishment) can help accomplish that objective. As noted by Deci et al. (1999, p. 657): "There is no lack of agreement between our viewpoint and that of operant and neo-operant theorists about the power of rewards to control behavior. It is clear that rewards can be used as a technique of control; indeed CET [Cognitive Evaluation Theory] specifically proposes that it is because people are controlled by rewards that they become less intrinsically motivated."

3. *The debate is not over whether or not the use of positive techniques, such as praise and rewards, is better than the use of punishment in motivating behavior.* All researchers on both sides of the debate would certainly concur that, given the choice of managing behavior with either rewards or punishment (assuming that this is one's aim), the use of rewards is preferred.

4. *The debate is not over the appropriateness of using praise and rewards to motivate behavior that is not occurring, or not occurring to the extent desired.* When a lack of intrinsic motivation is clearly evident, extrinsic rewards are appropriate. This generalization applies to students who frequently exhibit behavior problems, such as those who demonstrate little or no interest in what is being taught and who consistently violate school rules. Those students should be rewarded when they do not exhibit the problem behaviors but instead alternative, or replacement, behaviors. The observation also applies to students who seldom exhibit prosocial behaviors, such as socially withdrawn ones or those lacking social skills. The observation would also apply more to younger than older students who have not yet learned appropriate social skills.

The View of One Side of the Debate: Tangible Rewards Can Harm Intrinsic Motivation

Upon reviewing over 100 studies on the impact of rewards on intrinsic motivation, Deci et al. (1999, 2001) found that tangible rewards, not praise, more likely harm intrinsic motivation—*but only under certain conditions.* The two most common ones are when rewards are perceived to be controlling and when social comparisons are made.

> **The greatest concern among some researchers is the overuse of rewards to manage or control student behavior.**

Informational or Controlling?

In explaining their findings, Deci et al. (1999, 2001) make the educationally meaningful distinction between interpersonal contexts that are *informational* and those that are *controlling.* When used in interpersonal contexts that are informational, praise and rewards communicate to students that they are performing well, affirming to them that their behaviors measure up to important standards that they value and exhibit under their own volition. Delivered in this context, the message increases intrinsic motivation and perceptions of autonomy, leading them to believe that "I'm responsible, competent, and in control of my own behavior."

It is when tangible rewards are experienced in an interpersonal context that is controlling that intrinsic motivation is likely to be undermined and its development stifled. This is largely because the message conveyed in controlling interpersonal contexts is that it is not the self who is determining one's own behavior but rather those who control the rewards (or punishment). That is, the interpersonal context is perceived as one in which rewards are being used to bring about obedience and to make one "think, feel, or behave in particular ways" (Deci et al., 2001, p. 4). As such, when rewards are perceived to be used in this way in school settings, students come to learn that "I behaved that way to earn rewards" (controlled by others) or "I was successful in earning rewards." Examples of rewards being used deliberately, or interpreted by students as being used in this manner, might include "If you don't tease Lashaun today, I'll give you a choice of prizes from the box" or "If the entire school earns 500 tokens, there will be a school dance."

Deci et al. (1999, 2001) note that a negative effect on intrinsic motivation is much more specific to tangible rewards than to praise—owing to the fact that praise is rarely used in a controlling manner. For example, rarely do teachers inform students in advance that if they behave they will receive praise. In contrast, tangible rewards, including tokens, are often delivered in a manner intended to manage or control student behavior; thus, the potential for harm is much greater.

The Harm in Social Comparisons

Deci et al. (1999, 2001) also found that the potential for tangible rewards to negatively affect intrinsic motivation is greatest when social comparisons are made and students recognize that they receive fewer rewards than others (e.g., posting reward charts on the wall, announcing who earned the most points or tokens). Apparently, under those conditions some students take to heart that their performance is less deserving or not good enough. Henderlong and Lepper (2002) reached a similar conclusion in their comprehensive review of the literature on praise and intrinsic motivation. However, they concluded that social comparisons might be harmful *regardless of whether* the interpersonal context in which praise and rewards are used is informational or controlling. They argue that, by referencing a student's behavior to the behavior of others ("You did better than Jessica and Kandia") and not to objective mastery of skills ("You showed that you are able to get to class on time"), educators run the risk of merely encouraging students to base their behavior on the norm and not strive for mastery of valued skills for its own sake. In situations in which students calculate that their peers are receiving more praise or rewards than they are (or where praise, rewards, or punishment are not salient for anyone), their motivation to behave well is likely to diminish. By focusing on social comparisons, thereby implying that students should act like their peers, educators also run the risk of having students infer that their inappropriate behavior is likewise okay so long as it is the norm or when the same behavior is exhibited by others.

Conclusion: Student Attributions Mediate the Effects of Rewards

Deci et al.'s (1999; 2001) findings are consistent with their cognitive evaluation theory and other social cognitive theories that emphasize the development and importance of autonomy and the critical role of attributions in mediating behavior. Those theories include social cognitive learning theory (Bandura, 1986; 2001), social information processing theory (Crick & Dodge, 1994), attribution theory (Weiner, 2006), and achievement goal theory (Ames, 1992; Pintrich, 2000). Each of these theories, and especially attribution theory, emphasizes that motivation and behavior are greatly influenced by attributions students make as to the causes of their successes and failures. Students often ask themselves why they performed well or poorly on a given task. How they answer this question mediates their future behavior on similar tasks. Studies (Henderlong & Lepper, 2002; Morrone & Pintrich, 2006; Weiner, 2006) show that when students experience failure their motivation and performance are more likely to improve if they attribute such failure to a lack of effort rather than a lack of ability (e.g., "I didn't try hard enough," as opposed to "I'm not smart" or "I'm an angry person"). This is particularly true if they view their ability level as stable, or fixed, since it is easier to change the effort expended than one's relatively fixed ability. Similarly, motivation and performance also are unlikely to improve if students attribute their failure to external factors over which they believe they have little or no control (e.g., a teacher who is always unfair).

While attributions that focus on ability are likely to undermine motivation in situations in which *failure* is experienced, the reverse is often found in situations in which *success* is experienced—that is, motivation is likely to be enhanced. This phenomenon is seen in the effectiveness of *dispositional* praise, in which children are praised for relatively stable dispositions, to which they are encouraged to attribute their behavior (e.g., "You're the kind of person who likes to help others" or "Good sharing is important to you, isn't it?"). When given dispositional praise, students tend to be more generous and helpful even weeks after receiving the praise (Grusec & Redler, 1980). Dispositional praise encourages a prosocial image or a moral identity and communicates that continued effort is required to maintain it (Eisenberg, Cialdini, MaCreath, & Shell, 1989; Grusec & Redler, 1980). Dispositional praise is especially effective, in both the short term and long term, when it encourages internal attributions *and* also targets effort, or the process involved in succeeding on the given task (e.g., "You worked hard" or "You used your problem-solving skills") (Henderlong & Lepper, 2002). Most students recognize that effort, problem-solving skills, and to a certain degree dispositions are alterable and under their control. By using all three, teachers help to foster motivation and perseverance when students are faced with difficult tasks or failure in the future.

Social comparisons and attributions determine not only one's own behavior but also how one perceives others. That is, with respect to the systematic use of rewards in school-wide discipline, such use can have a significant impact on peer acceptance, rejection, and respect. This phenomenon occurs when students observe that their peers are receiving more rewards than they are—and for such "easy" tasks as not hitting others, coming to class on time, walking rather than running in the hallways, and other common behaviors that they believe should be exhibited by anyone their age. Research shows that students—especially after the third grade—are inclined to conclude that frequent praise and rewards for really simple tasks are given primarily to those "who need it," that is, those lacking in ability (or self-discipline) (Barker & Graham, 1987).

The Other Side of the Debate: Don't Worry

Not all researchers agree that teachers need to worry about the potential harm of tangible rewards (and certainly not about their use of praise). In contrast to the arguments of researchers cited in the preceding section, other researchers (e.g., Akin-Little, Eckert, Lovett, & Little, 2004; Baumrind, 1996; Cameron, 2001; Cameron & Pierce, 1994; Evertson & Emmer, 2008) point out that not all reviews of the literature on the use of rewards have reached the same conclusions as those reached by Deci et al. (2001). Indeed, other researchers have concluded that praise and rewards almost always increase desired behaviors and decrease undesired behaviors and only rarely have a negative impact on intrinsic motivation (Akin-Little et al., 2004; Cameron, 2001; Cameron & Pierce, 1994). Contrary to Deci et al. (1999, 2001), these researchers found that when tangible rewards are linked to explicit and clear standards of performance, they have *positive* effects on intrinsic motivation, regardless of whether or not students already prefer to engage in the targeted behavior. They concluded that the only conditions under which tangible rewards have a (reportedly small) negative effect is when they are used to reward students for behavior which they already prefer to engage in (e.g., completion of high-interest tasks, helping others) *and* for which the rewards are given either without any informational feedback or with feedback that is not clear with respect to the level of performance or standards expected or achieved (e.g., rewarding students for completing assignments regardless of their quality). These researchers argue that, since rewards are rarely used in this way, there is little reason to worry about any potential negative impact from their use.

> **Other researchers believe that although rewards are not always effective in improving behavior, rarely are they harmful as commonly used in classrooms.**

Summary of the Potential Negative Impact on Intrinsic Motivation

From the perspective of cognitive theorists, it is important to distinguish informative from controlling contexts because it is under informative conditions that praise and rewards are most effective in fostering intrinsic motivation and autonomy. Within controlling interpersonal contexts, however, tangible rewards are likely to undermine intrinsic motivation. From the perspective of behavioral theorists, the distinction between informative and controlling contexts does not matter much. Their focus is on the management of student behavior as reflected in short-term changes in observable behavior, not in autonomy. Their research supports the use of praise, rewards, and punishment in controlling behavior in the short term. The importance of nonobservable constructs such as intrinsic motivation and autonomy as well as the long-term aim of developing self-discipline are generally ignored. Although they recognize that some studies have shown that under certain controlling contexts rewards might not be effective and might actually harm intrinsic motivation, they dismiss the practical importance of such findings.

Most cognitive and behavioral psychologists would agree that several conclusions can be drawn from the research on the potential for praise and rewards to harm intrinsic motivation: (1) although praise is not always as *effective* in motivating behavior (either intrinsically or extrinsically), it rarely ever does any harm, including to intrinsic motivation; and (2) when used in an informative interpersonal context, neither praise nor tangible rewards undermine intrinsic motivation, and both are likely to improve behavior. Where cognitive and behavioral psychologists are always likely to disagree is over the use of rewards in controlling interpersonal contexts.

SUMMARY AND CONCLUSION: BEYOND PRAISE AND REWARDS FOR CONTROL

Overall, research indicates that how *often* students are praised and rewarded is much less important than the *manner* in which it occurs. That is, both the interpersonal context (Deci et al., 2001) and the quality of praise and rewards (Bandura, 1986; Brophy, 1981) are more important than the frequency that they are used (assuming, of course, that they *are* used at least occasionally and enough to be effective). Praise and rewards are most effective when they are used strategically in ways that are responsive to their limitations, as reviewed in this chapter. Perhaps most importantly, however, is the aim of their use. Educators should question whether the best way to develop intrinsic motivation and self-discipline is through the adults' managing student behavior by praising and rewarding the behavior they desire. Too often, this means compliance with their behavioral expectations and rules (as observed and measured by ODRs and suspensions). Praise and rewards become the *positive* alternative to punishment for effectively managing student behavior. To be sure, if (and when) one's aim *is* to manage student behavior externally, it makes sense to use praise and rewards in the most effective manner. But if educators truly expect to develop intrinsic motivation and self-discipline, they need to use praise and rewards differently than as used for management and control (as well as in combination with other techniques presented in this book for developing self-discipline). That is, they need to use praise and rewards more strategically—to gain short-term compliance (and preferably committed, as opposed to unwilling, compliance) but also to develop the social, emotional, and behavioral competencies of self-discipline. Such committed compliance and competencies enhance the prospects that, in the absence of external praise and rewards (and the absence of adult supervision and fear of punishment), students nonetheless act in a socially and morally responsible manner. How praise and rewards should be used to achieve both aims—committed compliance and the development of self-discipline—is the focus of the next chapter.

CHAPTER 7

Strategic Use of Praise and Rewards for Developing Self-Discipline and a Positive School Climate

Educators should be well aware of the limitations of praise and rewards, as discussed in the preceding chapter. Such limitations include the potential harm of tangible rewards on intrinsic motivation when employed in a controlling interpersonal context—as often done in many schools. However, when praise and rewards are not used—or not *perceived* by students to be used—in a controlling manner, educators need not be overly concerned. Although perhaps "oversold" with respect to their influence on classroom and schoolwide discipline (Brophy, 1981, p. 21), they still serve many worthwhile functions. Increasing student motivation and maintaining a positive teacher–student relationship and school climate are primary among them. Classrooms and schools would be dull and boring without praise, privileges, preferred activities, and other rewards. Less learning and more misbehavior would likely occur, and teacher–student relationships and school climate would certainly be less positive. Development of self-discipline also would likely suffer.

As discussed in Chapter 6, praise and rewards are not always effective in actually reinforcing desired behavior, but at times they are, and there are multiple reasons to use them other than for the purpose of reinforcement. Punitive techniques, including verbal reprimands and the "evil eye," also are not always effective in decreasing undesired behaviors, but it would be equally foolish for educators to should stop using them. Instead of refraining from using positive reinforcement and punishment, educators should think about how to use both positive and punitive techniques *wisely and strategically*, which means avoiding their limitations and enhancing their effectiveness. Perhaps more important, it includes capitalizing on their usefulness in developing self-discipline and in fostering positive teacher–student relationships and school climate. In this chapter, strategies for the use of praise and rewards are presented for achieving these multiple aims in the context of schoolwide discipline. The recommended strategies are based largely on research reviews on the effective use of praise and rewards by Bandura (1997), Brophy (1981, 2004), Cameron (2001), Deci et al. (1999, 2001), Hattie and Timperley (2007), Henderlong and Lepper (2002), O'Leary and O'Leary (1977), Ryan and Deci (2000), and Stipek (2002).

RECOMMENDATIONS FOR THE STRATEGIC USE OF PRAISE AND REWARDS

1. *Use praise and rewards for reasons other than positive reinforcement.* As noted above and reviewed in Chapter 6, praise and rewards serve multiple functions, other than that of positive reinforcement, in the teaching of social and emotional competencies. Foremost among them is that they help create and maintain positive teacher–student relationships and school climate. Students value teachers and staff who demonstrate warmth, care, and support. Praising and rewarding students—and not just for targeted desired behaviors—is one of many ways of demonstrating those qualities (see Chapter 5). For example, such praise as "Cool haircut!" or "I heard you had an excellent soccer game this weekend—congratulations on the win!" is offered not to elicit any particular desired behavior, but simply to show interest and care. Such praise should be freely offered to students schoolwide—in classrooms, hallways, and upon entering and leaving school each day. Moreover, although it certainly may be used for "catching kids being good" by reinforcing behaviors consistent with the school's rules and behavioral expectations, it should not be limited solely to those situations.

Likewise, privileges, preferred activities, and even tangible rewards should be used (albeit sparingly and much less often than praise) not only to recognize and acknowledge desired behavior but also to strengthen teacher–student relationships and promote a more positive school climate. For example, an entire school might be rewarded with free time or an ice cream party to celebrate the school's achieving a particular goal (preferably one set by the students). Entertaining schoolwide assemblies, field trips, school dances, ice cream socials, and other enjoyable activities also serve the worthwhile function of maintaining and improving school climate and do not need to be made contingent upon everyone's good behavior or the accumulation of a given number of points or tokens. When systematic reward systems are established in which school officials become obsessed with assuring that all "rewards" and positive actions are contingent upon targeted behaviors and given in a consistent manner throughout the school, the spontaneity and sincerity of teacher support and warmth are likely to suffer. Moreover, many teachers are likely to resist a cumbersome system designed to manipulate their *own* behavior (as observed by the author in numerous SWPBS schools, especially at the middle and high school levels).

As noted in the preceding chapter, praise and rewards also serve another valuable function, namely, to help children learn desired behaviors vicariously—by seeing others (in real life, role play, video, stories, etc.) praised or rewarded. To strengthen the effectiveness of vicarious reinforcement, however, educators should strive to make the models attractive to the students (see Form 4.3, pp. 77–78, in Chapter 4 for recommendations).

2. *Focus on the message: Emphasize the informative rather than the controlling function of praise and rewards.* Praise and rewards should not be viewed simply as the "positive" way to manage and control student behavior. The message intended, communicated, and received should be "There are many good reasons why [the targeted behavior] is important. Praise or a reward is simply used to help you and others recognize, learn, and appreciate the importance of that behavior and inform you how you're doing." This approach is in contrast to the message being perceived as "Here's what you must do for me to give you tokens, rewards, or praise" or "If you behave, I'll reward you." Such heavily controlling messages should be avoided, as well as more subtle messages of social control. For example, it is recommended that instead of *rewards* and *reinforcers* being distributed to students contingent upon their demonstrating behavior consistent with schoolwide rules and expectations, *recognition* and *acknowledgment* should be given to students for demonstrating self-discipline.

> For developing self-discipline, it often helps to think of ways to *recognize* and *acknowledge* desired behavior, rather than ways to reinforce or reward it.

3. *Avoid teaching students that the most important reason to act in a morally and socially responsible manner is to earn rewards or to be praised.* While the preceding recommendation concerns the targeted behavior and why praise and rewards are used—to inform and not to control—this recommendation concerns the impact of informative and controlling messages on students' thinking. As discussed in Chapters 3 and 4, in emphasizing rewards and punishment, school officials promote the most immature kind of moral reasoning and the lowest type of extrinsic motivation—a hedonistic, self-centered perspective based on rewards and punishment. To help avoid this perception from forming, educators must consistently ask themselves, "Are we teaching and reinforcing a self-centered perspective of 'be good when you think you might be rewarded and don't be bad when you might get caught'?" A similar guiding question should be "Are we simply teaching that 'the best people are those who earn the most external rewards'?"

4. *Praise and reward the cognitive and emotional processes and dispositions associated with self-discipline.* Too often, educators are instructed to target observable behaviors that are specific and operationally defined. Such a limited focus typically excludes how students think and feel, consisting of the cognitive and emotional processes that often underlie student behavior, as reviewed in Chapter 3. In teaching those processes, praise and to a much lesser extent rewards should be among the multiple techniques used. As noted by Kazdin (1981, pp. 47–48), using techniques of positive reinforcement to develop desired cognitive and emotional processes is "not necessarily incompatible with behavior modification interventions. Indeed, the behavioral approach can be readily applied." Such use is highly encouraged in this book.

> Just as good behavior should be recognized, so too should the thoughts and feelings that underlie the behavior be recognized.

Thus, in addition to praising and rewarding students for exhibiting specific, observable, and operationally defined motoric behaviors (e.g., sharing, complying with a teacher's request, etc.), educators also should use praise and rewards to recognize, acknowledge, and reinforce desired cognitive and emotional processes expressed by students. They should do so either verbally, in writing, or physically (e.g., a smile, a pat on the back). The social and emotional processes would include those commonly targeted in social and emotional learning programs, such as taking the perspective of others, thinking of alternative solutions, evaluating solutions, empathy, anger regulation, and assuming responsibility for one's actions. The processes would also include more global dispositions, such as caring, kindness, and honesty. As discussed in Chapter 6, research clearly shows that praise and rewards can be used effectively in reinforcing not only specific behaviors but also more global dispositions.

5. *Use rewards only occasionally for behavior that is intrinsically motivated and more often for behavior that is not intrinsically motivated.* This recommendation pertains particularly to the use of rewards and much less so to praise, since there is little risk of teachers using praise too often and students perceiving it as controlling. However, with respect to rewards, it makes little sense to implement an extensive and demanding schoolwide intervention that relies on external rewards when most students already exhibit behaviors that meet the school's standards and expectations. From the perspective of cognitive theory, such a strategy stifles moral development and intrinsic motivation. From the perspective of behaviorism, it simply is unnecessary and likely to even be counterproductive. That is, once the rewards are withdrawn, the behavior is likely to return to its prereward state or even become worse in the short term (Akin-Little et al., 2004). Although programming for maintenance and generalization of the behavior may help avoid this outcome from occurring, few programs have demonstrated effectiveness in doing so. Finally, from the practical perspective of school reformers, such a "one-size-fits-all" strategy is likely to be met with resistance and not be implemented with fidelity (as will be discussed further in Chapter 11).

In determining the extent to which external rewards should be used, educators should be guided by what cognitive theorists refer to as the *principle of minimal sufficiency* (Lepper, 1983) and behaviorists refer to as the *least restrictive alternative* (Barton, Brulle, & Repp, 1983). The principle of minimal sufficiency is grounded in the belief that the least amount of external pressure (via either rewards *or* punishment) does the least amount of harm to intrinsic motivation. The least restrictive alternative is based more on the rights and the freedom of students not to be coerced unnecessarily. The end message is the same however (Bear, 2005), namely, do not use more external control than necessary to produce the desired behavior. In practice, for the majority of individual students, this means to rely primarily on praise and to use rewards that are the most naturally occurring, such as rewarding them with preferred activities. It also means avoiding rewards that are contrived, such as tokens and tangibles (trinkets and prizes for good behavior), especially when given in a structured and contingent fashion (e.g., requiring a certain number of tokens to earn a prize).

However, when students are not intrinsically motivated, and the use of praise and rewards, as recommended above, is insufficient in motivating desired behavior, then educators should consider implementing a more structured positive reinforcement system. Under those circumstances, praise and rewards would be administered more specifically, frequently, and contingently, but their use would be *faded* or gradually reduced as the desired behavior increases. Again, if the desired behaviors are already being exhibited by the majority of students, it makes little sense to implement a schoolwide reward system contingent upon the desired behaviors. It would make greater sense, however, to implement such a systematic reward system in classrooms characterized by frequent discipline problems as well as with individual students who fail to exhibit self-discipline.

6. *Specify what is being praised and rewarded. Specificity* refers to two things, (1) the specific behavior that is subject to praise or reward and (2) how well the behavior is performed. Behavior should include effort. Praising or rewarding effort—not just the targeted behavior—is important from a motivational perspective because effort, unlike a fixed ability, is controlled by the student. Praising or rewarding effort also is critical from the standpoint of behaviorism. That is, it is important to reinforce progress, or *successive approximations*, toward achieving a targeted goal or behavior. Such progress may be seen visibly in student behavior, or sincere efforts might be verbalized by the student. How well the behavior is performed and whether sufficient effort was expended are determined by the student's meeting (or demonstrating an attempt to meet) a given expectation or standard. The expectation or standard should be based on one of the following: (1) a comparison to others who exhibit the desired behavior (e.g., "Thank you for doing what Erica and Joan did—raising your hand before speaking"); (2) a comparison to oneself over time that shows improvement (e.g., "Jeffrey, yesterday you blurted out three times during social studies, and today you didn't do it even once. Nice job! I appreciate that"); or (3) a set expectation or standard that is not tied to previous behavior or the behavior of others (e.g., "Excellent, Maurice! You demonstrated respect by raising your hand and waiting to be called on before speaking"). The second two types of expectations are preferable because they give students a benchmark by which they can evaluate their behavior when peers are either not present or are misbehaving.

> Whereas specificity is important, there are times when it is quite appropriate and effective to recognize more global dispositions, such as someone being a kind or caring person.

Regardless how the expectation or standard is determined, it should be clear, fair, and reasonable—and perceived as such by students. As noted by Henderlong and Lepper (2002, p. 786), "Learning what it takes to reach some standard of excellence—whether it be exerting a certain amount of effort, using a particular problem-solving approach, or answering a given percentage of questions correctly—may help children know where to focus their energies in the future; this may be a powerful source of motivation."

To be fair and reasonable, expectations and standards should be neither too high nor too low. As discussed in the preceding chapter, when expectations and standards are too low and students are praised or rewarded for "easy" behaviors, there is a risk that attributions of low ability are likely to follow. Praising or rewarding minor achievements also can be embarrassing or even humiliating to the student, and is likely to be perceived as controlling, such as when an adolescent is given a token in front of peers for an act of compliance.

Similar risks exist when standards and expectations are perceived by students as unrealistic, or too high. Under those conditions, they create anxiety, pressure, and a sense of helplessness. Students are likely to think "Why bother, since I'm not going to meet what the teacher expects?" (now and in the future). Standards that are too high also may lead to low self-perceptions of competence and self-worth in the future when students fail to meet those standards (Covington, 1984; Henderlong & Lepper, 2002).

In many cases, and particularly when behavior needs improvement, expectations and standards should change as behavior improves (Akin-Little et al., 2004). For example, if the class earns a free homework pass as a result of 80% of the students completing their homework that week, then the following week the criterion would be raised to 85%. The ultimate targeted goal might be 90%, and effort (or successive approximations) toward reaching that goal, as indicated in meeting the changing criterion, should be reinforced. To minimize external control and foster self-discipline, students should actively participate in setting the standards and be encouraged to develop and adopt personal goals and standards.

As noted earlier, recognizing and acknowledging more global dispositions also is effective in improving behavior. For most students, "Thanks for being so kind" is sufficient when praising them for assisting a peer with an assignment. They know what their kind behavior was. What matters the most is that the information communicated in praise or rewards helps students understand and appreciate what deserves recognition and acknowledgment, which includes both effort and not just behavior, and also the underlying emotions and cognitions. Obviously, greater specificity is necessary for younger children and those students who do not understand what a disposition means, such as being kind or honest. Greater specificity also is appropriate when one desires to help develop, reinforce, or recognize particular skills that exemplify more general competencies or dispositions (Henderlong & Lepper, 2002). For example, one might say (privately), "Juanita, an important part of a discussion is showing that you can listen and respect the perspectives of others. You demonstrated that by not interrupting when Alfonso was disagreeing with you."

7. *When used for purposes of reinforcement, make praise and rewards contingent on the success in demonstrating desired behavior or the effort expended.* If one's aim is to positively reinforce the target behavior, praise and rewards should follow only when students perform the targeted behavior well or demonstrate sufficient effort and progress toward the desired level of performance. Students should not be praised or rewarded for poor performance or effort. Although this may sound obvious, it is not uncommon for teachers to praise students, particularly low-achieving students, for *poor* performance and lack of effort, perhaps because they fear damaging the students' self-esteem (Brophy, 1981). Such praise conveys low expectations, may actually reinforce poor performance, and often results in, rather than avoids, lower self-esteem.

Likewise, one must be careful not to praise and reward students for behavior that they believe is not worthy of praise or rewards, including success on easy tasks or tasks performed well but "not well enough." Although such use of praise or rewards may be intended to protect students' self-esteem and reinforce their continued efforts, most likely it has little effect on self-esteem and may actually backfire. That is, students may interpret such praise or rewards as conveying that the one praising them thinks less of them than others, that they are not capable of doing well, or that praise and rewards are given indiscriminately and thus are not meaningful.

8. *Communicate sincerity.* The effectiveness of praise and rewards often hinges on whether students perceive the praise and rewards as being sincere and credible. For these incentives to be most effective, students must believe that the person praising and rewarding the behavior or effort truly appreciates it. This is particularly true with praise, since the attractiveness of a reward—especially if highly valued—hinges much less on who gives it and how it is given. "Great job" can be voiced in different tones and with varying facial expressions—the words are the same, but the messages are not. Praise loses its effectiveness and can be harmful to the teacher–student relationship when offered with a snicker, sarcastically, or in a monotone voice with no expression. Faint praise can be particularly damning, as can be false promises (e.g., a reward promised but not delivered). Too much enthusiasm and exaggeration also can be interpreted as reflecting insincerity. Finally, timing is important. If an adult pauses a long time before finally saying "Great job!" there is a risk that the student and classmates will view the praise as insincere. To convey sincerity in the use of verbal praise, it helps to praise spontaneously, with variety (not repeating the same phrases), while conveying warmth with eye contact and a smile.

9. *Rely much more on praise than rewards, and particularly on private praise after the early elementary grades.* As noted in Chapter 6, one of the major advantages of praise is that its use is much less likely to be perceived as controlling than the use of rewards, especially when administered privately. Many older students prefer that they be praised privately instead of publicly (Brophy, 1981; Burnett, 2002; Elwell & Tiberio, 1994). For example, Elwell and Tiberio found that 60% of high school students preferred private praise or no praise at all over public praise. Likewise, in a survey of students ages 8–12, Burnett found that 52% preferred to be praised privately and individually (17% preferred not to be praised at all). Burnett attributed the finding that 69% of the students did not desire public praise to the students not wanting to be singled out in front of their peers as being better than others. He also suggested that doing so may encourage teasing and bullying. Public praise is more likely to be perceived as controlling, and embarrassing in front of peers, among adolescents than among young children. By praising privately, one also enhances the perception of sincerity and decreases social comparisons. Regardless of whether praise is given publicly or privately, it should be more common than rewards and much more common than criticism. A ratio of four positive comments for every one corrective comment is commonly recommended (Cameron & Pierce, 1994; Epstein et al., 2008).

> **Private praise is often more effective than public praise, especially among older students. Regardless of the student's age, however, the praise must be perceived to be sincere to be effective.**

10. *Highlight the present and future usefulness of the behavior praised or rewarded.* One way to divert attention from the praise or reward itself and toward the importance of the behavior is to highlight the usefulness and significance of the target behavior, including

both its present and future usefulness and significance. For example, when praising a student for completing an assignment on time, praise might be worded as "Excellent, Ahmed. People really appreciate it when you demonstrate responsibility by completing things on time. That will help you a lot next year in high school, as well as in college and when you get your first job."

11. *Encourage students to self-evaluate and self-reinforce their prosocial behavior and to take pride in their own behavior.* Praise and rewards serve the function of acknowledging or verifying significant and worthwhile actions, choices, achievements, efforts, or dispositions, which in turn should foster feelings of pride (Brophy, 2004; Cameron, 2001). To help foster intrinsic instead of extrinsic motivation, however, it is important to direct the feeling of pride toward the targeted action or some more global disposition (being kind, responsible, caring) and not toward the reward per se (e.g., "Excellent choice, Vivian, you should feel proud of yourself for not pushing Evan back").

A sense of pride should be encouraged not as a result of external praise and rewards but, more important, as a result of self-evaluation. Where appropriate and feasible (i.e., given students' developmental level and previous history, circumstances surrounding the behavior, and time available), students should be challenged to reflect upon, evaluate, and reinforce their own behavior. This challenge would include the self-evaluation and self-reinforcement of social problem-solving skills, such as thinking of alternatives, considering the perspective of others, and so forth. Self-evaluation should be based on standards conveyed in schoolwide expectations and rules and taught in lessons integrated throughout the curriculum. Over time, most students come to internalize these standards as their own. To facilitate this process and foster intrinsic motivation, with increasing age students should be increasingly encouraged to evaluate their behavior based on their "own" standards (when they are socially and morally responsible). A good time to require self-evaluation is when particular attention, via private praise or rewards, is given in recognition of a desired behavior. This self-evaluation diverts the focus from pleasing others and earning rewards and encourages intrinsic motivation. Of course, students should be encouraged to evaluate both desired and undesired behaviors, but the focus of this chapter is on positive behavior (see Chapters 9 and 10 for self-evaluation used in the correction of misbehavior).

12. *Actively involve students in determining the rewards, the behaviors to be rewarded, and in praising and rewarding others.* Students should be actively involved in determining behaviors to be targeted and what types of recognition and rewards should be given. Considerable care must be taken, however, in students' participating in the distribution of rewards, as perceptions of unfairness can quickly lead to resentment, bullying, and an undermining of the system. However, especially in the early grades, students should be encouraged to praise one another (and should be praised by adults when observed doing so). Several studies have found peers' praising and the reporting of peers' positive behavior to the teacher (who in turn, praises or rewards the student who did the praising or report-

> **Teachers should not be the only ones praising students for good behavior. Students should take pride in their own behavior. Praise also should come from peers, parents, and other adults in schools.**

ing while also highlighting the positive behavior to the class) to be effective in improving peer interactions and perceptions of those rejected or neglected by their peers (Skinner, Neddenrief, Robinson, Ervin, & Jones, 2002). For example, Skinner, Cashwell, and Skinner (2000) found students' reporting of positive behaviors to the teacher, or "tootling," to be an effective means of improving student behavior by reducing tattling (it also likely improved the classroom climate, though not measured).

The advantages of active participation of students are that it increases "buy in," minimizes perceptions of adult control, and enhances the likelihood that the rewards used may actually function as positive reinforcers. Active student participation can come from a student government body, in class meetings, or in special student committees.

13. *Administer rewards in an unexpected, or surprise, fashion.* A major finding of the review of the literature on rewards and intrinsic motivation conducted by Deci et al. (1999) was that tangible rewards did not harm intrinsic motivation when given spontaneously or unexpectedly. In the classroom, this would be similar to a teacher surprising the class with the reward of 15 minutes of free time on Friday after the students exhibited behavior consistent with the teacher's and school officials' expectations throughout the week. Although the students "earned" the reward, they were not told beforehand that they would earn it by meeting the teacher's expectations, nor were they given a specific level of performance they had to achieve. Used in this manner, the appearance of rewards as controlling is greatly minimized, and the focus of the students' efforts is not on earning extrinsic rewards.

14. *When rewards are used, make sure that all students have an equal opportunity to earn them.* Rewards have little or no motivational value if students believe they have little or no chance of earning them (Brophy, 2004). Students are likely to believe this if the expectations are too high. However, this is likely to occur when token economies or other programmed reward systems are used, and students recognize that teachers tend to disseminate tokens or rewards to two types of students: to the "really good ones," or "the teacher's pets"; and to "bad ones," or those who misbehave often but are rewarded when they are "caught being good." Recall in Chapter 6 that Brophy (1981) found that teachers tended to use praise in a similar fashion, praising mostly those students who sought it and those perceived by the teacher as needing it the most. Such practices are likely to lead other students to view the rewards as unfair.

15. *Recognize and be sensitive to developmental, cultural, and individual differences.* Programs that treat all students the same, irrespective of age, culture, or individual differences, are likely to fail. Adolescents do not generally think in the same way as preschoolers. For example, they cherish their peers' regard much more than their teacher's attention, they understand that gaining rewards is only one of multiple reasons to act in a certain way, and they have a strong desire to exert their autonomy and question authority, especially in response to actions they perceive to be unfair or unjust. These and other differences also exist among individual students of the same age. That is, some children mature faster than others, and not all share the same values, interests, and goals or are interested in the same rewards. As noted earlier, 60% of high school students prefer private praise or no praise over public praise. At this age, sincerity and the quality of the message are especially critical: one

sincere and credible private message from a respected teacher is likely to have much more impact than a dozen praises in front of the class.

In addition to sensitivity to developmental and individual differences in the preference for private versus public praise, one must also be sensitive to cultural differences. For example, deLuque and Sommer (2000) found that students of Asian collectivist cultures, compared to those of Western individualist cultures, preferred more group-focused feedback than individual-focused feedback. In both cultures, however, private feedback was preferred over public feedback. Henderlong and Lepper (2002) suggest that a preference for private over public praise might be particularly strong among ethnic minority students who do not want to be called out by adults (especially of the ethnic majority) in front of their peers.

16. *When using tokens or other rewards in a programmed manner, directly address issues of social control.* One way to help avoid the potential harm that praise and rewards might do to intrinsic motivation is by inoculating students with healthy attributions as to the reasons they are punished and rewarded (Henderlong & Lepper, 2002). To foster autonomy, intrinsic motivation, and self-discipline, students should be encouraged to attribute success (e.g., earning a token) to cognitions, emotions, and behaviors that they can readily control. They should understand that rewards are determined primarily by the students themselves and not by those disseminating them. However, in some situations of perceived failure (i.e., not earning rewards despite good behavior), students should be encouraged to understand that factors beyond their control can account for their not earning rewards, such as luck and the unpredictable perceptions of the person controlling the rewards. They also should understand that mistakes are a part of the learning process and can be corrected, and a "failure" to earn rewards or recognition is likely only to be temporary (Henderlong & Lepper, 2002). They should not interpret their failure to earn tokens to a lack of ability on their part, or even necessarily to a lack of effort. Learning to make such attributions can help avoid the potentially harmful indirect effects of rewards.

When rewards are used in a deliberate and systematic manner to manage schoolwide behavior, the reasons for such use should be given. Because students become gradually more aware of the motives and situations of others with age (Eisenberg, 2006), this advice would apply in the upper elementary grades (e.g., grades 4 and 5) and in all middle and high schools. It would particularly apply in schools that decide upon the schoolwide use of tokens, because tokens and tangible rewards are much more likely to be perceived as controlling than praise or the occasional use of privileges and preferred activities. At the very beginning of the school year, and preferably when school officials' expectations and the school's code of conduct are discussed, teachers, administrators, school staff, and students should discuss *why* rules are important, while emphasizing the school's dual mission (and teacher's role and responsibility) of maintaining order and safety *and* helping students develop self-discipline. Such discussions should occur in each classroom and be reviewed in grade-level or schoolwide assemblies, where appropriate. The rationale and various reasons for systematically using tokens and other rewards should be emphasized (assuming the reasons are valid), including their capacity to recognize, acknowledge, and show appreciation of desired behaviors; to promote positive school climate; to lessen the need for criticism and punitive techniques; to motivate students to perform tasks that they sometimes fail to perform well; and most importantly to foster self-discipline. It should also be emphasized that, just as educators would prefer that punitive techniques not be necessary, so too they prefer not to use rewards to *manage* student behavior—ideally, students should manage *their own* behavior. However, social control with punishment and rewards is appropriate when students choose not to control their own behavior, and it is definitely needed more for certain students than others.

17. *Use variety and novelty.* As widely noted in the behavioral literature (e.g., Alberto & Troutman, 2006), using the same reinforcers over and over is likely to be become satiating. Thus, educators are encouraged to provide variety and novelty in their use of both praise and rewards. Numerous textbooks on classroom management and intervention websites offer reinforcement menus for this purpose. Motivational theorists also strongly encourage teachers to use variety and novelty in their teaching methods to gain and retain students' interest and to increase both intrinsic and extrinsic motivation (Brophy, 2004).

18. *Plan for the generalization of the desired behavior that is praised or rewarded.* Programs for teaching social skills to students have a poor record of showing that skills learned in training sessions generalize to other settings and are maintained after the training (includ-

> If rewards are used in a systematic, programmed fashion, it is important that one plans for generalization and maintenance of the targeted behaviors.

ing the use of praise and rewards) has ended (Gresham, Sugai, & Horner, 2004; Kavale, Mathur, & Mostert, 2004; DuPaul & Eckert, 1994). Many programs attempt to address this lack of generalization by providing training in social skills throughout the school setting where the targeted behaviors naturally occur (as opposed to training in a small group or during a specific classroom period where behaviors are contrived) (e.g., Lewis, Sugai, & Colvin, 1998). For example, to foster generalization many SWPBS programs disseminate tokens for good behavior in the hallways and cafeteria, on the playground, and in all the classrooms. Unfortunately, while this approach may promote generalization of the behavior changes sought to those settings, there is little evidence that this reward distribution strategy facilitates the generalization of newly learned skills to settings in which rewards continue to not be salient.

When an SEL rather than SWPBS approach is used, other strategies for promoting generalization are usually employed, as reviewed in Chapter 4. They include (1) emphasizing the real-life applications of all social, emotional, and moral competencies taught in curriculum lessons infused throughout the curriculum and (2) providing ample planned opportunities for students to practice those skills across multiple settings (and praised or rewarded for doing so), including during disciplinary encounters and at home.

19. *If a schoolwide program systematically using tokens and/or rewards is implemented, be sure to fade its implementation shortly after the expectations and standards for the rewarded behavior have been met.* The goal here is for the desired behaviors sought through the reward system to continue to be exhibited even after the external rewards are

withdrawn or no longer given. In fading out the use of rewards, one gradually reduces or *thins* the reinforcement schedule. For example, if the school disseminates 1,000 tokens during September, much fewer would be disseminated during succeeding months and (hopefully) as behavior improves. The reinforcement schedule would become more and more intermittent. Indeed, eventually the programmed use of tokens and rewards should be replaced by the administration of rewards in an unexpected or surprise fashion, as recommended above when the lack of extrinsic motivation is not a concern. The goal of fading is for the desired behavior(s) to occur in the absence of contrived rewards, such as tokens, and to be motivated intrinsically or reinforced by more naturally occurring external reinforcers. More naturally occurring reinforcers include teacher praise, grades (especially if a grade or comment is given on a report card for behavior), praise from parents, privileges, and preferred activities. The challenge with regard to fading is properly calibrating the rate that one should withdraw rewards—neither too quickly nor too slowly (Alberto & Troutman, 2006). If rewards are withdrawn too quickly, the behavior may either never improve or very quickly return to its prerewarded state level. Conversely, if rewards are withdrawn too slowly, students might become dependent on the extrinsic rewards and fail to learn other reasons for engaging in the desired behaviors.

In addition to fading, several recommended strategies listed previously also should help foster maintenance of the desired behaviors, provided that an SEL approach is used. They are relying more on praise than rewards (one also should increase the frequency of praise—especially as the rewards are withdrawn); targeting not only the behavior but also cognitive and emotional processes and dispositions; highlighting the importance and usefulness of the targeted behavior; encouraging a sense of pride about the desired behaviors exhibited; and challenging students to evaluate and reinforce their own behavior. Not only should each of those strategies be used in combination with the fading of extrinsic rewards, but also each one should be subject to fading, itself. That is, as each desired supporting skill or understanding evolves, the emphasis on that skill and supports for its use should be gradually reduced.

SUMMARY

When used strategically and wisely, praise and rewards can do much more than simply reinforce targeted behaviors. They are particularly valuable in developing self-discipline, teacher–student relationships, and positive climates in classrooms and schools. But, these happen only when praise and rewards are used strategically and wisely. Unfortunately, this is often not done. In this chapter, 19 strategies were presented to help guide educators in the strategic and wise use of praise and rewards. Each is based on supporting research and theory, and each can be found among teachers and schools that are the most effective ones in using praise not only to manage student behavior, when needed, but more importantly to develop self-discipline. Form 7.1 provides a checklist for educators to use in reflecting on the extent to which they are following each of the 19 strategies for the strategic and wise use of praise and rewards.

Checklist to Guide the Strategic Use of Praise and Rewards

	Yes	No	Not applicable
1. Praise and/or rewards are used often, not only to reinforce specific behaviors but also to maintain a positive classroom or school climate.			
2. The informative, rather than the controlling, function of praise and rewards is emphasized.			
3. Deliberate efforts are made to avoid teaching students that the most important reason to act in a morally and socially responsible manner is to earn rewards or to be praised.			
4. Praise and rewards are used to recognize and acknowledge the cognitive and emotional processes and dispositions associated with self-discipline.			
5. Rewards are used only occasionally for behavior that is intrinsically motivated, and used more often for behavior that is not intrinsically motivated.			
6. Specific behaviors are praised or rewarded, and students know what they are.			
7. Praise and rewards are made contingent upon success in demonstrating the desired behavior or the effort expended.			
8. Praise and rewards are used in a sincere and credible manner.			
9. Praise is much more common than rewards. After elementary grades, private praise receives emphasis.			
10. The present and future usefulness of the behavior praised or rewarded is highlighted.			
11. Students are encouraged to self-evaluate and self-reinforce their prosocial behavior and to take pride in their own behavior.			
12. Students are actively involved in determining rewards, the behaviors to be rewarded, and in praising and rewarding others.			
13. Rewards are often administered in an unexpected, or surprise, fashion.			
14. When rewards are used, all students have an equal opportunity to earn them.			
15. Developmental, cultural, and individual differences are recognized in the use of rewards.			
16. When using tokens or other rewards in a programmed manner, issues of social control are directly addressed.			
17. Variety and novelty characterize the use of rewards.			
18. Deliberate plans are made for the generalization of the desired behavior that is praised or rewarded.			
19. If a schoolwide program of systematically using tokens and/or rewards is implemented, its implementation is faded shortly after the expectations and standards for the rewarded behavior have been met.			

CHAPTER 8

When Extrinsic Rewards Are Needed
Implementing the Good Behavior Game (While Developing Self-Discipline)

A main message throughout this book is that in many schools—and especially in those adopting the schoolwide positive behavior supports approach—rewards are used too frequently and often for the wrong reasons. They are used to manage student behavior, as observed in students' compliance with adult expectations and rules. When this use is the school's primary aim, it is a shortsighted one that neglects the development of self-discipline. However, it also has been stated repeatedly that at times students fail to exhibit self-discipline, and during those times it would be unwise for educators not to use external techniques (albeit preferably positive ones, including praise and rewards) to manage student behavior. In those situations, the immediate aim is to establish a classroom or schoolwide climate that is conducive to learning—one that is orderly but that also motivates students to learn and develop self-discipline. Although the aim is short-term, it is not shortsighted. That is, the long-term aim of developing self-discipline is not forgotten. All strategies presented in this book for developing self-discipline would continue to be used, although in the short run (and for as long as necessary) there would be greater use of teacher-centered strategies and techniques than student-centered ones.

This chapter and the two that follow are more about teacher-centered strategies and techniques than student-centered ones. The current chapter focuses on preventing behavior problems when self-discipline is lacking, while Chapters 9 and 10 focus more on correcting behavior problems. In all three chapters, however, the long-term aim of developing self-discipline is paramount. Indeed, the strategies and techniques presented are those designed to help achieve both the short-term goal of managing students' behavior and the long-term goal of having students manage their own behavior.

This chapter presents the Good Behavior Game (GBG; Barrish et al., 1969; Dolan, Turkan, Werthamer, Larsson, & Kellam, 1989). The GBG is a behavioral intervention (often referred to as an *interdependent group contingency system*) for managing student behavior at the classroom and schoolwide levels through the use of praise and rewards. GBG is most

> The Good Behavior Game (GBG) has been referred to as a "universal behavioral vaccine" (Embry, 2002). When used wisely, it is likely not only to result in short-term improvements in student behavior, but also foster the long-term development of self-discipline.

appropriate whenever students are lacking in self-discipline and/or when behavior problems at the classroom level interfere with learning. First, evidence supporting the effectiveness of the GBG is reviewed. Next, specific steps are presented for implementing the GBG in a manner that not only increases rule-compliant behavior in the short term but also helps educators achieve the long-term aim of developing self-discipline. Implementation is best accomplished by applying the knowledge and strategies presented in the preceding two chapters on the use of praise and rewards to the GBG.

THE GBG: SUPPORTING RESEARCH

The GBG was developed to "socialize children into the role of student and to teach them to regulate their own and their classmates' behavior" (Kellam et al., 2008, p. S7). It does this in two major ways: (1) by clearly defining behavioral expectations and rewarding self-discipline and prosocial behavior, and (2) by facilitating cooperation and positive interactions among peers (van Lier et al., 2005). Rewards are administered to individual groups, or *teams* within classes, contingent upon the behavior of *all* students on each team. For example, if all six members of the Eagles team follow the rules of the game while it is being played, then everyone on that team "wins" and is given a reward (e.g., a party). To earn the reward, however, each team has to earn a certain number of points by exhibiting behaviors desired by the teacher (or school officials).

Multiple studies have demonstrated the effectiveness of the GBG in improving student behavior (see Embry, 2002, and Tingstrom, Sterling-Turner, & Wilczynski, 2006, for reviews). However, most of those studies involved a small number of students and failed to employ a comparison group. Two major research projects are exceptions. In those projects, which have involved a number of separately published studies, large sample sizes and randomized control groups have been employed. The first project is the Baltimore City Public Schools project, conducted by Kellam and colleagues (Dolan et al., 1993; Ialongo, Pduska, Werthamer, & Kellam, 2001; Ialongo et al., 1999; Kellam & Anthony, 1998; Kellam, Brown, et al., 2008; Kellam, Rebok, Ialongo, & Mayer, 1994; Petras et al., 2008; Poduska, Kellam, Wang, Brown, Ialongo, & Toyinbo, 2008; Storr, Ialongo, Kellam, & Anthony, 2002). The second project is the Netherlands project, conducted by van Lier and colleagues (van Lier, Muthén, van der Sar, & Crijnen, 2004; van Lier et al., 2005). How the game was played in these studies and its impact on student behavior are discussed below.

Studies of the GBG in the Baltimore City Public Schools

In these studies, the majority of children were African American and lived in poor to lower-middle class urban areas, with a large percentage being at great risk of aggression and antisocial behavior or currently exhibiting such characteristics. The original intention of the researchers was not to study the effectiveness of the GBG but rather to investigate multiple factors that predict aggression and antisocial behavior. However, the researchers quickly discovered that nearly half of the first-grade teachers in their study were ineffective in managing their classrooms. These teachers required training in effective classroom management tools, and the GBG was implemented to meet that need.

The GBG was implemented in first- and second-grade classrooms during periods of the day when learning activities were less structured, such as when the teacher was working with individual students or small groups. When teachers first implemented the game, it was played for 10 minutes each day, three times per week. Over the course of 3 weeks, the time period was increased up to 3 hours. In an excellent example of avoiding satiation and using fading wisely, tangible rewards (e.g., stickers, erasers) were given immediately after the game was played but only during the first few months of the game's implementation. Over time, and as the behavior of the students improved, teachers shifted from the use of tangible rewards to preferred activities such as extra recess or a class party. They also shifted from rewarding those activities at the end of the day when the game was played to the end of the week. Moreover, as the year progressed, teachers no longer used the GBG on a regular basis but in a surprise or unpredictable fashion—that is, at varying times and for different activities.

Although results of the effectiveness of the GBG were not always consistent and varied largely as a function of respondents' gender, the outcome measure used, and the specific sample included in the study, the GBG decreased aggression and antisocial behavior in both the short term and long term (Dolan et al., 1993; Petras et al., 2008). During the first year the game was introduced, it reduced student aggression, antisocial behavior, and off-task behavior. In tracking those students into middle schools, decreased aggression and antisocial behavior continued to be found, but only among students who had evidenced the greatest amount of aggression in the early grades (Kellam, Ling, Merisca, Brown, & Ialongo, 1998; Kellam et al., 1994).

First graders participating in the GBG, as compared to controls, evidenced less drug use (except for marijuana use) during the subsequent course of their schooling (Poduska et al., 2008; Storr et al., 2002). Male first graders, in particular, also had less need for school-based mental health services (Poduska et al., 2008). When students were followed up in early adulthood and compared to students in the control group, fewer males (but not females)—especially among those who were the most aggressive and disruptive in the first grade—had drug and alcohol abuse/dependence disorders, antisocial personality disorders, and were regular smokers (Kellam et al., 2008). Moreover, those participating in the GBG in the first grade and who exhibited a consistent pattern of aggressive and disruptive behavior throughout their schooling were significantly less likely to have an antisocial personality disorder and to exhibit violent and criminal behavior in young adulthood (Petras et al., 2008). It should be noted that the findings in early adulthood were not replicated in a second cohort of students that was included in the two studies above. The researchers attributed this finding to the program not being implemented as well as it was with the first cohort group, noting that teachers received no additional training in the second year and were provided much less mentoring and monitoring.

GBG in The Netherlands

A major limitation of the Baltimore City Schools studies was that the sample was restricted to urban children, most of whom were African American and lived in poverty. Thus, it was unclear whether the results were truly generalizable. Studies by van Lier and colleagues (2004, 2005) addressed this limitation by implementing the GBG with a group of students in the second grade and again in the third grade in 13 "ordinary" elementary schools in the Netherlands, where only 33% of the respondents were from low socioeconomic homes). The GBG was implemented basically the same way as it was in Baltimore, but with a couple of interesting differences that reflected the Dutch culture (and which are consistent with many SEL programs): the teachers and the students developed the rules jointly, the teams did not compete against one another, and the names of the students who violated the rules were not called out in the class.

Over a period of 4 years the behavior of students participating in the GBG was compared to that of students in a randomly assigned control group. As found in the Baltimore studies, the students who benefited the greatest were those who were the most disruptive and aggressive. Over a period of several years they were found to have less aggression (based on self-reports), less relational bullying (reported by peers), and less delinquent behavior (van Lier et al., 2004, 2005). Students with moderate and low levels of antisocial behavior also benefited, although not in all of those areas. The moderately antisocial students evidenced less subsequent relational bullying and victimization, and those initially characterized as having a low level of antisocial group behavior also evidenced less subsequent victimization and anxious/depressed problems. In sum, as concluded by the researchers, the results showed that the GBG helped create a climate in which all students were safer over the long term.

Why Does the GBG Work?

The effectiveness of the GBG has been attributed to various aspects of the game (Dolan et al., 1993; Kellam et al., 2008; van Lier et al., 2005), including:

- Group cohesiveness and positive peer pressure
- A game-like atmosphere that is fun and motivational
- Students learning appropriate social skills early
- Students being more actively engaged in learning as a result of reduced off-task behavior

- The contingent use of rewards
- Teachers having more time to teach instead of correcting misbehavior
- Increased self-efficacy among students in their social competence which continues even after rewards are no longer used
- Less negative influence attributable to peers

Of these various reasons for improved behavior, van Lier et al. (2005) emphasized the last one—less negative influence attributable to students' peers. They argued that mixing aggressive and prosocial students together on teams not only increased the vicarious learning of prosocial behavior but also influenced peer relations at an early age. They surmised that such mixing, especially under GBG conditions, decreased the likelihood that disruptive and aggressive first and second graders would affiliate with deviant peers at that time but also in subsequent years. In turn, less affiliation with deviant peers

> **The GBG works not only because of the use of rewards per se, but also for various other reasons.**

may well have decreased the risk of rejection by the general peer group. Peer rejection is an important factor that has been shown to be related to multiple additional negative outcomes, including academic failure, aggression, and juvenile delinquency (Dodge et al., 2006). Perhaps what is most impressive about these findings is that they demonstrate that a relatively simply environmental intervention implemented classwide, and in some cases schoolwide (e.g., in some classes, teams were held accountable for their behavior in the hallways and cafeteria), can have a lasting impact on the life course of highly disruptive and aggressive students. Educators should be aware, however, that evidence of the effectiveness of the GBG is largely limited to its use in elementary school and particularly with highly disruptive and aggressive students. Just because an intervention works with one population of students does not mean that it would work with or should be applied to all other students. However, the GBG certainly fits the need of classes and schools in which intrinsic motivation is clearly lacking among students and where teachers have poor classroom management skills.

WHEN *NOT* TO PLAY THE GAME

Before explaining how the GBG is played, it should to be emphasized that the game should *not* be played, at least not on an ongoing basis, when students are already demonstrating the desired behavior without extrinsic rewards. Given the young age and disruptive behavior of the students in the cited research studies, and the lack of classroom management in many of their classrooms, the short-term goal of seeking compliance through external controls was quite appropriate.

> **When students are not disruptive, it makes little sense to use the GBG.**

However, irrespective of the age of students, the GBG should be considered, especially as an alternative to punitive techniques, for managing classes with disruptive students. It also should be a technique of choice for managing classes during those occasions when students who are generally well behaved need more than frequent external reminders and common motivational strategies used by most teachers.

PLAYING THE GBG TO MANAGE STUDENTS' BEHAVIOR AND DEVELOP SELF-DISCIPLINE

A very attractive feature of the GBG is that the rules and procedures for playing it are flexible and can be easily adapted to suit the individual preferences, needs, and aims of a teacher (or school). For example, those implementing the game determine whether positive points are awarded for exhibiting behavior consistent with the rules of the GBG or negative marks are given for violations of the rules. They also determine how many points or marks are needed to determine rewards, when and for how long the game is to be played, what behaviors are to be targeted, and what the rewards are.

Another attractive feature of the GBG is that it requires few if any new materials and little preparation and training. As shown in Figure 8.1, the GBG consists of three basic components: (1) participants, consisting of the students as players on teams of similar composition and the teacher acting as referee and coach; (2) five systems for play (rules, the reward system, the scoring system, the strategic use of praise, and a system for expansion, general-

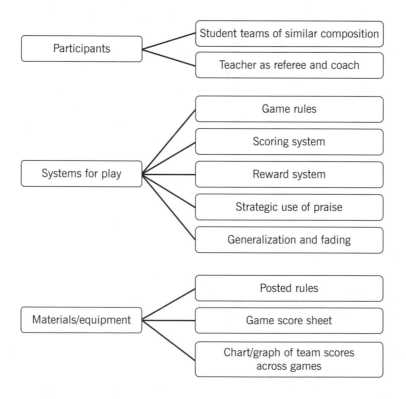

FIGURE 8.1. Components of the GBG.

ization, and fading); and (3) materials/equipment for posting the rules, keeping score, and tracking team standings (note that use of the chalkboard or a computer with a charting/graphing program or other existing materials is usually sufficient). Those basic components are described below, together with more specific procedures for implementing the GBG in a manner designed to improve student behavior in both the short and long term. Implementation is accomplished by balancing the teacher's need for effective management of student behavior with the students' need to develop self-discipline. Educators implementing the game, either in their classroom or schoolwide, should not hesitate to adapt the procedures to their own preferences and needs, so long as such adaptations are consistent with both the teacher's and the students' needs.

PREPARING FOR THE GAME

Step 1: Create Teams and Pick Their Membership

Divide the Class into Two or More Teams

Kellam and colleagues used three teams in each class and recommended that teams consist of four to seven players each (Dolan, Turkan, Werthamer-Larsson, & Kellam, 1989). To give no unfair advantage to one team over another and to foster positive student relationships and cooperation across various types of students, each team should be roughly comparable in composition, including diversity in gender, race, and behavior. Regarding the latter, it is especially important that each team include a similar number of students who are disruptive, who are shy, and those who are good role models. Teachers should not place all students with behavior problems on the same team, thinking that it might be easier to manage them by seating them together.

Be Prepared to Change Team Members

Although team composition should remain the same for a given game, and preferably when played on multiple occasions throughout the same "game season" (e.g., fall, winter, spring), there are several good reasons for occasionally changing a team's membership. One common reason is that a team may continually not earn points or rewards owing to the misbehavior of a particular team member or members. More often than not, the problem may be attributable to a single member of the team failing to exhibit self-discipline. When this situation arises, the teacher should make every effort to eliminate the behavior problems by using the preventive techniques discussed in Chapter 5 (e.g., eye contact and physical proximity) and asking peers to frequently remind the student of the game's rules. The teacher also should consider relaxing the rules a bit for some students where appropriate (e.g., a child with ADHD), especially when it is clear that he or she is exerting much effort and the violations are minor, such as when a student begins to get out of his seat but stops immediately when the teacher makes eye contact.

Occasionally there is another type of student who keeps a team from winning, namely, those who refuse to "play the game." Worse yet, instead of simply refusing to play, some students deliberately attempt to completely sabotage their team by preventing them from winning. This phenomenon occurs most frequently when students are not on the team of their choice and/or are on a team with peers they do not like.

A final circumstance for shifting team members is when certain members are *too* competitive and place undue pressure on their teammates. Although competition certainly has its motivational purposes, excessive peer pressure can be a shortcoming of the GBG (Skinner, Cashwell, & Bunn, 1996). For example, excesses can be observed whenever a teammate is bullied or ostracized for costing the team points.

When routine disciplinary measures (e.g., verbal and nonverbal warnings, physical proximity, problem solving with the student) fail to resolve the difficulties with chronic misbehavior, teams should either be reformed and rebalanced or the problematic students should be reassigned to their own "teams" (consisting of only one player).

Consider Assigning a Team Leader (Recommended for Elementary Grades Only)

Although seldom seen in other studies, in the Baltimore studies each team was assigned a team leader, primarily because the researchers were interested in addressing the social and emotional needs of first and second graders who were shy and withdrawn. Although other students were used as team leaders on a rotating basis, especially as a reward for good behavior, teachers were encouraged to use shy or withdrawn students initially as team leaders. It was hoped that the social status of these children would be enhanced and peers would interact with them more often if they were perceived as being associated with rewards and the teacher's favor. Research yielded mixed support for the GBG's reducing shy or withdrawn behavior: Although teacher ratings of behavior indicated some improvement, peer ratings did not (Dolan et al., 1993).

While some elementary teachers find the team leader function useful, it is not necessary to have a team leader. Moreover, it is strongly recommended that team leaders not be chosen at ages when students prefer not to serve in this role and when their peers are likely to tease them about it.

Step 2: Tentatively Define the Rules of the Game

Three to five rules should be created, with clear examples given of behaviors that fall under each rule. For example, in the Baltimore studies the following rules were recommended for the first- and second-grade classes (Dolan et al., 1989):

Rule 1: We will work quietly.

- Violations of the rule = talking without permission and making sounds such as humming or whistling.

Rule 2: We will get out of our seats only with permission.

- Violations of the rule = getting out of one's seat without permission.

Rule 3: We will follow directions.

- Violations of the rule = disobeying the teacher and not doing what the teacher says.

Rule 4: We will be polite to others.

- Violations of the rule = physically contacting or disrupting others, such as hitting, kicking, pushing, tripping, touching others, throwing objects, or taking or destroying someone else's property.

The rules do not have be exactly the same each time the game is played. Indeed, they should vary, based on the nature of the learning activity or the context in which the rules are applied. For example, when playing the GBG while teaching social and emotional lessons, I have always included the rule that everyone on each team must contribute to discussion: he or she must answer at least one question or offer a viewpoint during each class. All students also are to respect the opinions and perspectives of others by showing they are listening when others are speaking and not personally criticizing what they have to say. Such rules would not be appropriate for other learning activities.

At this point in time in the playing of the GBG, rules should not yet be set but only be tentative, allowing for appropriate recommendations and input from students before the games begin. Where feasible, rules should be directly linked to schoolwide behavioral expectations that might apply (e.g., respect others, be responsible, do your best).

Step 3: Determine What Rewards Will Be Used and When They Will Be Given

As with the rules, the list of possible rewards to be given to each winning team should also be tentative at this point to enable players to have an opportunity to provide input. Such input from students may well increase the prospects of the reward actually serving as a true reinforcer of behavior. In addition to the strategic use of praise throughout the game, both immediate and delayed rewards should be considered. Immediate rewards, given at the end of a game (e.g., 5 minutes of extra recess for young children, free time for any age), are most appropriate when the game is played the first few times, especially for younger students who find it difficult to delay gratification. Delayed rewards are awarded after multiple games are played, ranging from the end of a week of daily play to the end of an entire game season (e.g., 4–10 weeks). Examples of delayed rewards are an extra 15 minutes of recess, extra credit on an assignment, no-homework passes, a popcorn party, a movie, and going outside for 1 hour. Obviously, the size of the reward should vary as a function of the number of games played. For example, extra recess or no-homework passes might be awarded at the end of 1 or 2 weeks, and a party at the end of the season. If immediate rewards are used, which generally are not necessary beyond the early grades, they should gradually be phased out and replaced by delayed rewards, as explained later.

Step 4: Determine How the Score Will Be Kept and What Score Is Needed to Win

Different methods and criteria, ranging from the simple to the complex, can be used to determine a winning score. They depend on the personal preferences of the teacher but also should be based on the developmental level and behavior of the students. The Baltimore study used a simple recording method in which a mark was placed beside the team's name for each rule infraction (Dolan et al., 1989). The total score, consisting of the number of marks, was calculated for each team at the end of the game. A team earned a reward if it received less than five marks during the period that the game was played. Game times ranged from 10 minutes to over an hour. Interestingly, this format is very similar to the old "name on the board" (with checks) technique used in the early versions of Assertive Discipline (Canter & Canter, 2001). After receiving much criticism, Canter dropped this punitive technique and replaced it with more positive ones, including rewarding points for good behavior that could be exchanged for rewards. It is recommended that a similar positive behavior system be used with the GBG. That is, instead of giving marks based on the presence of inappropriate behavior, points should be given on the basis of the presence of appropriate behavior. Awarding points for good behavior helps to engender a positive rather than punitive atmosphere and enables the teacher to highlight *appropriate* behaviors. Of course, inappropriate behaviors that *cost* a team points also are noted, but emphasis is placed on appropriate behaviors that *earn* points.

> It is generally better to give students positive points for desired behavior than to give them punitive checkmarks for undesired behavior. Such use highlights the desired behaviors more than the undesired behaviors.

Points should be awarded either at the end of short games (e.g., 10 minutes) or at intervals throughout longer games (a more common strategy). For example, if the game is to be played during a 40-minute class period, scores for each team might be recorded on the board four times during that period, or roughly every 10 minutes apart once the game begins with the final recording concluding the game. It is better to use random times than fixed times to record the scores because it often is difficult to stop at a given time for that purpose.

The score given at the end of each interval might range from 0 to 5, as suggested below:

5 = PERFECT. The team followed all rules during 100% of the time interval.

4 = EXCELLENT. The team had only one minor infraction of the rules.

3 = GOOD. The team had two to three minor infractions of the rules.

2 = NEEDS MUCH PRACTICE. The team tried but still needs much practice, as seen in the three to five minor infractions observed.

1 = TEAM PROBLEMS. It is unclear whether the team even tried hard, as seen in more than five minor infractions.

0 = MAJOR VIOLATION. Disciplinary action necessary, as seen in one or more major violations of the rules (e.g., refusal to follow the rules even after several reminders; violation of the school's code of conduct). As discussed previously, team members with the violations would be eliminated from the game if the behavior continues across games.

Using the foregoing scoring system, each team could score a maximum of 20 points during the 40-minute game (5 points maximum x 4 intervals of 10 minutes each). The teacher would decide on the score needed to "win" (e.g., 80% of the maximum score possible, or at least 16 points, depending on what the teacher believes to be reasonable, given the behavior of the class). To be consistent across games, and easier for students to recognize low and high scores, the same 20 points-maximum score system would be used regardless of the length of the game. For example, if played for 60 minutes, a score would still be given only four times—three times during the game and once at the end, with scores being approximately 15 minutes apart. Or, with older students who understand percentages, the teacher could simply apply the 80% criterion irrespective of the number of points possible. In this way, the teacher does not have to worry about how points and intervals are used but simply records 1–5 points at any number of intervals as long as the game is being played. At the end of the game, it is determined whether 80% or more of the possible points were earned (i.e., the average score was 4 or higher across recorded scores).

One potential problem to avoid, especially with older students, is students settling for a less than perfect score because they figured out that they can misbehave several times but still earn the reward. One way to avoid this is by offering a bonus reward to those teams scoring above 90% of the points possible.

Game times, or intervals within a game, should be shorter when the game is first played, and then gradually lengthened as each team gains more "practice" and improves its skills. Likewise, intervals (and the length of games) should be shorter in classes in which behavior problems are common and more frequent monitoring and feedback are needed. Shorter intervals and game lengths are often necessary to ensure success when the game is first played. Without initial success, it is unlikely that students will desire to continue to play the GBG. These situations would include most early grades in elementary school, but also disruptive classes at any grade. The length of both the scoring intervals and the games would be increased as the behavior of the class improves and students demonstrate that they can manage their own behavior for longer periods of time. The criterion for winning also might be increased, especially if a relatively low criterion was set initially and easily met.

Decide When to Play the Game and When You Might Stop Playing It

As emphasized previously, the game should not be played when it is not needed—when there are few if any behavior problems that disrupt learning or when such problems are easily addressed with other preventive techniques. Also, it is recommended that it not be played too often or for too long. This is because it is likely to lose its effectiveness when the novelty of the game wears off. Playing the GBG often or for long periods when it is not needed also increases the risk of it being perceived as socially controlling, especially among older students. Furthermore, most students simply need a break from concentrating on playing the game.

The GBG is best suited for classes with a sizable number of disruptive students (e.g., more than 25% of the class), and it can be used in those classrooms any time of the day. However, it also is useful for "normal" classrooms in which violations of classroom rules occur less often but nevertheless interfere with learning. The latter circumstance is more likely to occur at certain (often predictable) times than others. For example, students are likely to be off-task when their teacher is working with another student individually or with a small group. This is a good time to play the GBG, provided that the teacher can continue to monitor the behavior of all teams to keep accurate score.

As done in the Baltimore and Netherlands studies, when the GBG is new to students, it should be implemented in three stages: introduction, expansion, and generalization. In the introduction stage, the GBG is played for a brief period of time with the aim of the students' learning and practicing how to play it. In the two studies, the *introduction* stage lasted about 2 months and started with three sessions per week during which the game was played for only 10 minutes. In the *expansion* stage, intervals are expanded (e.g., from 10 to 50 minutes, 3 games per week). Additionally, the game is expanded to other settings and behaviors when needed—for example, to behavior in the hallways. In the two cited studies, the expansion phase lasted 3–4 months.

Finally, during the *generalization* stage rewards are faded, with praise largely replacing rewards in their function. There also is an increased emphasis on self-regulation of behavior, or self-discipline, especially when the game is *not* played. On occasion, the GBG would still be played; however, it would be played less often, as a surprise and with smaller rewards. How long each stage or the game lasts should depend on the developmental level of the students. For example, the introduction stage should last much longer for younger than older students. Beyond the early elementary grades, the introduction stage should be very brief, entailing only one or two sessions, and the game times should be longer.

PLAYING THE GAME

The greatest challenge to teachers and schools in the use of techniques designed for the purpose of external management of student behavior, including the GBG, is using them in a manner that develops rather than stifles intrinsic motivation and self-discipline. Using external reinforcement techniques to help develop self-discipline might sound contradictory, but it does not have to be. When used wisely, the GBG can help manage student behavior while simultaneously fostering self-discipline by not only encouraging students to learn and practice desired ways of thinking and acting but also by fostering positive teacher–

student relationships and positive classroom and school climates. As shown below, these aims can be achieved by applying each of the 19 recommendations on the strategic use of praise and rewards that were presented in the preceding chapter specifically to the GBG. In the steps and recommendations for the GBG below, each of those recommendations is applied. Although they are applied specifically to the GBG, they can and should be applied similarly to other behavioral systems designed to manage student behavior. The intent is to redirect or balance the common teacher-centered goal of teaching and controlling specific observable behaviors with the use of extrinsic rewards to the more student-centered goal of developing self-discipline. For the recommendations below, each of the 19 recommendations in Chapter 7 is cited in parentheses below to show how it applies to the GBG.

Preseason Practice

When first introducing the game to students, it might help to use the analogy of a preseason game (or scrimmages) in many sports, with the purpose of teams getting ready for the real games by practicing rules and helping teammates. Several preseason games might be necessary. Have a trial run, or practice the game, before the first official game is played. At that time, explain or develop the following:

Explain the Purpose of the Game and When It Will Be Played

Avoid messages that might lead students to perceive the game as being used for the primary purpose of controlling their behavior. To do so:

- Present the game in a fun, game-like atmosphere. Keep in mind that, although reinforcement of desired behavior is one function of the game, another is to improve classroom and schoolwide climate. (*Recommendation 1: Use praise and rewards for reasons other than positive reinforcement.*)
- Explain that the game will be played at certain times at your discretion, but especially when the class might benefit from frequent reminders of classroom rules and when they might most appreciate something new and fun. (*Recommendation 2: Use rewards only occasionally for behavior that is intrinsically motivated and more often for behavior that is not intrinsically motivated. Recommendation 17: Use variety and novelty.*)
- Emphasize the critical importance of self-discipline and group cooperation (in this game, as well as in sports and other games) and that the players of the game, not the referee (i.e., you), determine who wins. Note that it is the job of the referee to remind players of the rules and to enforce them. This function assures that rules are applied fairly, that no one team has an unfair advantage during the game, and that bedlam does not occur during the game. Fairness and the safety of all players is always a concern of referees. Try to avoid statements, however, that might be perceived as overly controlling (e.g., "I'm using this game to make sure you follow the rules," "I decide

who wins," or "I will give rewards if I think you earned them"). *(Recommendation 16: When using tokens or other rewards in a programmed manner, directly address issues of social control.)*

Explain and Discuss the Rules of the Game

Ask the class what rules are needed to help establish and maintain order and respect during the time when the game is being played. Write their recommendations on the board, and add any rules (from the list of tentative rules that you developed earlier) that students might have overlooked. Remind them, however, that *all* school rules also apply during the games, which includes begin removed or "benched" for poor sportsmanship. *(Recommendation 12: Actively involve students in determining the rewards and the behaviors to be rewarded.)*

- *Decide upon three to five general rules or behavioral expectations.* Give examples of specific behaviors that each rule covers, and discuss the importance of those behaviors and rules. *(Recommendation 6: Specify what is being praised and rewarded. Recommendation 10: Highlight the present and future usefulness of the behavior praised or rewarded.)* I have found that students almost always come up with the same rules tentatively listed by the teacher, although they might need to be reminded of one or two of them.
- *Explain that rules might vary, depending on the learning activity or the time of the game.* For example, different rules might be needed during classroom discussions than during written assignments or when the game is played outside of the classroom, such as in the hallway. This is like shifting from playing football to playing volleyball—the rules are not the same (and it helps if the players are multitalented). Explain that when different rules apply they will be announced before the game begins.
- *Explain the point system and how it will be used to determine rewards.* Emphasize that each team can win by exhibiting certain behaviors that reflect self-discipline. Also emphasize that not just one team can win, but every team can. *(Recommendation 7: Make praise and rewards contingent upon success in demonstrating the desired behavior or the effort expended.)*
- *Explain your role as both coach and referee.* Make it clear that during the game you serve two roles as (1) coach and (2) referee, umpire, or field judge. You might shift from one role to the other. In the role of coach, you are there to help each team win by giving the members advice and at times having to model or teach the correct skill. Most of the time, however, you will serve as the referee. As referee, and for the sake of the players and the game, you must enforce the rules, which includes making sure that players regulate their own behavior. Emphasize that players should regulate their own behavior but that referees and coaches (or teachers) must step in when players fail to do so. Also note that, in the interest of fairness and not delaying the game, arguing with your "call" will not be allowed and may result in a penalty (the player's team losing a point). Continuing to argue with the referee will result in

removal of the offending player from the game. There are no challenges or instant replays!

Determine the Rewards

- *Solicit student preferences about rewards.* As done in the discussion of the rules, encourage student participation in creating the new game. Allow them to vote on reward choices offered by the teacher. Use different rewards during the course of the season. (*Recommendation 12: Actively involve students in determining the rewards and the behaviors to be rewarded. Recommendation 17: Use variety and novelty.*)

Announce the Players on Each Team and Where Each Team Will Be Placed

- Explain that teams were formed with the intent of making them similar in membership and giving each team an equal opportunity to win. Arrange seating in the classroom (or "field") such that team members are grouped together (e.g., front left quarter of seats = Team 1, back left = Team 2, etc.).

Practice the Game

The same rules and procedures should apply when playing for practice (i.e., in preseason) as when played thereafter (during the season). The only major difference, however, is that the teacher might need to serve more in the role of coach than referee in the first few games. During both the practice session(s) and all future games, apply the following:

> **As the saying goes, "practice makes perfect."**

Immediately before the Game Begins

- Post a game-day scoresheet with team names (see Figure 8.2). This can be done by using a computerized system (e.g., Smart Board, computer with LCD), portable erasable board or simply by writing the team names on the chalkboard and drawing a simple chart to record the scores each time the game is played.

- Post a list of agreed-upon rules for the game (see Table 8.1). Review each rule during the first few games and when otherwise needed, such as when violations are frequent. Remind students of the rules at the beginning of all games.

- If rewards are given only at the end of the season, as opposed to the end of the game, post a chart that shows each team's current scores for the season (see Figure 8.3). For example, if each team must earn a certain number of points over 5 or 10 games to earn a reward, post the scores for each of those games for each team to see the current standings. This can be done by using a poster board, a corner of the chalkboard, a portable erasable board, or a computerized scoring and charting system that can be viewed by the entire class.

Today's Scores					
Team	1st period	2nd period	3rd period	4th period	Total game points
Eagles	4	3	4	3	14
Barnacles	5	4	4	4	17
Red Fury	5	5	5	5	20
Jags	4	5	5	5	19

5—PERFECT
4—EXCELLENT
3—GOOD
2—NEEDS MUCH PRACTICE
1—TEAM PROBLEMS
0—MAJOR VIOLATIONS

FIGURE 8.2. Sample score sheet for each game.

TABLE 8.1. Example of Game Rules

1. *Respect others. This includes:*
   - Do not talk while others are speaking. Wait until you are called on.
   - Respect the opinions of others, even when you disagree.
   - Do not bother or disturb others when they are working.
   - Follow the Golden Rule: Treat others as you would like to be treated.

2. *Work as a team.*
   - Help others follow the rules.
   - Help others with assignments, as allowed.

3. *Be responsible for your own behavior.*
   - Control your impulses! Raise your hand before speaking. Stay in your seat. Keep your hands to yourself.
   - Accept correction from the referee (teacher). Do not argue.

Game Scores for Season											
Team	Game 1	Game 2	Game 3	Game 4	Game 5	Game 6	Game 7	Game 8	Game 9	Game 10	Total
Eagles	14	18*	18*	20**	16	18*	18*	19**	20**	19**	180
Barnacles	17*	20**	18*	19**	17	18*	20**	19**	18*	20**	186
Red Fury	20**	19**	20**	19**	18*	20**	18*	19**	20**	19**	192
Jags	19**	17*	18*	19**	17	19**	20**	18*	19**	20**	186

*Team met goal of 80%. **Team scored above 90%, earning bonus points.

FIGURE 8.3. Example of a score sheet completed across games.

• Remind the players of the reward for winning and that every team has the opportunity to win. Also, remind them of any bonuses for exceptional play.

During the Game

• Award points for self-discipline and team behavior at the end of each interval of play (or at the end of a very short game). At the end of the first interval, explain why the points were awarded, for example, "Team A received 5 points for each member demonstrating self-discipline and the team working cooperatively throughout the entire period. Team B also received a high score of 4 and lost only 1 point because a player was talking while I was. Overall, the class did very well." *(Recommendation 2: Focus on the* Message: *Emphasize the informative rather than the controlling function of praise and rewards. Recommendation 6: Specify what is being praised and rewarded. Recommendation 7: Make praise and rewards contingent upon success in demonstrating the behavior or the effort expended. Recommendation 8: Communicate sincerity. Recommendation 10: Highlight the present and future usefulness of the behavior praised or rewarded.)*

• Frequently praise individual students and teams for following the rules of the game, respecting others, helping others on their team (e.g., reminding teammates of the rules and encouraging them to follow them), and exhibiting other desired behaviors. *(Recommendations 2, 6, 7, 8, and 10 as immediately above.)*

• In addition to the above and when feasible, praise students privately, especially those students demonstrating team cooperation and leadership and improved self-discipline. *(Recommendation 9: Rely much more on praise than rewards, and particularly on private praise after the early elementary grades.)*

• Be sure to praise students for using problem-solving skills and for regulating their emotions and behavior. Where appropriate, praise general dispositions, such as being a kind person or a team player and remind them of their importance. *(Recommendation 4: Praise and reward the cognitive and emotional processes and dispositions associated with self-discipline.)*

• Motivate good behavior by reminding students throughout the game of the importance of self-discipline, the multiple rewards of self-discipline (and not just extrinsic ones), and that the game is a fun way to encourage self-discipline. Be sure to attribute their good behavior to self-discipline and motives other than earning rewards and winning the game. *(Recommendation 3: Avoid teaching students that the most important reason to act in a morally and socially responsible manner is to earn rewards or to be praised. Recommendation 11: Encourage students to self-evaluate and self-reinforce their personal behavior and to take pride in their own behavior.)*

• At the end of each game, total the points for each team, and record them on a chart where team scores can be tallied or graphed from game to game throughout the season. Post this chart where all players can keep track of the scores. Reward students or remind them of the reward that will be given in the future.

Expansion and Generalization/Fading

Once the GBG has been established, and assuming that it is effective in improving classroom behavior when it is played, consider extending the game's rules so that they apply to additional settings and/or to different behaviors. This should be done, however, *only if* the behaviors targeted are problematic and likely to improve with the GBG. Other behaviors might include participating in discussions, being prepared and organized for the learning activity in which the GBG is played, completing homework related to the activity, and coming to the class on time (especially in middle and high school, where there is a change of classes). Behavior in other settings might include cooperative and prosocial behavior on the playground during recess, safety in the hallway (e.g., no running, fighting), respect for others in the cafeteria during lunch, and cooperative and prosocial behavior during special activities such as music, arts, or physical education. Clearly, such expansion to other settings would be more appropriate and feasible in elementary schools than in middle and high schools, especially because students are more likely to be together in one class.

> When playing the GBG, be sure to evaluate how you are addressing each of the 19 recommendations in Chapter 7 on the strategic and wise use of praise and rewards.

Fading applies to both (1) rewards, including the type used and how long teams must wait to receive them, and (2) the use of the game. As noted previously, if tangible rewards are used to reward behavior when the game is first practiced and played (e.g., giving players a piece of candy or stickers in a fun, motivating manner), it is important that they be quickly replaced by preferred activities such as free time or a party. Eventually they are completely replaced by teacher praise and surprise rewards.

Fading of rewards also should include increasing the time students must wait before receiving a reward, such as the preferred activity. As rewards are faded, so too should the frequency with which the game is played. For example, while a fourth-grade class might play the game three times a week for 3 weeks in October before each team is given its reward of 30 minutes of free time, it might play it only once a week for 6 weeks during February and March before earning the same reward. Subsequently, the game might be played even less often over time, but only if all teams are consistently winning. In this manner, both rewards and game frequency are faded.

When and how quickly fading occurs should always be contingent upon improved behavior. Do not fade the rewards or the use of the game if it is clear that the students do not exhibit self-discipline without it. Indeed, if behavior does not improve, the duration of the game and the interval of time before receiving a reward should be shortened, not lengthened, and one should consider offering a different reward (as well as creating different teams). Nevertheless, for the teacher, students, and school officials to truly "win" in the use of the GBG, as seen in increased self-discipline and less need of extrinsic control, the game should be played much less—if at all—by the end of the year. (*Recommendation 19: If a schoolwide program systematically using tokens and/or rewards is implemented, be sure to fade its implementation shortly after the expectations and standards for the rewarded behavior have been met.*)

Of course, the game can always be reinstituted on occasions when it is needed, but such occasions should be much less frequent over time. When the game is not played, rewards should continue to be used; however, although still contingent upon good behavior, they should be given only occasionally and unexpectedly (i.e., as a surprise), as opposed to a programmed fashion. *(Recommendation 13: Administer rewards in an unexpected, or surprise, fashion.)*

Form 8.1 (at the end of the chapter) presents a useful checklist of the foregoing items for preparing and playing the GBG.

Developmental, Cultural, and Individual Differences

In planning and implementing the GBG, developmental, cultural, and individual differences should be considered. *(Recommendation 15: Recognize and be sensitive to developmental, cultural, and individual differences.)* As noted previously, the GBG is developmentally most appropriate for the early grades, when students are learning school rules and are lacking in social and moral maturity and self-regulation of behavior. However, it also is appropriate when students, irrespective of grade level, fail to demonstrate intrinsic motivation or self-discipline. At times, this shortcoming is seen at every age, albeit more so among some students than others. In general, however, the GBG should be played much less often with each increasing grade level. Likewise, the length of time the game is played, and as well as the intervals within sessions, should be shorter in the lower grades than in the upper grades.

Perhaps the greatest individual difference that needs to be addressed is that of reward preferences. Rarely does everyone in a class like the same reward. To avoid this problem, students should be actively involved in determining the most attractive rewards. However, consensus often fails to emerge from the class. Typically, free time with a choice of various activities is attractive to everyone.

Cultural differences specific to the GBG should be of minor concern, but nevertheless cultural differences should be considered. As discussed in the preceding chapter, while students of an Asian background may especially appreciate the cooperative aspects of the GBG as it operates within their team, they might not like the classwide emphasis on competition among class members. On the other hand, students with Western cultural backgrounds might like the competition but object to the fact that the behavior of others determines whether or not they will be rewarded themselves. Such cultural concerns can largely be addressed by emphasizing the value of both group and individual behavior, directly addressing issues of fairness, and noting that although the game entails some competition it depends mostly on cooperation.

SUMMARY

The GBG has consistently been shown to be an effective positive technique for the management of disruptive behavior. Although generally used at the classroom level, it also can be used schoolwide. In light of its demonstrated effectiveness and ease of use, the GBG has been recommended as an evidence-based intervention by multiple organizations and agencies, including the U.S. Surgeon General (2001) and the American Federation of Teachers (2000). Indeed, in a recent review of its effectiveness, it was adjudged a "universal behavioral vaccine" (Embry, 2002).

The greatest challenge to educators is using the GBG in a manner that effectively manages student behavior while simultaneously helping develop self-discipline. To help educators do so, the recommendations on the strategic and wise use of praise and rewards presented in Chapter 7 were applied to the GBG in this chapter. Although the regular and systematic use of the GBG is not a necessity in many classrooms and schools, it serves a valuable purpose when used in those classes and schools where either students lack sufficient self-discipline or classroom management and schoolwide discipline are deficient. The GBG may also be appealing on occasion to teachers who believe their students could benefit from a fun game designed to motivate self-discipline. When played, the GBG should always be combined with other strategies and techniques presented throughout this book for preventing and correcting behavior problems and developing self-discipline.

Good Behavior Game Implementation Checklist

Check items as they are completed in the planning and playing of the game.

Pregame Planning

____ Teams created (about four to seven members on each team).

____ Teams are similar in composition.

____ Three to five clear rules for the game drafted, such that students should know exactly what is required to earn points (might change with student input, but unlikely).

____ Potential rewards planned (might change with student input).

____ Scoring system planned, with criteria for "winning."

____ Chart for posting scores drafted (will need to fill in team names later).

____ Decide when the game will be played (which days, for how long).

Game Time

Before Playing the First Game

____ Explain purpose of the game—to motivate self-discipline.

____ Explain and discuss the rules, inviting input for possible changes (where appropriate). Note that rules might vary in the future, depending on the learning activity or time of the game.

____ Explain the point system and what is required for a team to "win."

____ Emphasize that all teams can "win"—there are not necessarily *any* losers.

____ Explain your role as coach and referee.

____ Discuss and determine rewards, linked to points for "winning."

____ Announce and form the teams.

____ Post the scoreboard (and chart, if one is used).

____ Post the rules.

____ Practice the game before playing the first "real" game.

During All Games

____ Combine praise with points, using praise often and more frequently than awarding points.

____ Award team points at the end of each scoring interval.

____ Post the final scores for each team.

____ Act as a coach—provide support and guidance to each team.

____ Act as a referee—enforce rules, don't argue, but *do* explain scoring decisions briefly when challenged.

(cont.)

Good Behavior Game Implementation Checklist (page 2 of 2)

____ Praise and rewards are used strategically to promote both compliance *and* self-discipline, as seen in the practices below.

____ The primary goal of praise and reward is self-discipline, not obedience, of each team and its individual members, which includes cognitive and emotional processes as well as dispositions (respecting the perspectives and rights of others, empathy, kindness) that are often seen in behavior that is consistent with the rules.

____ Praise and rewards are used in an informative rather than controlling manner.

____ Praise and rewards are contingent upon each team and its individual members demonstrating specific behaviors that reflect self-discipline (including following the rules). This requirement is made clear when points are awarded.

____ Praise and rewards are given to teams in a sincere and credible fashion.

____ Praise greatly exceeds negative feedback and constructive criticism.

____ Praise is given much more often than game points.

____ Both public and private praise are used, and public praise is directed more toward a team than an individual.

____ Cooperation is emphasized much more than competition (everyone is aware that all teams can "win" simultaneously).

____ Teams clearly know what behaviors are expected and recognized.

____ Occasionally mention is made of the present and future value of the behaviors demonstrated (i.e., self-discipline).

____ Students are encouraged to self-evaluate and reinforce and take pride in their positive behavior.

____ The use of praise and rewards is sensitive to any developmental and cultural differences.

Expansion, Generalization, and Maintenance

____ After the game continues to be successful, the game's rules are gradually expanded to include additional behaviors needing improvement (e.g., everyone's participation in discussion, tardiness for class, work completion).

____ The same social and emotional competencies recognized during the GBG game are recognized in non-GBG settings and by multiple adults (and peers, where appropriate).

____ Rewards are faded, both in type and how long it takes to earn them.

____ The number of times the game is played is faded.

____ Deliberate efforts are made to replace the rewards in the GBG with more natural rewards in the environment (social recognition, pride, surprise rewards).

CHAPTER 9

Authoritative Discipline
in the Correction of Misbehavior

Most educators recognize the important goal of developing self-discipline, but it is the *use* of discipline to correct misbehavior that typically comes to mind when one thinks of school discipline. There has never been a shortage of techniques used to correct misbehavior and to bring about short-term compliance. Indeed, ample research supports the use of common techniques of applied behavior analysis (see Alberto & Troutman, 2006) and more specifically five basic behavioral techniques found in nearly every classroom (Landrum & Kauffman, 2006): positive reinforcement, negative reinforcement, extinction, response cost punishment, and punishment involving aversive consequences. It is primarily because those techniques *are* effective (Stage & Quiroz, 1997) and easy to use that they are found in nearly every textbook on classroom management as well as in nearly every teacher's repertoire of techniques for managing student behavior (Brophy, 1996).

The purpose of this chapter, and the one that follows, is not to provide another review of those five behavioral techniques and others, and specific steps for implementing them (see Alberto & Troutman, 2006; Cangelosi, 2007; Kerr & Nelson, 2009; Scheuermann & Hall, 2008; Walker, Ramsey, & Gresham, 2004). Rather, the purpose is to offer recommendations, guided by theory and research, on how common behavioral techniques used by teachers and schools to correct misbehavior might be used in a manner to achieve not only the short-term goal of compliance but also the additional goals of developing self-discipline and maintaining a positive school climate. Research on authoritative discipline, reviewed in Chapter 5 on *prevention*, provides guidance on how to achieve all three of these goals in the context of *correction*. As discussed in that chapter, the most effective teachers (and parents) are both *responsive* and *demanding*. In both preventing and correcting behavior problems, authoritative adults are responsive to children's social and emotional needs, especially the need for autonomy. They demonstrate responsiveness and support through acceptance,

> "Within the authoritative model, behavioral compliance and psychological autonomy are viewed not as mutually exclusive but rather as interdependent objectives: children are encouraged to respond habitually in prosocial ways *and* to reason autonomously about moral problems, *and* to respect adult authorities *and* learn how to think independently." (Baumrind, 1996, p. 405)

respect, involvement, warmth, and caring. In influencing behavior, they prefer to guide with advice, modeling, persuasion, and moral reasoning rather than the use of punishment. However, authoritative adults also are demanding: they recognize that, just as autonomy is important, so too is compliance with rules and adult expectations. Demandingness, or structure, is provided through adult monitoring, supervision, clear and high expectations, and the firm and fair enforcement of rules and the

consequences of violating them, including the judicious use of punishment, where appropriate. By being both responsive and demanding, authoritative adults are effective not only in bringing about short-term compliance with preventive and corrective techniques but also in developing self-discipline with those and additional techniques. They do not see achieving both compliance and self-discipline, or autonomy, as being incompatible goals.

In sum, responsiveness and demandingness, as seen in authoritative discipline, not only help develop self-discipline but also help create and maintain a positive school climate characterized by prosocial behavior, few behavior problems, caring relations among staff and students, and safety (Gregory et al., in press).

It is important to emphasize that the authoritative approach stands in contrast to the authoritarian approach. The latter is commonly seen in schools that adopt a pervasive zero tolerance approach to school discipline. Typically, under the authoritarian approach punishment is perceived by students as overly harsh and unfair (Arum, 2003). Indeed, the primary aim of the authoritarian approach is social control and compliance, and punishment is seen to be the best way to achieve that aim. In correcting misbehavior, the greatest difference between the authoritative and authoritarian approaches is not the use of punishment per se but rather the manner in which it is used. In the authoritarian approach, punishment is used frequently and exclusively and without the support and caring inherent in the authoritative approach. Authoritarian adults rely on the frequent use of threats and scolding, are overly hasty in contacting other authorities (e.g., administrators, parents, police), and employ whatever punitive techniques are available in asserting their power and attempting to control student behavior.

In contrast, authoritative educators refrain from resorting to those techniques, using them sparingly and only after multiple preventive techniques, more positive techniques, and mildly punitive techniques have failed. However, authoritative educators are no pushovers: they clearly expect and demand appropriate behavior. In correcting misbehavior, they may give offenders a firm but not emotionally intense "lecture" that explains the social and moral inappropriateness of the students' behavior, prescribes better choices, and invokes fair and logical consequences that include types of punishment ranging from removing privileges to removing students from the classroom (Brophy, 1996). For certain, authoritative educators use punishment, but when doing so they recognize its many limitations (as discussed in Chapter 1) and use it only in combination with responsiveness.

GENERAL PRINCIPLES
TO GUIDE THE CORRECTION OF BEHAVIOR PROBLEMS

The primary goal of correction should be to reduce the likelihood that the behavior that is corrected will recur in the future—both in the short term and in the long term. Long-term effectiveness is the most challenging goal, and it is their response to this challenge that largely distinguishes authoritative from authoritarian educators. Unlike authoritarian teachers, who ask "What techniques can I use to stop the misbehavior?", authoritative teachers ask: "What techniques can I use to stop the misbehavior now, but also to develop self-discipline and thus help prevent the misbehavior from recurring when adults are no longer present?" They also ask: "How can I manage student misbehavior while also maintaining supportive teacher–student relations and a positive school climate that is not overly controlling?" The answer to both questions is that, in correcting misbehavior, authoritative adults combine common behavioral techniques (e.g., punishment and reinforcement of replacement behaviors) with those techniques—presented in previous chapters—for preventing misbehavior and developing self-discipline. The latter would include emphases on teaching social problem solving and other social and emotional competencies and providing guidance and support during disciplinary encounters. Recommendations for how these and other strategies and techniques might be used during disciplinary encounters to promote self-discipline are presented below as 11 guiding principles.

> **Managing student behavior is a lot easier than teaching students to manage their own behavior.**

1. *View disciplinary encounters as educational opportunities.* Disciplinary encounters should be viewed as opportunities for school officials to help students develop and practice social and emotional competencies related to self-discipline. Most educators understand that students learn to read while reading and learn math while doing math, and that students often make errors in reading and math that require correction. The teachers routinely and constructively correct those errors. Moreover, in fostering maintenance and generalization of reading and math skills outside of the lesson-specific context, effective teachers provide a variety of real-life opportunities for students to continue to learn and practice academic skills successfully. The same should hold true in teaching and developing social and emotional competencies: just as educators praise students for reading books or solving math problems, *correct their errors*, and provide ample practice, so too should they do the same with respect to developing social and emotional skills.

"Errors" in behavior, especially minor acts of misbehavior such as getting out of one's seat, talking without permission, not completing homework, teasing others, and running in the halls, are developmentally normal. Not only do nearly all children exhibit such behavior occasionally, but in the normal classroom teachers should expect about 20% of students to exhibit minor disruptive or off-task behavior, about 8% noncompliance, and about 5% aggression (Myers & Holland, 2000). Even more serious behavior problems (e.g., fighting, skipping school, stealing, cheating) are not abnormal among children and adolescents, especially when exhibited only rarely. Viewing rule violations as developmentally normal, however, does not mean they should go uncorrected. They clearly should be corrected, not only to help students learn the consequences of their behavior and for the desired behaviors to become habitual but also to deter other instances and to maintain order and safety. However, by viewing these behaviors as developmentally normal, educators are reminded that they are teaching children and adolescents, *not* adults. It also reminds them that correction should not be viewed as serving to punish deviant, reprehensible, or pathological behavior (or, worse yet, a deviant, reprehensible, or pathological *person*). In sum, correction should be viewed from the perspective of authoritative *educators* seeking to develop future adults who will be socially and morally responsible, not from the perspective of authoritarian *prosecutors* seeking criminal justice.

From the perspective of education, not criminal justice, it behooves educators to elicit the thoughts and feelings of students, to confront or challenge their thoughts or lack of emotions related to irresponsible behavior (e.g., lack of empathy, guilt), and to provide guidance and support that influences how they might think, feel, and act in the future. This approach includes using disciplinary encounters as opportunities to develop social and emotional competencies (as discussed in Chapter 3), especially those most directly related to the problem behavior being corrected. Those competencies would often serve as alternatives, or replacements, to the problem behaviors, thoughts, and emotions. They would include the five major social and emotional competencies that are commonly highlighted in social and emotional learning programs: self-awareness, self-management (including impulse control and goal setting), social awareness (including taking the perspective of others, empathic concern about others, respect for others), relationship skills (including communication, cooperation, negotiation, peer resistance, resolving interpersonal conflicts, and help seeking), and responsible decision making (including social and moral problem solving and responsibility). Specific techniques for helping develop those competencies during disciplinary encounters are presented in the next chapter.

2. *Be fair—not too lenient and not too harsh.* As discussed in Chapter 5 in the context of prevention, fairness of rules and their consequences—but especially as *perceived* by students—has consistently been shown to be a strong determinant of student behavior, school climate, and school safety (Arum, 2003; Benner et al., 2008; Brand et al., 2003; Gottfredson et al., 1993, 2005; Mayer & Leone, 1999; Welsh, 2000, 2003). If student perceptions of fairness are so important, how might adults communicate fairness? The most obvious answer, supported by the related research, is that the rules must be neither too lenient nor too strict. Punishment for rule violations should "fit the crime." As such, mild punishment is used for minor offenses, with harsher punishment reserved for the most serious infractions. Thus, if one's goal is a positive school climate, then it is important that educators not focus entirely on the *effectiveness* of an intervention (i.e., whether it stops or decreases the misbehavior) but also on its *fairness*, particularly as perceived by students, not the educators. In addition to making sure the punishment fits the crime, the following are suggested during disciplinary encounters to help increase the likelihood that a corrective action will be perceived by students as fair:

- *Be consistent.* Every effort should be made to be consistent in enforcing rules. However, being consistent should not be at the expense of being judicious, as discussed next.

- *Be judicious.* Judicious refers to wise and sensible judgment but also to practical expediency. Both are critical to perceptions of fairness. At times being wise and sensible means *not* being consistent, especially if one views consistency as meaning that the same punishment should always be administered for the same behavior, irrespective of the circumstances involved. For example, for the sake of consistency a principal might expel Kate for bringing a knife in her lunchbox to cut her birthday cake because he or she imposed the same punishment on Rachel, who brought a knife to harm someone. Unfortunately, this and similar cases abound in schools with an authoritarian zero tolerance approach to discipline. In fact, while writing this chapter, a second grader in a public school near my office was suspended for 5 days and faced expulsion for bringing a knife to school to cut her birthday cake. According to the report in the local newspaper, the teacher actually used the knife to slice the cake before sending the girl to the office. The school district officials and state department of education supported the consequences in the name of consistency and expediency, noting that school authorities do not have sufficient time to consider the specific circumstances or the alleged intentions of students. Such practices, while consistent, are unwise. Being consistent *and* wise would result in treating Kate and Rachel differently (and as one might wish one's own child would be treated under the circumstances).

> In being judicious and fair, one is not necessarily consistent in the use of punishment or rewards. Being judicious and fair means using discretion and considering the individual circumstances in a case. Given the same behavior *and* circumstances, consistency should be seen.

- *Ensure that the student who is punished is the one actually responsible for the accused misbehavior.* To do otherwise invites mistrust and causes all students to question the legitimacy of the adult's authority. Perceived moral authority is critical to willing compliance (Arum, 2003). When students deny or question their own responsibility, adults should present evidence supporting their claim. However, students also should be allowed to question or challenge such evidence, where appropriate. Indeed, it is not only fair and ethical, but often legally required that the due process rights of students be respected when the consequences or penalties are harsh, especially in cases of out-of-school suspension or expulsion.

3. *Examine the factors that help explain or contribute to the misbehavior, especially those factors that are most directly related to the misbehavior.* Unquestionably, multiple factors determine behavior, including factors within the student, the school, the classroom, peers, the home, and the community. Any one of those factors, either proximal (e.g., a mismatch between the curriculum and the student's abilities) or distal (e.g., stress at home influencing the student's mood in school), can help explain a student's misbehavior. Typically, it is a combination of factors that is responsible. Some of those factors are more malleable and

easy to change than others. For example, behavioral expectations and the fairness of rules are fairly easy to alter, but poor parenting is not. The purposes of reflecting on factors that might be influencing the student's misbehavior are (1) to gain insight as to why the behavior is occurring and (2) to target those influencing factors that are most directly related to the misbehavior and that hold the greatest promise for change in order to decrease the undesired behavior and replace it with desired behavior. One might refer to this, especially the purpose, as conducting a functional behavioral assessment (FBA). However, this would be appropriate only if an FBA is viewed broadly and not in a narrow manner. Unfortunately, too often an FBA is limited to a narrow focus on observable antecedents and consequences of the target behavior—what is seen in the environment before and after the behavior occurs. To be sure, often behavior is influenced heavily by antecedents and consequences in one's immediate environment, and in those cases it makes perfect sense to try to alter those antecedents and consequences in order to change behavior. By observing the environment in which a behavior occurs, one might see that certain antecedents trigger the behavior and certain consequences reinforce or punish it. Hypotheses about the behavior's function can then be developed that are linked to interventions (Stoiber, 2004).

The most common functions of behavior are positive reinforcement (get attention or a desired object or activity) and negative reinforcement (avoid demands, people, and undesired activities) (Crone & Horner, 2003; Crone, Horner, & Hawken, 2004). What is not seen in an FBA that focuses on observable antecedents and consequences, however, are the multiple additional factors that influence behavior or the thoughts and emotions underlying the observed behavior and its function. For example, other unobserved factors might be that the student simply hates the teacher, peers are encouraging the behavior outside of the classroom, the student did not take prescribed medication or slept too few hours the night before, the parents recently divorced, and so forth. How and what students think

> In emphasizing the importance of observable and alterable environmental factors, it is often said in books on behavior management that *behavior does not occur in a vacuum.* Although certainly true, it is equally true that *students' brains are not vacuums or empty* spaces. Neglecting students' thoughts and emotions when correcting misbehavior is just as irresponsible as neglecting environmental factors.

and will think in the future are important determinants of their present and future behavior. Thus, it is recommended that, although observable environment antecedents and consequences certainly should be reflected upon as possible determinants or contributors of student behavior, those factors should not be the only ones considered. The thoughts and feelings of students should always be considered as influencing factors. This is especially true if one's goal is to teach students that their decisions, choices, and self-regulating skills determine their behavior.

FBAs can be brief and informal, such as simply reflecting upon possible factors that might explain or contribute to the problem behavior, or recording observations of the antecedents, behavior, and consequences. They also can be formal and complex, such as developing a written report based on multiple methods of assessment that include behavioral observations, standardized rating scales, and an interview with the student and teacher.

For most behavior problems, educators should not be overly concerned about matching interventions to results of an FBA or the causes of a behavior. Research suggests that for most common behavior problems in school a formal FBA is of little value in increasing intervention effectiveness. That is, most evidence-based interventions that are appropriate for a given problem behavior—such as physical proximity, verbal warnings, taking away privileges, and reinforcement of appropriate behavior—are just as effective with or without a formal FBA (Gresham, 2004; Gresham et al., 2004; Schill et al., 1998). Formal FBAs should be reserved for more serious and complex behavior problems that are resistant to interventions, as typically found at Tiers 2 and 3 (Gresham, 2004; Gresham et al., 2004).

Nevertheless, whether or not a formal FBA is implemented, and irrespective of the complexity of the problem behavior (and the FBA, if one is conducted), effective classroom managers routinely reflect upon a broad range of factors that influence a student's misbehavior, and such reflection often guides their interventions (Brophy & McCaslin, 1992). The same types of considerations should apply at the schoolwide level. For example, if students who are referred to the office say that their work is too difficult, some consideration should be given to altering the instruction or materials. Likewise, if it is clear that students enjoy being sent to the office to get out of work, some modifications in the teaching, curriculum, or classroom environment should be considered, or the student's class work should be completed in the office (or in an in-school suspension room). If students report that their misbehavior is reinforced by peers, the adult should discuss the problem with the peers. The most common functions of misbehavior and their contributing factors are listed in Form 9.1 (at the end of the chapter). Whether or not a formal FBA takes place, those functions and the contributory factors should be reflected on when considering interventions, and the factors considered most malleable should receive the greatest priority for changing.

4. *Adhere to the principle of minimal sufficiency, where feasible.* This principle, as recommended in Chapter 6 on the use of rewards, refers to using the least amount of external pressure necessary to change behavior. Underlying this principle is the concept that the degree to which students are likely to *perceive* their behavior as determined externally or internally is directly related to the strength of the consequence of their behavior, whether the consequence is punishment or a tangible reward. The stronger the punishment (or reward), the more likely it will be perceived by students as controlling their behavior—and thus potentially harmful to intrinsic motivation and moral development. This perception occurs when students are led to believe that the only or primary reason to behave is to earn external rewards or avoid punishment. There are three other important reasons for following the principle of minimal sufficiency. First, harsher interventions often are no more effective—and sometimes less effective—than milder ones. For example, research has consistently shown that brief periods of time out are just as effective as long periods and that removing students from the classroom for long periods of time often increases, rather than decreases, academic and behavior problems (Kazdin, 1981). In the case of the second-grade girl mentioned earlier who was suspended 5 days for bringing a knife to school to cut her cake, it is extremely unlikely that 5 days of suspension served as a greater deterrent than 1 day.

A second reason for following the principle of minimal sufficiency is that multiple limitations to the use of punishment, as discussed in Chapter 1, are likely to be more pronounced with harsher forms of punishment. For example, in the above case, harsh punishment resulted in retaliation from the child's family (i.e., it contacted the school board and the media) as well as 5 days of lost academic time and likely harmed the teacher–student relationship. The third reason for following the principle of minimal sufficiency is that this is consistent with research on teacher acceptability of interventions. Such research shows that teachers prefer interventions that are positive, of brief duration, and are easy and inexpensive to implement, and that they also understand that more serious offenses require aversive and longer-lasting interventions (see Reimers, Wacker, & Koeppl, 1987). Thus, teachers prefer verbal reasoning (Rósen, Taylor, O'Leary, & Sanderson, 1990), redirection, and positive reinforcement to, alternatively, the use of harsh punishment when correcting most common behavior problems (Martens, Peterson, Witt, & Cirone, 1986).

5. *Recognize that there's a right and wrong time for confrontation and social problem solving.* It is extremely difficult to communicate with students—much less influence their thinking during a disciplinary encounter—when they are overly angry, upset, or depressed. It is unlikely that students will process any message other than "I'm in trouble." During such occasions one should either calm students or wait until they calm themselves before attempting to do anything other than invoke the necessary consequences for a rule violation (e.g., sending a student to the office or in-school suspension, removing a privilege). In some cases, where feasible, one should wait for the student to calm down before even invoking the consequences. At times it simply is not feasible or reasonable to do anything beyond simply invoking the consequences. For example, when a student is disruptive and needs to be removed from the class, the teacher should not be expected to stop teaching the class in order to help guide and support the student in social problem solving. When a student is uncooperative and unwilling to engage in social problem solving, it makes little sense to force it upon the student. Attempts to provide guidance and support should come later when the student has had an opportunity to cool down.

The foregoing advice applies equally to adults. They too should not engage in problem solving with students when they are angry, frustrated, or upset but, rather, should wait until they are calm.

6. *Don't use punishment solely, but always combined with positive techniques.* Among the many limitations of punishment discussed in Chapter 1 is that it typically teaches behaviors that can be performed by a dead person (Winett & Winkler, 1972); that is, instead of teaching students what they *should* do, punishment teaches them only what they *should not do.* To avoid this limitation, when punishment is used, efforts should be made to combine it with other techniques to teach desired behaviors, the intent being to develop replacement thoughts, feelings, and behaviors that the student might use when faced with a similar situation in the future. The choice of techniques should be determined by such considerations as (1) the behavior's severity (e.g., its impact on the learning of others, harm to oneself or others); (2) the student's developmental level; (3) the student's response to previous interventions; (4) the cognitive, emotional, and environmental factors contributing to the behavior; (5) the teacher's competencies in the use of various techniques; and (6) a host of practical

and situational factors (e.g., the immediacy of addressing the problem, the time available to devote to the behavior, the resources available, the student's acceptance of the intervention, school policies).

For sure, it is unreasonable to expect a teacher to stop teaching and engage in a private problem-solving meeting with a student every time a student gets out of a seat, talks without permission, or exhibits similar common behavior problems that often are responsive to mild forms of punishment. Likewise, it would make little sense to focus on developing social and emotional competencies

> **Over the course of disciplinary encounters, it is important to employ the strategy of combining a variety of techniques, where feasible, for developing self-discipline, preventing misbehavior, and correcting misbehavior.**

when it is clear that the student already possesses them—the problem being not one of "can't do" but "won't do." But, regardless of whether it is a can't-do or won't-do problem, it is very unlikely that punishment alone will be equally as effective as a combination of techniques.

7. *Emphasize the impact of the student's behavior on others and additional reasons why the behavior is wrong other than because of the adverse consequences.* In the developmental psychology literature *induction* refers to inducing empathy (and a reasonable amount of empathy-based guilt) during disciplinary encounters by emphasizing the impact of one's behavior *on others* (e.g., "How do you think Stan felt about what you said to him? What made him feel that way? How might you feel if others teased you?"). This approach contrasts with encouraging a student to focus solely on the consequences of the behavior on oneself (e.g., "You lost 10 minutes of recess for saying that"). With induction, the message learned is "When I tease others, they feel badly (even if I don't get caught)" instead of "If I get caught teasing others, *I* will feel badly about losing recess." There is no reason why both messages should not be conveyed, but if one's aim is to foster self-discipline in the absence of fear of external punishment, there is every reason not to focus on what happens only *if* one gets caught. Induction has been shown to be a common technique used by authoritative parents to foster internalization of the values of caring and concern about others and a sense of responsibility for one's own actions (Eisenberg et al., 2006; Hoffman, 2000). It also is highly recommended in schoolwide discipline programs that focus on caring and responsibility, such as Responsive Classrooms (Charney, 2002) and the Caring Schools Community (Watson & Battistich, 2006).

That one's behavior impacts on others should be the primary reason why the student should not repeat the misbehavior, but often additional reasons should be highlighted. As appropriate for the given disciplinary encounter, which often depends on the nature of the behavior and the time available, multiple reasons for alternative behaviors should be discussed. As presented in Form 10.1 in the next chapter, these reasons might include the impact on one's future, others' perceptions (parents, coach, friends) about the behavior, one's reputation, one's self-concept and moral identity, and class or school norms and desired reputation.

8. *Encourage acceptance of responsibility.* As discussed in Chapter 3, both theory and research show that perceptions of autonomy, self-control, and choice are critical to self-

discipline. The actions of individuals are more likely to be consistent with their own values and beliefs if they attribute those actions to being controlled by themselves rather than by others (Weiner, 2006). The concept of emphasizing responsibility and choice during disciplinary encounters is certainly not new. William Glasser posited this emphasis in his models of discipline, including reality therapy (Glasser, 1969), control theory (Glasser, 1986), and the Quality School (Glasser, 1998). Glasser believed that students choose to behave or misbehave, and thus they should assume responsibility for their actions, including any resulting negative consequences. Glasser clearly understood that a host of individual and environmental factors influence student misbehavior, but he maintained that misbehavior almost always reflects a personal choice (a common exception, however, occurs in many impulsive actions): students *choose* to tell the truth or lie, to respect or not respect the rights of others, to follow or not follow rules, to bully others, and so forth. He also recognized that, while students must accept responsibility for their behavior and make a commitment to change it, schools have a moral and social responsibility to help students develop social and emotional competencies that will lead them to make the right choices.

Disciplinary encounters present an excellent opportunity for students to learn that their own decision making and choices basically determine their behavior or conduct. Although clearly related to the above recommendation, this recommendation is different in an important way. It means that, in addition to highlighting reasons why a behavior is wrong, educators must encourage students to understand that *they are ultimately responsible for their own behavior*—that they have constant choices with respect to their behavior and that their choices affect others' well-being.

9. *Tactfully challenge students' denials and excuses used to avoid responsibility.* It is not uncommon for students (as well as adults) to try to avoid responsibility when they do something wrong by either denying what they did or admitting they did it while giving excuses for doing so. Denying their actions with the deliberate intention of deceiving others is simply lying. Nearly all children have lied occasionally, primarily to avoid punishment or to gain a reward. Among about 5% of boys and 2% of girls, lying is a persistent and serious problem (Hughes & Hill, 2006). In addition to lying to avoid punishment or to gain a reward, lying is often effective to allowing students (and adults) to escape feelings of responsibility (i.e., guilt) by convincing others (and themselves) that although they committed the wrongful act they were either not responsible or not deserving of punishment because they have a good excuse. Such excuses have been referred to as cognitive distortions (Gibbs, Potter, & Goldstein, 1995), faulty logic and biased perceptions (Dreikus & Grey, 1968), and mechanisms of moral disengagement (Bandura, 2002; Bandura, Caprara, Barbaranelli, Pastorelli, & Regalia, 2001). They serve not only to avoid punishment but also to protect one's self-esteem ("See, I'm not a bad person, because it wasn't my fault").

> **It is only natural for students to give excuses for their misbehavior; however, when they deflect responsibility for their own actions, those excuses should not go unchallenged.**

Although nearly all students (and adults) use them occasionally, denial and excuses have been shown to be most common among juvenile delinquents (Barriga, Landau, Stinson, Liau, & Gibbs, 2000). Indeed, denials and excuses, or mechanisms of moral disengagement, explain why many good people do bad things—not just students but nearly everyone (Bandura, 2002; Bandura et al., 2001), including even teachers and leaders in the highest offices. Several of the mechanisms of moral disengagement identified by Bandura certainly apply to students when they violate classroom and school rules. They are not always expressed verbally, although often they are. Those mechanisms are (1) moral or social justification, (2) euphemisms and convoluted language, (3) exonerative or advantageous comparison, (4) blaming as well as displacement and diffusion of responsibility (note that Bandura separates blaming from displacement and diffusion, but they are combined here since their differences are subtle and not important in the context of correction).

- *"I had a good reason!" (moral or social justification).* Students justify to themselves, and try to justify to others (especially the ones likely to impose punishment), that their behavior was the right thing to do. Common examples are "I had a good reason, "He deserved it," But I meant well," and "I didn't mean for that to happen."
- *"I was just kidding" (euphemisms and convoluted language).* "Convoluted and sanitizing verbiage" (Bandura, 1991, p. 67) is often used by students to convince others, and themselves, that their irresponsible behavior was not intentional. Common examples are "I was just kidding," "It was just clowning around," "I was just joking," "It was just horseplay," and "I didn't know."
- *"It wasn't that bad" (exonerative or advantageous comparison).* Here, students lessen or deflect assumptions of responsibility by comparing their behavior with the (worse) behavior of others or by arguing that their behavior wasn't really that bad and certainly not deserving of the punishment that is likely to be rendered. Common examples include "But others were worse," "Did you see what others did—why aren't they punished?," and "I can't believe I'm being punished just for that."
- *"It wasn't my fault" (blaming, and displacement and diffusion of responsibility).* It's easy to deny responsibility when you think others are to blame for what happened or for your actions or that your behavior was beyond your control. Common examples are "It wasn't my fault, she made me do it," "If she hadn't said that, I wouldn't have hit her," "You didn't say we couldn't do it," and "I didn't take my meds this morning." This gambit also would include blaming "a stupid rule" or the person enforcing it.

Typically, when denials and various excuses are employed, they are not used alone but in combination. That is, if denial does not work (e.g., the student sees there is too much evidence showing that he or she really *did* do it), students try various excuses. When such denials and excuses go unchallenged and are effective in avoiding punishment and feelings of guilt-based responsibility, they are negatively reinforced. Thus, students learn that those mechanisms are effective and use them again and again. It is difficult to develop a sense of social and moral responsibility among students when they rarely attribute their misbehavior to themselves. To prevent this misattribution from playing out, denials and excuses should be challenged or tactfully confronted during disciplinary encounters. Such challenging should not be done in an interrogative or authoritarian manner but, rather, in an authoritative way—one that strives to maintain the adult–student relationship while holding students accountable for their behavior.

10. *Encourage students to accept the consequences of their misbehavior and to repair any harm on others or in the relationship with others.* In assuming responsibility for misbehavior, one admits making a mistake and accepts the fair consequences, but also seeks to "fix" the mistake or solve the problem. Depending on the context, fixing the problem may entail repairing something that is physically broken (or buying a replacement), doing something one was supposed to do (e.g., completing an assignment or homework), or apologizing and attempting to repair any emotional harm done to another person as well as to regain that person's trust and respect. However, although adults might force students to apologize, they cannot force them to mean it. As one 10-year-old made very clear to me when I confronted him for teasing a classmate he strongly disliked, "You can make me say I'm sorry, but I won't mean it." This was a valuable lesson to me. It's wise to explain why an apology might help and why one should apologize (and to express your disappointment if the student chooses not to), but it makes little sense to force an apology if the student really does not mean it.

11. *Be demanding but also supportive and guiding in teacher–student relationships.* In demanding appropriate behavior, high expectations are made clear, fair consequences are invoked, and denials and excuses are confronted. All of this should occur in the context of support and guidance and in the context of education, not criminal justice. The demanding part is the easiest: almost all educators can assert their authority and invoke punishment. Doing so takes little training, as is suggested in the brief training of prison guards as compared to teachers. Likewise, educators can make their expectations clear regarding future behavior—and they should do so. The bigger challenge to educators is practicing both dimensions of authoritative discipline—being demanding while also providing the support and guidance needed to help students choose and exhibit more desirable behavior in the future. There are two key interrelated elements of effective support and guidance: relationship skills and process skills. The relationship skills are discussed here, while the process skills, consisting of the social problem-solving steps used during correction in which demandingness is combined with guidance and support, are discussed in the next chapter.

The importance of a strong teacher–student relationship was emphasized in previous chapters in the contexts of both preventing problem behaviors and developing self-discipline. The relationship is equally important in correcting misbehavior, especially if school officials' aim is not simply to invoke punishment but instead to decrease the likelihood that the same behavior will recur in the future. As noted earlier in this chapter, students are more likely to accept punishment from—and to respect, like, and listen to—those educators whom they view as demanding but also as fair and caring (Wubbels et al., 1999).

When correction of behavior occurs by the classroom teacher, and other adults are not involved, it is critical that the teacher exhibit both relationship and process skills. When multiple adults are involved, such as when a student is sent to the office by the classroom teacher and the principal suspends the student, one would hope that all adults involved exhibit the requisite skills. However, when this is not feasible, such as when the administrator has not developed a positive relationship with the student, some other adult should provide the necessary support and guidance. This should be the student's classroom teacher, but also might be another adult in the building, such as the guidance counselor, intervention specialist, or school psychologist. The importance of having at least one adult with whom the student has bonded is critical to student engagement in school (Osterman, 2000).

How might respect, guidance, and support be communicated during a disciplinary encounter? In addition to the recommendations above, especially those pertaining to fairness and emphasizing student responsibility, the following are suggested:

- Emphasize that it is an adult's responsibility in school to hold high behavioral expectations and that, although adults have to enforce the rules, they take no special pleasure in having to do so. Both the high expectations and the fair enforcement of rules are for the welfare of all students, including this one.
- Convey disappointment in the behavior of the student but also optimism that his or her behavior will improve. Point out that the same behavior is not always exhibited and that you trust that it will be exhibited much less, if at all, in the future. When feasible, point out the particular strengths of the student and how they might be used to help prevent the behavior's recurrence.
- Treat each student with dignity. Do not criticize the student per se but only his or her behavior. Saying "You are a bad person" is very different from saying "What you did was bad." In addition to protecting the student's sense of self-worth, respect the student's needs for autonomy and social belonging.
- Be firm, calm, and patient. Do not yell or argue, or humiliate and denigrate the student. Modeling aggression (physical or verbal) is hypocritical and should be avoided. The same advice applies to public humiliation, such as when reprimanding the student loudly in front of peers. Whenever feasible, handle major disciplinary problems privately. Be patient, especially if multiple factors are contributing to the misbehavior. It takes a long time to develop self-discipline.
- Save the lectures for special occasions! Although an occasional lecture about the misbehavior does little harm, and often conveys the message that the misbehavior is truly serious, students are likely to tune out those who give frequent lectures.
- Emphasize that you are trying to help students and are determined to see them succeed in improving their behavior. For example, you might say: "You remember how hard both of us worked in order for you to learn fractions. Well, we're going to work just as hard with you as you learn to control your anger when someone says or does something you don't like."
- Be sensitive to cultural and racial differences. This is a tough and complex issue with respect to the correction of misbehavior. Unquestionably, it is unfair, unjust, and discriminatory to treat any cultural or racial group differently based on culture or race alone. It is also clear, however, that high behavioral expectations and enforcement of

rules are critical elements of effective schoolwide discipline, as discussed previously. In many schools, consistency and high expectations are likely to result in a disproportionate percentage of students from certain cultural or racial groups being corrected for problem behaviors when factors related to those problem behaviors (e.g., poverty, frequent moving, poor parenting, and poor role models in the community) are more common among those groups than other groups in the same school who are subject to less correction. However, those factors do not fully account for the disproportionality. It is important for school officials to reflect on all factors that contribute to the problem behavior and disproportionality and to seek to minimize any biases or prejudices among educators.

With respect to techniques for correcting problem behavior, there is very little research showing that any particular style or technique of correction is more effective with one cultural or racial group than another (Gregory et al., in press; Kauffman, Conroy, Gardner, & Oswald, 2008). Research that does exist suggests that an authoritarian style might be more culturally appropriate for African American and Asian students, especially those living in poverty (Baumrind, 1996; Gonzales, Cauce, Friedman, & Mason, 1996; Kelley, Power, & Winbush, 1992). The implications are disturbing, however: Should schools therefore monitor and punish those students more? Fortunately, a larger number of studies show that the authoritative approach, characterized by demandingness and support, is best for everyone (Gorman-Smith, Tolan, & Henry, 2000; Gregory et al., in press; Mandara & Murray, 2002; Shumow, Vandell, & Posner, 1999; Taylor, Hinton, & Wilson, 1995).

SUMMARY

In correcting behavior problems, authoritarian adults use a combination of behavioral techniques, especially various forms of punishment, with the goal of managing and controlling student behavior, as seen in student compliance with rules and adult authority. In contrast, authoritative adults achieve the important outcome of short-term compliance—but much more. Like authoritarian adults, authoritative adults are demanding, but they also are very responsive to the psychological needs of students, as seen in the warmth, support, and guidance they provide when correcting behavior problems. In blending demandingness and responsiveness, authoritative adults foster the development of self-discipline. This chapter presented 11 general recommendations for schools to follow for applying the authoritative approach to correction. The more specific authoritative strategies and techniques to use during discipline encounters are presented in the next chapter.

Checklist of the Most Common Functions of Misbehavior and Factors That Contribute to Misbehior

Check the functions of misbehavior and other contributing factors that might help explain the student's behavior problem that you are targeting for intervention.

____ To gain adult attention

____ To gain peer attention (including responding to peer encouragement and peer pressure)

____ To get to do what he or she wants (e.g., seeking tangible rewards, preferred activities)

____ To avoid an activity that is too difficult or frustrating

____ To avoid work or a task that isn't necessarily too difficult, but one the student simply wishes not to complete

____ To avoid others

    ____ Dislikes the teacher or specific other adults in the school

    ____ Dislikes peer(s)

    ____ Is teased/bullied

____ To communicate one's feelings, thoughts, and needs

____ To express one's autonomy or self

____ To exert power or control over others

____ To help others

____ To seek justice (e.g., to protest what is perceived as an act of unfairness)

____ To seek revenge or retaliation

Other Common Factors That Contribute to Problem Behaviors
Individual Student Factors

____ Attention problems

____ Impulsivity, hyperactivity

____ Interfering emotions (e.g., anxiety, depression, anger, loneliness)

____ Lack of academic skills

____ Lack of motivation (knows what to do and can do it, but chooses not to or is not motivated to do so)

____ Negative perceptions toward the school and teachers

____ Deficits in social and emotional learning and social problem-solving skills:

    ____ Lack of knowledge (does not know the rule or desired behavior)

    ____ Lack of social or prosocial skills (knows what to do but does not have the skills to do it)

    ____ Lack of desired alternative solutions

    ____ Lack of emotion regulation

(cont.)

Checklist of the Most Common Functions of Misbehavior and Factors That Contribue to Misbehavior *(page 2 of 2)*

____ Difficulty in resisting peer pressure or encouragement

____ Fails to consider or respect perspectives of others; is self-centered, concerned only or primarily with him- or herself

____ Lacks self-confidence or self-efficacy. Thinks poorly of him or herself or his or her ability to exhibit desired behaviors.

____ Refuses to accept responsibility for his or her own actions

Classroom and School Factors

____ Lack of resources and supports (in classrooms, the school, and/or the community)

____ Instruction and curriculum lacking in motivation and effectiveness

____ Mismatch between the student's skill level and academic expectations (too much is expected of him or her)

____ Lack of sufficient monitoring and supervision of behavior

____ Poor classroom and schoolwide management of behavior

____ Unclear, unfair, or inconsistent schoolwide discipline (policies, expectations, practices, etc.)

____ Negative school climate and "sense of community"

____ Lack of caring and supportive adult–student relations

____ Unpleasant physical and learning environment (e.g., overcrowding, poor facilities)

____ Lack of close home–school communications and collaboration

____ Lack of training, ongoing staff development, and supervision

____ Programs not evidence-based

____ Lack of administrative leadership and supervision

____ Lack of planning and evaluation

Peer Factors

____ Role models of aggression, noncompliance, lack of motivation, and other undesirable behaviors and attitudes

____ Lack of friendships

____ Peer rejection or nonacceptance

____ Bullying and peer conflicts

Home and Community Factors

____ Lack of parental support (e.g., no help with homework, noninvolvement in school, dislike of school)

____ Nonsupportive relations with siblings and others

____ Stressors at home and in the community

____ Role models that do not foster learning or social and emotional competencies

____ Lack of community resources (e.g., after-school programs, mentors, etc.)

CHAPTER 10

Developing Self-Discipline
When Correcting Misbehavior

The goal of this chapter is to demonstrate how the general guiding principles of authoritative discipline presented in the preceding chapter on correcting behavior problems can be applied during disciplinary encounters. When applying those principles, the primary goals of educators are twofold: to reduce the recurrence of behavior problems and to develop self-discipline. For purposes of this chapter, a *disciplinary encounter* refers to a situation in which an adult corrects one or more students for either violating school rules or otherwise exhibiting behavior deemed inappropriate by school authorities. Correction is necessary when students fail to exhibit self-discipline, and the preventive techniques in Chapter 5 were either not used, ineffective, or inappropriate (i.e., due to either the behavior's severity, such as a fight, or the behavior's recurrent nature).

Several types of behavior tend to warrant more than routine techniques of classroom management (Epstein et al., 2008, p. 15):

- Behavior that interferes with teaching (or other responsibilities of school or with learning
- Behavior that harms classroom climate or school climate
- Behavior that is significantly deviant and developmentally inappropriate
- Behavior that causes others to avoid or reject the student
- Behavior that threatens the safety of others
- Behavior that typically is not much of a problem but becomes problematic because it persists or becomes contagious (i.e., spreads to others)

When these types of behavior occur, some form of punishment is usually rendered, ranging from a verbal reprimand to suspension or removal from school. Punishment is the easy, albeit often necessary, part to correction. The more challenging part of correction is using disciplinary encounters as educational opportunities to identify and target for intervention those factors within students and their environments that contribute to their problem behavior. This intervention is necessary to achieve the goals of both reducing the behavior problem and developing self-discipline. To take full advantage of disciplinary encounters as educational opportunities and achieve these two goals, it is important that both the student *and* the adult(s) who is(are) correcting the misbehavior play active and reflective roles during the corrective process. This joint involvement is achieved in the context of a two-part social problem-solving process presented in this chapter. The two parts are *student problem solving* and *school problem solving*. Both parts are guided by the principles for correction presented in the preceding chapter.

Part 1, student problem solving, occurs in the context of the actual disciplinary encounter. A private problem-solving meeting is held with the student and a member of the school staff who is responsible for handling the disciplinary infraction. The school staff member might be the student's classroom teacher, an administrator, or a member of the support staff in an office to which the student is sent, or an intervention specialist in charge of in-school suspension. During the problem-solving meeting the adult guides students to reflect on their problem behavior (e.g., why it was wrong, what contributed to it, why the student was responsible for any negative outcomes) and to determine how they will respond differently when faced with similar problem situations in the future. A *student reflective action plan* is developed, either verbally or in writing.

While Part 1 of the problem-solving process focuses on how the *student* might think and act differently, Part 2 focuses on what the *teacher or school* should do, beyond punishment, to prevent the behavior problem from recurring and to foster self-discipline. Part

> It helps to think of correction as having two parts: student problem solving and school problem solving.

2 entails implementing techniques and practices that are both demanding and responsive to the student's needs, which includes supporting the individual student's reflective action plan under Part 1 but also making changes in the classroom or school environment, as needed. These changes, which likely affect not only the student being corrected but other students in the school, include changes in classroom management, school policies, schoolwide monitoring, teacher–student relationships, home communications, peer relationships, and providing additional supports beyond those specific to the individual student's reflective action plan.

PROBLEM SOLVING DURING CORRECTION: PART 1. THE PROBLEM-SOLVING MEETING AND REFLECTIVE ACTION PLAN

The Problem-Solving Meeting

The problem-solving meeting with the student has three primary goals: (1) to encourage reasoning and behavior that is not centered solely on punishment and rewards; (2) to encourage responsibility for one's choices and behaviors; and (3) to encourage the valuing of relationships with others. Regarding the first goal, in order to promote the development of self-discipline during disciplinary encounters students must be challenged to reflect upon their behavior and its consequences not only to oneself but especially to others. That is, they should learn something other than "next time don't get caught or you'll get punished" and "be good to get rewards." They should learn there are good reasons not to misbehave even when one doesn't get caught or is not rewarded for being "good." As emphasized in Chapter 9, students also need to be encouraged to act in a manner consistent with those reasons when faced with similar situations in the future.

Regarding the second goal, if the school truly values responsibility as part of self-discipline, students should learn to *assume* responsibility, or at least share responsibility, for their actions. That is, they should learn that, while the school environment (including rewards, punishments, teachers, and peers) certainly *influences* their behavior, it does not *determine* their behavior.

> **One's greatest aim when correcting misbehavior should be developing responsibility for one's own behavior, or self-discipline. This is not done by simply teaching students "don't get caught next time" or "if you're good, someone might give you a reward."**

Students should learn that, although multiple factors influence their behavior, they almost always have a choice about their behavior and are responsible for that choice. Their own responsibility includes learning how to influence those factors, such as negotiating with or avoiding certain peers and complying with adult requests. Moreover, it includes learning and accepting the consequences of their choices and behavior, both good and bad. Finally, addressing the third goal, if supportive and caring relationships are valued not only for promoting a positive school climate but also for helping to instill self-discipline, students should learn that it is important to maintain such relationships. Doing so entails "fixing" interpersonal problems, which often includes repairing harm done to relationships with others, either peers or adults, and exhibiting prosocial behaviors.

These three goals lead to four action steps during the meeting.

Step 1: Identify the Problem Behavior and Explore Why It Occurred

It should be clear to students why they are being corrected, whether for a violation of a specific school rule or a behavior that otherwise harms others or is deemed inappropriate by school authorities. When applicable, supporting evidence should be presented (e.g., "Here's what I saw," "Here's what _____ [teacher, peer] reported to me," or "Here's what I know happened"), but the student's perspective also should be solicited regarding what happened and *why*. For example, the adult might ask some of the following questions:

- "Is my account of the event correct? If not, what do you think happened?"
- "Help me understand why this incident occurred?"
- "What led up to the problem?"
- "What were you thinking or feeling when the incident occurred?"
- "Why were you thinking and feeling that way?"
- "What was your goal or intention? Was there something you wanted, wanted to do, or something you didn't want to do?"

To be sure, the adult should begin thinking about multiple factors that might have contributed to the problem behavior, but at this point the focus should be limited to those factors that the adult might address and share with the student specific to the problem situation (e.g., "I'll speak to Carol and Latoya about their teasing, but let's talk now about how you responded to it."). Environmental factors that contributed to the problem—especially those that are subject to change by the school but outside of the student's control—are addressed during Part 2 of the problem-solving process.

Step 2: Discuss Why the Behavior Is Indeed a Problem

Upon identifying the problem and soliciting the student's perspective, the dialogue should quickly turn to why the behavior is wrong, that is, why one should not do what he or she did. Avoid the simple and common reasons "because it's against the rules" or because "I said so" unless the rationales underlying the reasons also are spelled out. It is quite likely that the student already knows the rule and understands that adults do not desire the behavior.

First, the consequence or punishment of the behavior, if any, should be invoked and discussed. As noted in Chapter 5, rules should be grounded in basic constitutional rights or the need and legal right of school officials to maintain a safe and orderly environment that is conducive to academic, social, and emotional learning. During disciplinary encounters, and where appropriate, students should be reminded that the punishment meted out does not reflect an arbitrary exercise of power but rather an educator's duty and responsibility to enforce rules. The reasons for rules and enforcing them should be discussed (e.g., "Why do think we have a rule against what you did and the consequence of 2 hours of in-school suspension?"). Depending on the behavior, those reasons might include safety and order, respect for the rights of others, respect for authority, maintaining a positive school climate, and deterring others from similar misbehavior. It also should be emphasized that consequences are a part of learning and must be invoked when students choose not to regulate their own behavior or when they make poor choices.

Next, additional reasons why the behavior presents a problem, or why it is wrong, should be discussed while highlighting the impact of the behavior on the student and others. Form 10.1 (at the end of the chapter) presents various "tests" that might be used to help guide this discussion during dialoguing. The student might respond to the questions in writing before the meeting and/or verbally during the meeting.

Step 3: Encourage Responsibility for One's Actions, Including Accepting Consequences and "Fixing" the Problem, Where Appropriate

Responsibility should be inculcated not only with respect to the students' choices, their behavior, and their acceptance of the consequences of poor choices and inappropriate behavior but also with respect to fixing or correcting their mistakes. Once the punishment is explained and the reasons why the behavior is a problem are discussed, attention should quickly turn to how the student might repair any harm done to others, including any damage to interpersonal relations. An appeal to a sense of integrity and honor often helps (e.g., "I believe you usually mean well, but you made a mistake this time. Other than accepting the consequences, what is the responsible or honorable thing to do now to fix the problem and make Felicia feel better or view you more favorably?").

> **Responsibility often includes not only accepting the consequences, but fixing the problems. It also includes actions to prevent the problem from recurring.**

Fixing the problem may entail repairing something that is physically broken (or buying a replacement), doing something one was supposed to do but did not (e.g., completing an assignment or homework), or apologizing in an attempt to repair any emotional harm to another person or to regain that person's trust and respect. As noted earlier, while adults can force a student to apologize, they cannot force the student to mean it, and therefore it makes little sense to require an apology if the student really does not mean it. It's wise, however, to explain why an apology might help and why the student should apologize. It also often helps to express your disappointment if the student chooses not to apologize and to express optimism that the student will eventually reconsider and seek to restore the broken relationship, which applies to apologies to both peers and adults.

Step 4: Help the Student Determine How to Avoid Repeating the Behavior

During this final step, the student is guided to generate, evaluate, and choose appropriate alternative behaviors to the misbehavior for which he or she is being corrected. Although often referred to as *replacement behaviors*, the replacement "behaviors" should also include alternative ways of thinking, or replacement ways of thinking *and* feeling. This is especially true if certain thoughts and feelings—or the lack thereof—are associated with the misbehavior, including a self-centered perspective of seeking rewards and avoiding punishment (e.g., "I wanted what he had and didn't think I would get caught"), a lack of empathy (e.g., "I wasn't thinking about how he would feel" or "I don't care how others feel"), or the lack of social problem-solving skills (e.g., a failure to think of alternatives or a hostile attribution bias). Where appropriate, those and other social cognitive and emotional deficits and deficiencies commonly associated with aggression and antisocial behavior should be addressed during this step. The following common social problem-solving steps would be used to guide both alternative behaviors and thoughts:

- *Generate alternative solutions.* For example, ask: "The next time you're in the same situation, or the same problem behavior might occur, what are some things you might think and do that might help avoid getting into trouble?" "What do others do in similar situations that you *should* do?"

- *Evaluate each solution.* As each solution is generated, it should be evaluated, particularly with respect to whether or not the solution is (1) morally and socially responsible and (2) likely to work. To assist in reflecting upon the first criterion, the 12 tests in Form 10.1 should be used, as appropriate, with greatest emphasis on the solution's impact on others. Evaluating whether each solution will work should be tied to moral and social criteria linked to personal goals and the likely outcomes of each solution.

- *Choose the best solution(s) and commit to it.* Students should be asked to choose what they consider the best solutions and commit to trying them. Where appropriate (unlikely to be the case with many adolescents), students should be asked to role-play the situation, exhibiting the desired thinking skills and actions. Students also should consider what others might do to help them succeed with the solutions they choose, which helps set the stage for Part 2 of the process, in which adults reflect upon what they can do.

Finally, a sense of self-efficacy, which refers to students believing that they will be able to avoid the problem in the future by thinking and acting differently, should be strongly encouraged. This aim can be accomplished by making sure students have the necessary skills, with the adults voicing optimism that they will succeed, giving examples of valued others who improved their behavior, and noting occasions in the past when the students exhibited the desired behavior.

The Reflective Action Plan

Form 10.2 (at the end of the chapter) presents a reflective action plan that students might complete either immediately before or during the problem-solving meeting. It can be completed either orally or in writing. For students who are unable to read the items or write responses, the questions could be read aloud by the adult and the responses recorded. It is recommended that the plan *not* be completed when students are overly angry or noncompliant.

If completed during the problem-solving meeting, the reflective action plan would be developed either during Step 4 or at a time soon thereafter. Steps of the plan should align with the four steps above, as seen in Form 10.2. Defining the behavior should refer to both the undesired behavior to be reduced and the desired behavior to replace it. Both behaviors should be sufficiently clear and concise such that both the student and the adult agree as to what those behaviors are and so that one or both can easily record when the behavior occurs, if needed.

Where appropriate, the reflective action plan can easily be converted to a more traditional written behavioral contract in which behavior is to be recorded and the consequences (positive and punitive) are specified (see Anderson, 2002). If the behavior is to be recorded, this commitment should be spelled out as to when, where, how, and by whom. Both the starting and renegotiation dates would be included. When appropriate (i.e., given the student's age and following the principle of minimal sufficiency), the commitment would include the use of any external rewards contingent upon improved behavior.

SELF-MANAGEMENT TECHNIQUES

As part of the reflective action plan, or in addition to it, educators should consider employing one or more of six common types of self-management techniques, specifically, goal setting, self-instruction, self-recording, self-evaluation, self-reinforcement, and/or self-punishment (Alberto & Troutman, 2006).

In *goal setting*, students set their own goals rather than relying on adults to do it for them. This technique can easily be incorporated into the reflective action plan by asking the student, "What is a good (i.e., realistic and doable) goal for you to set in improving [the specific behavior]?" In *self-instruction*, students verbally instruct or guide themselves on how to think, act, or feel. For example, following cues taped to her desk, Madison reminds herself to pay attention to the teacher and to raise her hand before talking. Or, while talking to herself, she prompts herself through social problem-solving or anger control steps such as: "OK, what is the problem? First, I need to calm down and think. What are some solutions? Which one is the best? Can I do it? I feel confident I can."

Self-recording refers to simply recording one's own behavior. For example, a student might record on an index card or chart (taped to the desk or carried with the student) each time the target behavior occurs. Self-recording alone has been shown to be associated with improvements in behavior (Shapiro & Cole, 1994). In *self-evaluation*, the student monitors his or her behavior and judges or evaluates it (e.g., "I followed the problem steps and correctly, and they worked"). Although self-recording is not required for self-monitoring and self-evaluation, it often increases the accuracy of self-evaluation (Alberto & Troutman, 2006). Self-evaluation is used in the reflective action plan when students are asked to respond to each of the 12 tests for guiding behavior and decision making.

Self-reinforcement consists of rewarding oneself with positive statements (e.g., "I'm doing a great job"), material rewards, or preferred activities contingent upon one's own actions. In contrast, *self-punishment* consists of self-imposing negative consequences (e.g., taking away a privilege, self-criticizing). When used, self-reinforcement or self-punishment should follow self-evaluation. For those two techniques to be most effective, the self-evaluation should be correct (O'Leary & O'Leary, 1977); that is, the students judge their behavior to be appropriate, and it actually is. To enhance correct self-evaluation, the teacher, or other adult or peer, should check the accuracy of the self-evaluation by comparing his or her evaluation with that of the student (Peterson, Young, Salzberg, West, & Hill, 2006; Shapiro, Durnan, Post, & Levinson, 2002). Correct self-evaluation is important because, if students fail to evaluate their behavior correctly, they are likely to reinforce their behavior inappropriately (e.g., reinforcing themselves although their behavior failed to meet an acceptable criterion).

Typically, these self-management techniques are used in combination with one another. For example, Shauib might set a goal of being tardy for class only once per week (as compared to the current three to five times). He then self-records each time he is late for class by marking on an index card whether he is late each day of the week, self-evaluates the record against a specific criterion ("I was on time 4 of 5 days, or 80% of the time, which is much better than the 60% I exhibited before self-recording"), and self-reinforces with praise ("I feel good about meeting my criterion of 80%, and it will probably improve my grade") or a reward ("I deserve to buy myself something"). In addition to combining various self-management techniques, educators also should consider combining self-management techniques with external techniques when self-management techniques alone are not sufficient, as part of a multicomponent intervention.

Advantages

There are three good reasons for using self-management techniques. First, they are evidence-based. A large number of studies have found them to be effective in reducing disruptive behavior (see Briesch & Cahfouleas, 2009; Hoff & Sawka-Miller, 2010; Shapiro & Cole, 1994; Shapiro et al., 2002, for reviews). Second, the use of self-management techniques is consistent with the important principle of minimal sufficiency in developing self-discipline, as discussed in Chapters 4 and 9. That is, students are likely to perceive self-management techniques (although they are often externally imposed), as less socially controlling than external techniques, unless they are required and the student does not want to use them. Third, educators generally like self-management techniques, because they often are more practical and convenient than many other behavioral techniques, and their use demonstrates to adults that students are making efforts to improve their own behavior (Shapiro et al., 2002).

Limitations

Self-management techniques do have their limitations, however. Chief among them is that, similar to the use of external behavioral techniques, self-management techniques tend to produce improvements that are short-term or nonlasting. That is, their effects often end when the technique ends, and their effectiveness often typically fails to generalize to other settings, times of day, and behaviors (Ardoin & Martens, 2004; Nelson et al., 1991). Another major limitation is their lack of effectiveness when students are not motivated to change their behavior (Hughes & Lloyd, 1993). Finally, self-management techniques alone are seldom sufficient for students with recurrent behavior problems (Hoff & Sawka-Miller, 2010). Despite these limitations, self-management techniques should be included as part of the action plan for most students, but especially those students motivated to improve their behavior. Although self-management techniques are appropriate for students of all ages, their application always should be adapted to the developmental level of each student.

PROBLEM SOLVING DURING CORRECTION: PART 2. THE SCHOOL'S RESPONSIBILITY

Although Part 2 of the problem-solving process is discussed separately to focus on the responsibility of the teacher or school, this ordering is not meant to suggest that Part 1 is completed before Part 2 begins. Actually the two parts of the process should occur simultaneously or closely together. Part 2 recognizes that the responsibility for student behavior should always be a *shared* responsibility. It should be shared by the student, school officials, the parents, and at times also peers. Thus, the student's teacher and the school staff should demonstrate the same or a comparable commitment as the student to improving his or her behavior. Part 2 of the problem-solving process entails two steps: (1) directly supporting the student in implementing the reflective action plan and (2) reflecting on and altering, as needed, current preventive and corrective policies or practices.

Directly Supporting the Student's Reflective Action Plan

Although multiple adults might be involved, depending on the severity of the behavior and the number of settings in which it occurs, one adult should assume *primary* responsibility for helping the student implement his or her reflective action plan. This individual is likely to be the student's classroom teacher but also might be a member of the school support staff (e.g., school counselor,

> **In Part 2, the onus is not on the student, but on adults. The responsibility for improving student behavior should be shared.**

school psychologist, interventionist, assistant principal), with whom the student checks in or reports to daily or as often as needed. To avoid being perceived as overly controlling, the adult(s) should act as an authoritative educator (rather than a correctional official), challenged with the goal of helping the student to improve his or her behavior, sharing responsibility for the success of the reflective action plan, and providing a balance of support and structure. Responsibilities include:

• *Frequently reminding the student of the reflective action plan, the skills to be developed or exhibited, and his or her commitment to improve.* Depending on the given behavior's severity, this reminding function might consist of direct or indirect prompts or cues in settings where the behavior occurs, ranging from direct verbal reminders to praising others for engaging in the desired behavior. The function might also be part of a self-management intervention in which the adult monitors the accuracy of self-recording and self-evaluation.

• *Modeling the desired social, emotional, and behavioral competencies.* As a direct teaching technique, modeling is most appropriate when it is clear that the student actually lacks the given skill needed (i.e., has a "can't-do" as opposed to "won't-do" problem). In such cases, which are more common in early than in later grades, modeling should be used as the primary method of directly teaching the desired or replacement competencies. However, modeling also is an appropriate way of reminding students of desired skills (e.g., "Jackson, remember: here's what we're looking for. Watch me! See—it's not that difficult, and you know how to do it"). This function would certainly include the modeling of thinking skills by "thinking aloud," such as: "Here's what I would think in this situation. Hmm, I agreed to try really hard to improve my behavior. I don't want to get into trouble again, and it's unfair for others and disruptive to the class to get out of my seat whenever I want to. And I should not expect my teacher to have to always be the one controlling my behavior—I should do it myself." Modeling should be provided directly by the teacher or other adult but also indirectly via peers, where feasible (e.g., placing the student near good role models), and via curriculum materials (e.g., stories that highlight the target behavior).

• *Helping to ensure that the desired competencies, and efforts made to apply them, are reinforced.* This function would include reminding students to self-reinforce but would also include the frequent and strategic use of external praise. It also should include the strategic use of rewards when intrinsic motivation is lacking. As such, the techniques for the strategic use of external praise, presented in Chapter 7, should be applicable to this function.

• *Ongoing monitoring and evaluation of the effectiveness of the student's reflective action plan.* As is true with all other interventions, success depends largely on the degree to which the intervention is implemented with fidelity. One way to help ensure fidelity is by monitoring and evaluating the student's implementation of the reflective action plan. Minimally, this function requires systematic follow-up and feedback on the student's implementation and progress. However, for behaviors that are recurrent and resistant to previous interventions, the responsibility should include actually recording the target behavior and analyzing the data. As noted previously, if self-recording and self-evaluation are used, this function also entails cross-checking with the student on the accuracy of his or her self-assessment techniques—that is, seeing whether the adult's recording and evaluation match those of the student. Whenever improvement in behavior is not satisfactory, changes in the intervention plan should be made, which entails either altering the existing plan or developing a new one.

Altering Current Preventive and Corrective Practices

It is the responsibility of adults in the school to help students succeed in implementing their reflective action plans. Those plans focus on how *students* are to change their behaviors as well as the thoughts and feelings underlying them. It also is the responsibility of *adults* to reflect upon changes in the student's environment, which include adults' *own* behavior, and making efforts to implement those changes, where appropriate. This requirement includes reflecting upon all factors that contribute to the student's problem behavior and targeting those that are subject to change. Common contributing factors were listed in the preceding chapter (see Form 9.1 in Chapter 9), categorized as student, classroom/school, peer, and home/community factors. Those factors should be considered as targets for school-based interventions. The specific factors and the degree to which they should be targeted depend on (1) whether there are evidence-based techniques for changing the target behavior that school officials can either implement or use in facilitating their implementation and (2) whether such techniques are perceived as appropriate by those who are implementing them. Appropriateness is determined by such variables as the student's age, the perceived feasibility of implementing the techniques (e.g., sufficient time, the requisite skills, and adequate resources available to significantly impact the given factor), and the frequency and severity of the problem behavior (problem behaviors that are more frequent and severe tend to justify more demanding interventions). As used here, *appropriateness* incorporates the concept of acceptability. Acceptability is critical because when educators perceive interventions as inappropriate, or unacceptable, they are either unlikely to implement them or to do so with insufficient fidelity for success (Fullan, 2007).

Form 10.3 (at the end of the chapter) presents a comprehensive checklist for educators to use to help determine which intervention techniques should be implemented in light of their acceptability, prior use, past effectiveness, and likely future effectiveness. In judging past effectiveness, educators should consider both the short-term and long-term effectiveness. Short-term effectiveness would be seen as immediate compliance or the cessation or decreased frequency of the behavior when adults are present. Long-term effectiveness would be seen as the same improved behavior over time, even in the absence of close adult supervision and when external rewards and the fear of punishment are not salient considerations.

As emphasized earlier, improving student behavior is a *shared* responsibility. Although the student being corrected and his or her teacher should be the parties primarily responsible, both the student's parents and his or her peers also should provide much needed support, as appropriate for the situation. And if their support is not sufficient, additional sources of support may need to be called upon, as discussed below.

SUPPORT FROM PARENTS AND PEERS

Support from Parents

The extent to which parents should be contacted about the student's misbehavior and be part of any intervention plan depends primarily on the seriousness of the misbehavior. Clearly, parents can be an invaluable source of support and should share responsibility in a student's behavior at school.

> Teachers shouldn't be the only ones providing support to a student with behavior problems. Help also should come from parents, peers, and other staff members.

Often, contacting parents—or warning that one might do so—is an intervention in itself that decreases the misbehavior. However, contacting parents about relatively minor acts of misbehavior that should be responsive to everyday techniques of classroom management is inconsistent with the message that students should regulate their own behavior. If done frequently, this is likely to undermine not only self-discipline, but also the teacher–student relationship, especially among adolescents, who generally greatly value their autonomy. Nevertheless, the student's parents should be contacted, and collaboratively involved in interventions, when problem behaviors are either serious (e.g., stealing, cheating, fighting) or are resistant to routine techniques of classroom management. Home-related techniques of demonstrated effectiveness in improving student behavior include:

- School–home notes and report cards (Riley-Tillman, Chafouleas, & Briesch, 2007)
- Parent–teacher conferences (Minke, 2006)
- Conjoint teacher–parent consultation (Sheridan & Kratochwill, 2008)

Support from Peers

At all ages, peers exert a powerful influence on student behavior. With respect to school discipline, that influence is often viewed as negative, such as in the context of bullying, peer reinforcement of misbehavior, peer pressure, poor role models, and deviant peer groups. Clearly, in those contexts, efforts should be made to curtail the negative effects as a means of supporting the student's action plan, such as by confronting peers directly, holding a peer mediation meeting, or moving the student within the classroom. In the current context of supporting the student's reflection action plan and making changes in the classroom or school environment, peers should be viewed not as a source of the problem but as a potential source of support in improving the student's behavior. Peer-focused actions that might be considered are:

- Hold class discussions that focus on the behavior (though not on the individual student), with the entire class engaging in social and moral problem solving. This alternative would include discussing the impact of the behaviors (desired and undesired) on the class and brainstorming and evaluating solutions. Note, however, that whole-class interventions, based on punishment and rewards for the behavior of an individual (e.g., the entire class is punished for the behavior of one or a few students), are not normally preferred by students (Lovegrove, Lewis, Fall, & Lovegrove, 1985).

- If the behavior problem(s) is schoolwide and not specific to a small number of students or classrooms, the school's student council, or a newly appointed social problem-solving group, should meet to discuss the behavior and to develop possible actions for preventing and correcting it.

- Institute a a "buddy" or peer coaching arrangement in which a same-age or older student serves as a mentor (see Chapter 4).

- Train peers to reinforce the desired behavior. For example, several studies have combined self-monitoring and positive reinforcement with teacher–peer mediated support to successfully improve socially appropriate behavior of at-risk children (Coogan, Kehle, Bray, & Chafouleas, 2007).

When These Solutions Are Not Sufficient

The foregoing strategies and techniques apply to *all* students, including those considered to be at tiers 2 or 3 of intervention due to the severity or chronic nature of their behavior problems, or the risk thereof. For the most part, those strategies and techniques per se are not what distinguish interventions at Tier 1 from those at Tiers 2 and 3 so much as it is the number of interventions, whether they are used in combination, and the intensiveness of their application. For example, at all three tiers the basic techniques of prevention, correction, and developing self-discipline apply, although they may be implemented more frequently and systematically with students at Tiers 2 and 3. The full panoply of options would include the use of praise, rewards, punishment, clear and fair rules and expectations, positive teacher–student relationships, and home–school communications and collaboration; teaching social and emotional competencies and providing ample opportunities to practice them; motivating instruction and curriculum; and close monitoring and supervision. It also would include reflective action plans, altering the classroom and school environments, and garnering support for teachers, parents, and peers.

Some evidence-based interventions, however, are more specific to students with the most serious and chronic problem behaviors, such as parent management training (Kazdin, 2003), family therapy (Valdez, Carlson, & Zanger, 2005), and anger control training (Lochman et al., 2006). Those interventions are generally provided outside of school and would be most appropriate for students whose behavior problems continue to adversely impact their own and others' learning despite the use of school-based evidence-based interventions (Gresham, 2004).

The following features characterize the most effective programs for students with serious problem behaviors (Bear, Webster-Stratton, Furlong, & Rhee, 2000).

- They are *comprehensive* (i.e., they address multiple risk and protective factors).
- They are *broad-based* (i.e., they adopt a "systems" perspective, in which it is understood that schools, families, and community agencies must work together).
- They are *guided by research and theory*.
- They are *intensive and sustained* over time.
- They are *delivered early* (i.e., delivered at an early age, but also when problems first warrant intervention, irrespective of the age of the student).
- They are *individualized* (developmentally and culturally appropriate and based on the student's strengths and needs).

These features describe what is often referred to in the positive behavior support literature as "wraparound" interventions, supports, and services (Burchard, Burns, & Burchard, 2002; Epstein et al., 2005). These interventions, supports, and services are provided by a team of educators, mental health specialists, family members, and others (e.g., social workers, school nurses, school resource officers), as needed. The team generally employs a network of supports and services that extend beyond the school to the home and community.

SUMMARY

At one time or another, nearly all students exhibit some inappropriate behavior, either minor or serious, during school hours that requires correction by a teacher or another school staff member. When these disciplinary encounters occur, they should be viewed as educational opportunities to help students develop self-discipline—not as occasions to simply correct the behavior by using such external techniques as punishing the bad behavior and promising rewards for future good behavior. Guided by the authoritative principles of school discipline presented in the preceding chapter for both correcting misbehavior and developing self-discipline, a two-part process of correction involving both student problem solving and school problem solving was presented in this chapter.

The two-part process emphasizes the need to view correction as a shared responsibility, chiefly between the student and the teacher (or other adult). During the first part, the student problem-solving meeting, the student is encouraged to complete a student reflective plan to help guide his or her social problem solving and decision making. The teacher facilitates the plan by providing dialoguing and scaffolding, but the responsibility for the plan lies primarily with the student. In the second part of the process, school problem solving, the primary responsibility shifts to the teacher. This part of the process is designed for two purposes: first, to enable teachers to provide the supports students need to successfully implement their corrective plan; and second, perhaps more importantly, to challenge teachers to reflect upon changes they might make to help prevent the behavior problem from recurring—including changes in their current teaching practices and relationships with students—as well as obtaining support from the students' parents and peers.

Multiple "Tests" for Guiding Behavior and Decision Making

1. *School Rules Test:* Did my behavior follow all school rules and expectations? Which rule(s) were not followed?	Yes	No	Not sure
2. *Respect for Others Test:* Was my behavior respectful of others, including both students and adults?	Yes	No	Not sure
3. *Impact on Teaching and Learning Test:* Did my behavior help the teacher teach or help me and other students learn?	Yes	No	Not sure
4. *Golden Rule Test:* Would I want others to do the same to me?	Yes	No	Not sure
5. *Fairness test:* Was it fair to do what I did?	Yes	No	Not sure
6. *Current Consequences Test:* Will the consequences of my behavior be good?	Yes	No	Not sure
7. *Future Test:* Will this behavior help me in the future?	Yes	No	Not sure
8. *Parent Perception Test:* Would my parents approve of this behavior?	Yes	No	Not sure
9. *Teacher Perception Test:* If I were a teacher, would I want students to do the same?	Yes	No	Not sure
10. *Guilt or Pride Test:* Should I feel good about what I did?	Yes	No	Not sure
11. *Self-Perception and Self-Identity Test:* Was my behavior consistent with the kind of person I want to be?	Yes	No	Not sure
12. *School Climate Test:* Was my behavior consistent with the kind of school that the school staff and most students desire?	Yes	No	Not sure

Student Reflective Action Plan

This Reflective Action Plan is written to help _____ [student's name] to be responsible for his or her own behavior and not to _____
[the problem behavior].

This is why I did it: _____.

It is understood that there are several good reasons why it is important not to _____
_____ [the problem behavior]. They are:

- The punishment this time is: _____.
- The punishment next time will be: _____.
- What are three more good reasons why this behavior is wrong?
    1. _____
    2. _____
    3. _____

To correct or fix the problem now I will: _____

Instead of doing the same thing next time I will:

Think this: _____

Do this: _____

Please check one of the following:

_____ I need to be taught or shown how to do this.

_____ I already know how to do this.

Other than not getting into trouble again, here's why it is important not to do what I did before and instead do the following:

_____

_____

Here's what others might do to help me:

_____

_____

_____

Checklist to Help Determine Intervention to Be Implemented

On a scale of 1–5, please rate:

1. The *appropriateness* of this intervention for the given problem behavior. In rating each intervention technique, consider the student's age, the severity and frequency of the behavior (generally, demanding techniques are more acceptable for more severe and frequent problem behaviors), and the feasibility of the intervention.
2. The *frequency* with which the technique already *has been used.*
3. The *general effectiveness* of the intervention, if used already, in bringing about *short-term* compliance (i.e., the behavior stops or decreases immediately).
4. The general effectiveness of the intervention, if used already, in bringing about more *long-term improvement* (i.e., the behavior improved and improvements continued to be seen weeks after the intervention was implemented). Leave blank, if not used.
5. The *extent to which the technique should be used* with this student. High ratings should be assigned to those techniques of demonstrated effectiveness (short-term or long-term) and those deemed appropriate and likely to be effective regardless of previous use.

Appropriateness:	1 = Not at all	3 = Somewhat	5 = Very appropriate
Frequency:	1 = Never used	3 = Used sometimes	5 = Used very often
Short-term effectiveness:	1 = Never worked	3 = Worked sometimes	5 = Always worked
Long-term effectiveness:	1 = Not effective	3 = Somewhat effective	5 = Highly effective
Recommended use:	1 = Not recommended	3 = Recommended	5 = Highly recommended

	Appropriateness for this behavior	Extent to which technique has been used	Effectiveness to date for this technique		Recommended use
			Short-term	Long-term	
Preventive/Corrective Techniques					
Praise the student for desired behavior more than criticizing or correcting him or her for undesired behavior.					
Praise other students nearby more for desired behaviors than criticizing or correcting them for undesired behavior.					
Ignore the problem behavior.					
Verbal redirection and foreshadowing (e.g., state the student's name or reminding the student or class what is expected of him or her; remind the student or class of what will be coming soon, such as a transition or a more challenging task).					

(cont.)

Checklist to Help Determine Intervention to Be Implemented

	Appropriateness for this behavior	Extent to which technique has been used	Effectiveness to date for this technique		Recommended use
			Short-term	Long-term	
Verbal warnings (remind the student of behavioral expectations, rules, and consequences).					
Nonverbal redirection (e.g., use eye contact or a facial expression that conveys displeasure; use hand signals or other visual/auditory prompts such as hand claps).					
Reward the student for the desired behavior (other than with praise).					
Physical proximity (stand near the student or circulate around the room and near student(s) prone to problem behavior).					
Deliberately spend time in *positive interactions* with the student (e.g., talking privately to the student at times when no misbehavior is seen while showing a sincere interest in the student's life).					
Frequently monitor the student and respond immediately to signs of misbehavior.					
Review the rules and behavioral expectations with the student and the class. Make sure that they are clear and fair.					
Change the *physical environment* to make it more conducive to learning for the student, less distractible, and more supportive (e.g., move the student's desk, remove distractions, place the student near desired role models).					
Provide *predictable procedures and routines* (and practice them frequently).					
Adjust the curriculum materials and teaching strategies to match the student's ability and achievement level (e.g., so that the student can readily read materials and understand lessons and so that there are no cultural and linguistic barriers).					
Provide instruction and materials that are *motivating* to students (e.g., use variety, novelty, and topics and materials of high interest).					
Provide *supportive student relations* (e.g., situate the student near peers who are good role models, provide greater peer assistance).					

(cont.)

Checklist to Help Determine Intervention to Be Implemented
(page 3 of 3)

	Appropriateness for this behavior	Extent to which technique has been used	Effectiveness to date for this technique		Recommended use
			Short-term	Long-term	
Positive home–school communication (contact parent[s] via phone call, e-mail, or notes about something positive about the student and his or her behavior; this positive feedback may be combined with expression of concern about minor behavior problems).					
Additional Corrective Techniques (needed when the above techniques are not sufficient)					
Privately discuss the problem with the student, including its impact on others, its consequences, and how to "solve the problem" (e.g., use the Reflective Action Plan form).					
Discuss the problem behavior with the class (but not referencing any specific student). This technique is appropriate when the behavior problem is wide-spread.					
Take away privilege(s) (e.g., recess, free time, lunch with others).					
Write out a behavioral contract (i.e., a written agreement that specifies behaviors to improve and their positive and punitive consequences).					
Use a self-management technique (e.g., help the student develop personal goals and monitor, record, evaluate, and reinforce his or her own behavior).					
Use home–school communications and collaboration (e.g., employ home–school notes or weekly report card on behavior, hold a teacher–parent–student conference).					
Remove the student from the class.					
Refer the student to the office or to an interventionist.					
Refer the student to a school team for a consultation or assessment.					
Other—please list:					
Other—please list:					

CHAPTER 11

Implementing Schoolwide Change

> System-level change must be planned and pursued in a systematic manner over time. It does not just happen. Furthermore, it is not an event or activity, but an on-going process that should never end.
> —CURTIS, CASTILLO, AND COHEN (2008, p. 892)

Change is difficult. As noted above, "It does not just happen." It entails an ongoing process that requires considerable reflection and in-depth discussion, commitment, planning, leadership, supports and resources, staff development and training, implementation and institutionalization of new practices, and ongoing evaluation. It requires time, which is a precious commodity in schools, where an ever increasing number of demands and requirements are added to the plates of educators while little is ever removed. True and lasting change requires much more than just "tinkering" (Fullan, 2007), or minor changes in policies and practices that might produce small short-term effects (e.g., reduced office disciplinary referrals) but not more meaningful and long-term changes (e.g., self-discipline and an improved school climate). As Fullan (2007) concluded, upon reviewing the school reform literature: "In summary, simple changes may be easier to carry out, but they may not make much of a difference" (p. 91).

> **True and lasting change requires much more than just "tinkering" (Fullan, 2007).**

TINKERING VERSUS MEANINGFUL CHANGE?

Meaningful change requires that educators question their current knowledge and practices—knowledge and practices that may be correct or incorrect, effective or ineffective. When such questioning results in the determination that change is needed, educators must then commit themselves to *new* (and often unknown) practices, ones usually promised by others to be more effective than the current ones. It is no wonder then that change is often met with resistance, and while many ineffective schools never seriously embark upon systems change others do so only half-heartedly.

Too often school officials jump on the latest schoolwide discipline or mental health "bandwagon" with little reflection and planning. With the usual goal of reducing behavior problems, improving mental health, or improving school safety, they hastily implement simple and easy "fixes." Popular bandwagons in the past have included values clarification (Raths, Harmin, & Simon, 1966), the development approach to moral education (Power, Higgins, & Kohlberg, 1989), the self-esteem movement (California Task Force to Promote Self-Esteem and Personal and Social Responsibility, 1990), and behavior modification using punishment and assertive discipline (Canter, 1976). Today, in response to fears of increasing school violence, many schools have adopted zero tolerance policies, while others have posted behavioral expectations and implemented token economies (and little more) to manage or control student behavior. As argued throughout this book, those techniques may be of value for a specific, limited, and perhaps justified short-term purpose. However, implementing social control techniques is "tinkering," or attempting to provide a quick fix to a complex problem. It is analogous to placing a Band-Aid on a cancerous sore: it covers the problem and looks good, especially to others, but the Band-Aid soon falls off and the cancer remains. Sadly, too often school officials claim that their change efforts are effective in spite of a lack of data or only limited data (e.g., subjective opinions of administrators and staff, reduced office disciplinary referrals). In such cases, their "success" is fleeting, the transparency of the approach or program is soon discovered, and several years later the school begins searching for another easy fix to the complex problem of schoolwide discipline.

This chapter presents recommendations and strategies for system change designed to prevent this outlined scenario from continually recurring in your school. The recommendations are based on both my own personal experiences working with schools in implementing school violence prevention and SWPBS programs (Bear, Blank, & Pell, 2009; Bear, Giancola, Veach, & Goetz, 2006; Giancola & Bear, 2003) and on research on school reform and systems change (e.g., Center for Mental Health in Schools, 2008; Chinman, Imm, & Wandersman, 2004; Curtis et al., 2008; Desimone, 2002; Fullan, 2007; George, White, & Schlaffer, 2007; Knoff, 2008; Sugai & Horner, 2008, 2009). Before presenting recommendations and strategies for change, however, it is important to emphasize that many schools and teachers *are* effective, as reflected in the first recommendation, below.

DON'T CHANGE, OR CHANGE VERY LITTLE, IF YOU'RE ALREADY EFFECTIVE!

Many advocates of school reform, including advocates of SWPBS, strongly imply that *all* schools, and teachers within them, need to change, that is, that they need to change from what they are currently doing to what others think they *should* be doing. For example, the attitude commonly is: "If you're not a SWPBS school or classroom, then you need to be one," or "If other schools in your district are doing it, so should you." The author saw this scenario played out in Delaware over the past decade as the state department of education jumped on the SWPBS bandwagon and embraced the goal of all public schools quickly becoming SWPBS schools. Unlike in Texas, where SWPBS is actually mandated by law, in Delaware the schools were only *encouraged* to adopt SWPBS. Several school districts quickly joined the "positive" bandwagon, with central office administrators informing all schools in their district that they too would join. Consistent with recommended SWPBS practices, preschools to high schools quickly posted behavioral expectations and disseminated tokens schoolwide to students contingent upon their good behavior.

The absurdity of this "one-size-fits-all" statewide initiative became clear (though not to everyone) when the principal and staff of one elementary school protested the district's pressure to adopt SWPBS. In that school, teachers and staff had been trained in an evidence-based SEL program, Responsive Classroom (Brock, Nishida, Chiong, Grimm, & Rimm-Kaurman, 2008; Charney, 2002), which the school had been fully implementing for several years. There was no evidence that the school needed to change its current practices, much less adopt a systematic extrinsic system of rewards that was in conflict with the student-centered philosophy of the Responsive Classroom approach. No evidence was provided by the state or district (and none existed in the research literature) that SWPBS was the more effective of the two approaches or that SWPBS was effective in any way other than in reducing office disciplinary referrals (which wasn't even a major issue of concern at that school). Nevertheless, the school was expected to join all other schools in the district to become a SWPBS school, and thus all teachers were to be trained in functional behavioral assessment, positive reinforcement, and other techniques of applied behavior analysis.

> **It makes little sense to think that the same SWPBS or SEL program is best for every school or needed by every teacher and student.**

This stand-pat recommendation also means that school officials should not require the most effective teachers in their school to change classroom practices when they already are quite effective (and often more effective than those they are being asked to switch to). If one does so, expect resistance—and justifiably so! This mistake is perhaps more common than that of requiring all schools to adopt one particular approach. That is, often it does not seem to matter whether a teacher is experienced or inexperienced, or effective or ineffective, in classroom management and in promoting self-discipline. Instead, often for the sake of schoolwide consistency, *all* teachers are required to complete the same training and to implement the same "new" practices. To be sure, *ineffective* schools and teachers should be encouraged, if not required, to change their existing practices. But, it makes little sense to ask *effective* schools and classroom teachers to replace their existing practices with new ones not yet shown to be any more effective.

DETERMINING THE NEED FOR CHANGE

School officials should not embark upon an extensive school reform effort before first determining and justifying the need to do so. If this is not done, officials may have difficulty persuading key stakeholders that they need to change what they are doing. It also is foolish to try to do so. Unfortunately, however, this scenario plays out too often. When reform is not justified in advance, the result often is resistance, as seen in a lack of commitment to change and the failure to implement the program with fidelity or as its developers intended. Resistance to change is the most common reason for the failure of most school reform efforts (Curtis et al., 2008; Fullan, 2007). To avoid making this mistake, the first step in any change effort relating to schoolwide discipline should be to conduct a strengths-and-needs assessment, which is a systematic process of gathering information to determine the need for change and the specific areas where it is most needed. The assessment should include the identification not only of needs but also of strengths or assets that might be useful in addressing those needs. For this reason, and because many schools should credit themselves for already being effective in addressing at least some areas of schoolwide discipline, the term *strengths-and-needs assessment* is used instead of the more common term *needs assessment*.

A strengths-and-needs assessment should be comprehensive and broad-based, covering the full range of needs related to schoolwide discipline for a school's given population (Doll & Cummings, 2007). Thus, it should include all four components of comprehensive schoolwide discipline: developing self-discipline, preventing behavior problems, correcting behavior problems, and addressing the more challenging needs of students at Tiers 2 and 3.

The responsibility for conducting a strengths-and-needs assessment should be assigned to a schoolwide discipline committee, team, or work group. However, all members of the school staff should participate in its completion and, more importantly, in the analysis of the results. As with all other aspects of systemic change, it is critical that key stakeholders be included or represented on the committee (e.g., the principal, several regular education teachers, a special education teacher, the school psychologist, the school counselor, the school nurse—even parents and students, where appropriate). Three methods should be used in conducting the strengths-and-needs assessment: (1) examine existing schoolwide data; (2) survey the school's strengths and needs, as currently viewed by major stakeholders; and (3) administer additional measures, as needed. Each of these methods is described below.

> **Before adopting a new program or making major changes in an existing one be sure to assess your school's strengths and needs.**

Examine Existing Schoolwide Data

The schoolwide discipline committee should always begin the assessment of the school's strengths and needs by reviewing the data already available. It is important, however, that the data be current, be viewed by major stakeholders as valid and reliable, and be indicators of all four components of comprehensive school discipline. Because all three of these conditions seldom hold true, most committees end up not limiting themselves to existing data but rather collecting additional information and data, such as:

- Number of ODRs
- Suspension rates (in school and out of school)
- Expulsion rates
- Truancy rates
- School completion rates (high school)
- Absenteeism rates (for both the students and staff)
- Achievement scores
- Number and percentage of students referred to the school's student support team (e.g., the instructional support team or student intervention team)
- Number and percentage of students referred for special education and support services (e.g., school counselor, school psychologist, school social worker)
- Number and percentage of students receiving mental health services in or outside of school
- Previously collected information on perceptions of school climate by school staff, parents, and students
- Reports of previous schoolwide evaluations or improvement plans
- Information on staff training and development (e.g., surveys of needs, descriptions of training provided)
- Information on the availability of resources and supports, both in and outside of the school (e.g., counseling, school psychology social services)

Survey Strengths and Needs, as Currently Viewed by Major Stakeholders

This survey would include teachers, administrators and other school staff, parents, and students. Their perceptions and evaluations would be gathered, using one of two common methods or both: (1) a survey consisting of general, open-ended items and (2) a survey with multiple items designed to pinpoint specific strengths and needs.

Open-Ended Survey

Form 11.1 (at the end of the chapter) presents sample items that might be included in a general, open-ended survey of strengths and needs.

Itemized Survey

Instead of or in addition to a general survey, a more detailed survey consisting of specific items assessing school discipline should be considered. The Schoolwide and Classroom Strengths-and-Needs Assessment: From Schoolwide Discipline to Self-Discipline, which appears in Appendix A, was designed for this purpose. Forty items on this assessment tool tap the four components of comprehensive schoolwide discipline: (1) developing self-discipline, (2) preventing misbehavior, (3) correcting misbehavior, and (4) addressing serious and chronic misbehavior and preparing for possible crises. An additional 10 items assess staff development and program evaluation. The strengths-and-needs assessment is designed to be completed by all teachers and school staff members who have sufficient knowledge to evaluate the majority of the items. Those completing it rate each item as to (1) to extent to which it is believed to be a current strength or weakness at the schoolwide and/or classroom level and (2) its perceived importance. This format allows raters to pinpoint areas of strength and need by examining differences in what they are currently *doing* and what they believe they *should be doing*. A large discrepancy in scores between the two ratings would suggest an important area of need that should be targeted for improvement.

After this assessment is completed, it is recommended that results be compiled by a schoolwide discipline committee and presented for reflection and discussion by the entire school faculty (and others, as appropriate). A guide for administering the assessment, interpreting and discussing the results, and translating the results into improved practices is available free from *www.delawarepbs.org*.

Administer Additional Measures, as Needed, That Assess Important Outcomes and Might Help to Identify Areas of Specific Need

Many schools lack sufficient existing data to identify their strengths and needs adequately in all areas of schoolwide discipline. Moreover, stakeholders' surveys of the school's strengths and needs do not always make up for the lack of existing data. Because such surveys are also subject to social desirability bias, the results can be misleading, especially when those completing the surveys have a vested interest in the results and desire that their classroom, school, or an existing current program look good, especially to others. Thus, for a more accurate assessment of the school's strengths and needs, it is often necessary to administer additional measures, especially in areas of particular concern. Those areas of concern should be indicated from the two sources already mentioned, existing data and survey results.

School Climate

One important measure that is often missing in most schools' information is a measure of school climate. School climate refers to how teachers, staff, students, and parents perceive the school's environment, including teacher–student relationships, student peer relationships, and school safety. The results of measures of school climate are valuable in their own right, but without assessing school climate it is often difficult to know if changes in other measures, including reduced ODRs and school suspensions, are related to anything more than tinkering, or simple changed policies and practices. For example, if directed by their principal, teachers may refer fewer stu-

> It's difficult to know if schoolwide discipline is sufficiently comprehensive and effective without assessing student and teacher perceptions of school climate, especially teacher–student and student–student relationships.

dents to the office; yet, the atmosphere of both the classrooms and the overall school may remain unchanged and unpleasant.

Supporting the importance of measuring school climate, research shows that a positive school climate is clearly related to multiple positive social, emotional, and academic outcomes (Cohen et al., 2009). Although several measures of school climate exist, few are of demonstrated validity and reliability, free to schools to use, and sufficiently brief yet comprehensive enough for widespread acceptance and use by many schools. One exception is the Delaware School Climate Surveys (Bear, 2008; Bear, Smith, Blank, & Chen, in review), which are presented in Appendices B, C, and D. The surveys are completed by students, teachers and staff and the home. Table 11.1 shows the areas assessed by each survey and

TABLE 11.1. Delaware School Climate Surveys

Subscales of Delaware School Climate Surveys		
Student Survey	**Teacher/Staff Survey**	**Home Survey**
Part I		
Student–Student Relations (8 items: 1, 6, 9*, 11, 14*, 16, 21, 26)	Student–Student Relations (8 items: 1, 6, 9*, 11, 14*, 16, 21, 26)	Student–Student Relations (8 items: 1, 6, 9*, 11, 14*, 16, 21, 26)
Teacher–Student Relations (7 items: 2, 7, 12, 17, 22, 27, 28)	Teacher–Student Relations (7 items: 2, 7, 12, 17, 22, 27, 28)	Teacher–Student Relations (7 items: 2, 7, 12, 17, 22, 27, 28)
Fairness of Rules (5 items: 3, 8, 13*, 18, 23*)	Fairness of Rules (5 items: 3, 8, 13*, 18, 23*)	Fairness of Rules (5 items: 3, 8, 13*, 18, 23*)
Clarity of Rules and Expectations (5 items: 5, 10, 15, 20, 25*)	Clarity of Rules and Expectations (5 items: 5, 10, 15, 20, 25*)	Clarity of Rules and Expectations (5 items: 5, 10, 15, 20, 25*)
School Safety (3 items: 4, 19, 24)	School Safety (3 items: 4, 19, 24)	School Safety (3 items: 4, 19, 24)
	School–Home Relations (5 items: 30, 31, 32, 33, 34)	School–Home Relations (5 items: 30, 31, 32, 33, 34)
Total School Climate (28 items: sum of above items)	Total School Climate (33 items: sum of above items)	Total School Climate (33 items: sum of above items)

*Item is reversed scored: 4 = 1, 3 = 2, 2 = 3, 1 = 4.
Note. Item 29 on each survey is not included on any subscale.

Part II		
Punitive Techniques (4 items: 1, 4, 7, 10)	PunitiveTechniques (4 items: 1, 3, 5, 7)	Punitive Techniques (4 items: 1, 4, 7, 10)
Positive Techniques (4 items: 2, 5, 8, 11)	Positive Techniques (5 items: 2, 4, 6, 8, 9)	Positive Techniques (4 items: 2, 5, 8, 11)
SEL Techniques (5 items: 3, 6, 9, 12, 13)	SEL Techniques (5 items: 10, 11, 12, 13, 14)	SEL Techniques (5 items: 3, 6, 9, 12, 13)

the number of items in each section. Guidelines for the use of the Delaware School Climate Surveys are available from *www.delawarepbs.org*.

Reflect on the Result of the Assessment of Strengths and Needs

Information and data from the above sources should be collated and summarized by a schoolwide discipline committee, represented by all major stakeholders, and presented to the entire school faculty for thorough reflection and discussion. Only after this has been done—which often requires numerous meetings—should a decision should be made to embark upon efforts for systems change.

WHEN CHANGES ARE NEEDED: THE FIVE PHASES OF SYSTEMIC CHANGE

Results from the above methods for conducting a strengths-and-needs assessment should indicate the need for changes in existing practices as well as the possible need for *new* practices or a new approach to schoolwide discipline. A new approach might be shifting from an authoritarian zero tolerance approach to a more positive authoritative approach. Weaknesses in a few specific areas may call for few changes that might be addressed through problem-solving discussion among school staff, staff development and training in targeted areas, changes in specific policies, or implementation of specific curriculum activities. More pervasive weaknesses, however, would call for intensive systemic change—extensive changes in the existing approach or the adoption of a new one. Assuming that the need for change is indicated, the next step is to begin the process of systemic change.

Upon reviewing the literature on school reform and mental health in the schools, the Center for Mental Health in Schools (2008) identified four overlapping phases of systemic change: (1) *creating readiness*, (2) *initial implementation*, (3) *institutionalization*, and (4) *ongoing evolution and creative renewal*. The first phase includes readiness, commitment, and the development of a plan. Given the amount of activity included in this phase and the length of time required to accomplish it, in this chapter the first phase of this model is treated as two separate phases: (1) creating readiness and (2) developing a plan. Thus, the five (slightly reconfigured) phases presented in this chapter provide a useful heuristic for guiding program development and implementation. They apply to schools focused on adopting an existing program or approach to schoolwide discipline. They also apply to schools engaged in creating their own program while drawing from key features of existing approaches or programs, including SWPBS and SEL. The phases also apply to those schools that have already implemented a schoolwide program but are engaged in expanding, renewing, or replacing aspects of it. The five phases of developing and implementing a comprehensive approach to schoolwide discipline, with more specific action steps and guiding questions, are described below.

Phase 1: Create Readiness and Commitment to Change

In short, it is possible, indeed necessary, to combine ambitious change and quality. I have maintained that it is what people develop in their minds and actions that counts. People do not learn or accomplish complex changes by being told or shown what to do.
—FULLAN (2007, p. 92)

Failure in school reform most commonly occurs when educators adopt or develop a program before engaging in serious reflection and discussion of its underlying theory and philosophy and before devoting ample time to planning (Center for Mental Health in Schools, 2008; Fullan, 2007; Meyers, Meyers, Proctor, & Graybill, 2009). I witnessed a good example of failure as a member of the state's SWPBS committee in Delaware schools. That is, as recommended by Sugai and Horner (2009; Sugai et al., 2008), at least 80% of teachers and staff members in every SWPBS school in Delaware agreed to implement SWPBS. However, it was apparent that in many schools such "commitment" rarely evolved after any serious reflection about what the educators were agreeing to or about any alternatives to the state's SWPBS approach. Typically, the SWPBS approach was explained briefly by a districtwide SWPBS coach at the school's faculty meeting. Teachers and staff members were then either told by the principal (via the district office) that their workplace would become a SWPBS school or were asked to raise their hands if they supported the new positive approach to schoolwide discipline. The impermanence of such commitment frequently became apparent in many of those schools when the interest in SWPBS either waned after a year or two and/or it became evident that not much was actually implemented beyond the posting of rules and the dissemination of tokens. In addition to lacking in-depth discussion and reflection about what the school was actually embarking upon, little time was devoted to developing the school's *own* individualized plan based on a comprehensive assessment of its strengths and needs. Instead, time was spent on determining how the staff would implement someone else's approach (e.g., what expectations would be posted and what kind of token system would be used). In sum, the most critical phase of systemic change was shortchanged or given insufficient attention.

> A true commitment to change entails much more than simply raising one's hand at a faculty meeting and voting in favor of something new. Serious reflection underlies true commitment and this takes time.

To generate meaningful readiness and lasting commitment to systemic change, as well as to help sustain such change, the following issues must be thoroughly examined, discussed, and debated among major stakeholders during Phase 1. This elaborate preparation must occur *before* adopting or developing an approach or program and before writing a plan for its implementation. Guiding questions to help determine readiness for change are presented in Form 11.2 (at the end of the chapter).

Serious reflection about the questions in Form 11.2 cannot occur in just one or a few faculty meetings. Multiple meetings are required extending over a period of 2–6 months. These meetings should be immediately followed by additional meetings, over the course of 4–6 months, for the purpose of developing an implementation plan in Phase 2. Much of the information discussed during Phase 1 would be directly linked to Phase 2 planning. Meetings in both phases, which may extend up to a year, should include all major stakeholders involved in systemic change, such as administrators, teachers, support staff, and parents (and some discussions and planning sessions should include students, where appropriate).

During the meetings and prior to drafting a plan, alternative evidence-based programs, or elements thereof, should be reviewed. In addition to reviewing literature on evidence-based programs, the planners should include visits to other schools that are currently implementing programs of interest, e-mails or telephone conversations with those at other sites or with consultants, staff presentations and discussions of other programs and approaches, and attendance at relevant workshops. In addition to reviewing programs as to their likely effectiveness and feasibility of implementation, the school staff should also consider how one or more programs might be adapted to best fit the strengths and needs of the school. That is, school officials should not feel constrained to adopt all features of a given program, such as the use of tokens in SWPBS, especially if those features are not consistent with the school's philosophy or mission.

The most important outcomes of this phase should be a *shared vision* of what changes are needed, what they might entail, and how they will occur (Fullan, 2007). Educational leaders do not produce a shared vision by simply telling teachers and staff that they "will be a SWPBS school" but by successfully persuading them that change is important and needed and by helping them understand what change means and entails. A shared vision is best achieved by facilitating serious reflection upon the questions in Form 11.2. Only after serious reflection has occurred should stakeholders be asked to vote on whether or not they are committed to pursue their shared vision and embark upon the process of change. At least 80% of the school staff should vote that they are committed—not only to simply implementing the program but also to systematically doing so over a period of 3–4 years (Sugai et al., 2008).

Phase 2: Developing a Plan

Once a shared vision has emerged and a program or a combination of features of existing programs has been chosen for adoption or adaptation, a planning committee should be appointed to draft an implementation plan. The planning committee may consist of members of the previously formed committee. It is important that all major stakeholders be included or represented. Parents and students (as age appropriate) also should be members or otherwise have an ongoing voice in the decision-making process. If the plan is presented as an SWPBS program a substantial number of the committee members should be general education teachers, as opposed to special education teachers and support staff in order to avoid the program's being perceived as a special education initiative and thus creating resistance on part of many regular education teachers. Likewise, consistent with research on school reform (Fullan, 2007), including SWPBS (Sugai et al., 2008), it is important that building administrators be active participants in the planning process (as well as in all other aspects of the change). Their inclusion is likely to increase the likelihood that the program will be implemented as intended—with fidelity—and will be sustainable over time.

The school's implementation plan should include the core elements listed in Form 11.3 (at the end of the chapter). If the school elects to adopt a prepackaged program or approach, many of these elements may already be available. In such cases, however, the planning committee should thoroughly review and consider modifying those elements, as appropriate, to best fit the school's shared vision, strengths, and needs.

I will not take the time or space to discuss each item in Form 11.3. My experience, however, has been that school officials too often fail to make certain that the program's goals, objectives, and action steps are (1) *directly linked to the school's mission and philosophy*, (2) *guided by evidence-based research and theory*, (3) *neither too broad nor too narrow*, and (4) *measurable*. As noted earlier, the various existing evidence-based programs should be closely reviewed. Whether one particular program or approach is selected for adoption or selected components of various programs and approaches are chosen, the program and its components must be consistent with the philosophy and mission of the school and compatible with current research as to their effectiveness. Goals should not be too broad and idealistic (e.g., "improve the mental health of all children") or so narrow in focus that they are unlikely to result in meaningful change (e.g., "reduce the number of ODRs from the hallways," and "increase the number of acknowledgments or recognitions that students are given for good behavior").

It also is critical that program goals feature desired outcomes that can be measured. Desired outcomes might include changes in *knowledge* (e.g., knowledge of school rules, awareness of social problem-solving steps); *attitudes, values, and emotions* (e.g., student attitudes toward aggression, bullying, responsibility; empathy and anger; perceptions about school climate); *social cognitive skills* (e.g., anger control, resisting peer pressure, application of social problem skills); and *actions* (e.g., behavior problems, prosocial behavior, teacher–student interactions). Several websites for evidence-based approaches and programs offer reliable and valid measures that school officials can use to measure changes in these areas as well as guidance in developing goals and objectives (e.g., see *www.childdevelpment.org*; *www.committeeforchildren*; *www.CASEL.org*).

Each measurable goal should be translated into specific action steps that include timelines, assignment of responsibility for initiating the action step, the specific outcome that is expected to emerge (quantified), and the roles and responsibilities of the stakeholders involved.

Phase 3: Initial Implementation

Phase 3 largely overlaps with Phase 2, program planning. The primary difference is that Phase 3 involves actual implementation (either an intact program developed by others or selected components of other evidence-based programs). More specific to this phase is the importance of an existing infrastructure that provides necessary support and guidance to those implementing the changes, including the items listed in Form 11.3. The importance of the first item on that list cannot be emphasized enough—that is, schools must be assured that the leaders (e.g., principal, coaches) have advanced training in the program components to be implemented and that they support the program's theoretical perspective. For example, advocates of SWPBS advise that coaches and SWPBS teams have advanced training in ABA (McKevitt & Braaksma, 2008; Sugai et al., 2000), but it might be unwise to ask them to lead the implementation of an SEL program such as Responsive Classroom (Charney, 2002) that is inconsistent with the operant behavioral approach. Indeed, this type of mismatch might undermine the program's effectiveness.

Phase 4: Institutionalizing the Program through Policy, Curriculum, and the Culture of the School

A very common finding in the school reform literature is that many programs are no longer around after a few years, and many of the same schools then begin searching for another bandwagon (Fuller, 2007). At times this pattern reflects the fact that the program was found to be ineffective. Perhaps more frequently, however, it is because interest and enthusiasm about the program waned, and there was little or no effort made to plan and establish the program's sustainability and maintenance. This latter outcome is particularly true in schools where there is mobility or change in leadership and staff. Programs that are sustained over time (including where there are changes in leadership and staff) tend to be those in which sustainability is built into the school's infrastructure. Form 11.4 (at the end of the chapter) presents a checklist of items for sustaining and institutionalizing programs.

Phase 5: Ongoing Evolution and Creative Renewal

Not institutionalizing a program through policy, curriculum, and the culture of the school is a common reason why many programs fail or are not sustained over a long period of time. Another common reason is that the programs simply become stale. The latter is avoided in schools in which stakeholders continue to be engaged in in-depth discussion and exploration of how their program can evolve and achieve its long-term aim(s), such as developing self-discipline. As emphasized in Phase 1, *all* stakeholders should thoroughly discuss what changes are needed, what change means, what it entails, and how it is best achieved. But discussion, reflection, and planning do not end with the completion of that phase. Instead, they should be ongoing and recursive. Obstacles to change are continually anticipated and addressed, data on effectiveness are continually examined, and whatever is not working is modified or replaced. During this process, the school faculty operates as a *community of learners* or *professional learning community* (Fullan, 2007) and not as passive recipients of recommendations from an administrator, coach, or committee. As noted by Fullan (2007): "Under these conditions teachers learn how to use an innovation as well as to judge its desirability on more information-based grounds; they are in a better position to know whether they should accept, modify, or reject the change. This is the case with regard to both externally developed ideas and innovations

> Operating as a professional learning community, the school staff should continue to be actively involved in a program's evaluation and renewal in order to prevent a program from becoming stale.

decided upon or developed by other teachers. Purposeful interaction is essential for continuous improvement" (p. 139).

To be sure, active involvement and reflection should be seen during all five phases, but it is particularly important in Phase 5 in order to help ensure that a program does not become stale but, rather, continues to evolve. In operating as a community of learners, administrators, teachers, support staff, and other stakeholders work collaboratively to build a shared vision and to plan, implement, and institutionalize the program. A shared vision, which includes an agreed-upon mission and goals, fosters consistency in schoolwide practices and is critical to the effectiveness of schoolwide discipline programs. When planning, implementing, and institutionalizing the program, educators engage in collaborative problem solving and the sharing of knowledge, skills, resources, and technical assistance. There is no "coach"—as recommended in the SWPBS approach—who assumes the responsibility for disseminating knowledge and training others in the areas where they are deficient (e.g., functional behavioral assessment, use of positive reinforcement), and thus adheres to the direct behavioral consultation model (Watson & Sterling-Turner, 2008). Instead of telling and showing others what to do, the coach (or any other leader) acts consistently with the collaborative problem-solving model of consultation (Kratochwill, 2008; Sheridan & Kratochwill, 2008). In a community of learners, all stakeholders function as coaches, or more correctly, as collaborative team members who seek and offer support and technical assistance to and from one other. Achieving the program's goals is viewed as a shared responsibility, requiring collaboration and team work among all stakeholders (including students and parents). All stakeholders share not only responsibility but also accountability.

Functioning as a community of learners is important during *all* phases of systemic change. It is particularly important, however, when school officials choose not to simply implement what others tell them to do but rather to be creative in drawing evidence-based practices from multiple programs and applying these to their own situation. Their goal is not to implement someone else's program by the end of 3–5 years but to implement their own program—one that is constantly evolving and improving. To prevent staleness and foster evolution and renewal, stakeholders, functioning as a community of learners, should be guided by the following questions:

- What multiple forms of evidence do we have to indicate that the program is effective in helping to achieve the school's mission and the program's goals? Although this evidence might include ODRs (as commonly used in SWPBS), other measures should predominate (see list on p. 190), especially measures of school climate.
- Based on a current strengths-and-needs assessment, including a review of existing data, what have we done well, and what do we need to improve upon?
- Are there other important outcomes that we are not assessing or addressing that need to be added?
- Are there any unintended outcomes? If so, what are they? Do they need to be addressed? If so, how?
- Is our program best characterized as attempting to achieve meaningful and complex systemic change or as simply "tinkering"?

- Are we addressing the social, emotional, and behavioral needs of *all* children?
- How might we improve upon current practices? What new or additional evidence-based practices should be considered? What other practices are schools using that we should consider adopting?
- What obstacles lie in the way of the program's continual evolvement and improvement? How might they be avoided or minimized?
- Has the program been implemented as planned? How do we know this? How can we implement the program with greater fidelity?
- Should the program's goals and action steps be modified? Given what has occurred in the program, and evidence of the program's effectiveness, are the goals realistic, too narrow, or too broad?

SUMMARY

As emphasized by Fulton (2007), effective systems change and school reform require much more than tinkering—especially when the tinkering involves a limited number of techniques espoused in one particular approach that stakeholders have not truly reflected upon. Change is unlikely to occur or to be sustained when stakeholders blindly implement a "one-size-fits-all" approach dictated by others. Instead, resistance to change is likely to occur.

To help avoid resistance to change among stakeholders and to increase the likelihood that systems change efforts will be effective, five phases of systems change were discussed in this chapter: (1) creating readiness, (2) planning, (3) initial implementation, (4) institutionalization, and (5) ongoing evolution and creative renewal. Each phase is based on extensive research on systems change and school reform (e.g., Center for Mental Health in Schools, 2008). The main message conveyed throughout the five phases is that change is complex and requires considerable energy and time on the part of all major stakeholders, not just tinkering.

General Survey of Schoolwide Strengths and Needs

Please describe schoolwide strengths and needs in each of following areas of schoolwide discipline. Circle those items that you believe are major weaknesses and draw a star next to those that are relative strengths.

Developing self-discipline

Strengths: _____

_____

Weaknesses: _____

_____

Preventing behavior problems with effective classroom management.

Strengths: _____

_____

Weaknesses: _____

_____

Correcting behavior problems at the classroom level.

Strengths: _____

_____

Weaknesses: _____

_____

Preventing and correcting behavior problems outside of classroom.

Strengths: _____

_____

Weaknesses: _____

_____

Adult-Student Relationships.

Strengths: _____

_____

Weaknesses: _____

_____

(cont.)

General Survey of Schoolwide Strengths and Needs *(page 2 of 2)*

Student-Student Relationships.

Strengths: _____

_____

Weaknesses: _____

_____

Communications and collaboration with parents.

Strengths: _____

_____

Weaknesses: _____

_____

School Climate.

Strengths: _____

_____

Weaknesses: _____

_____

School Safety.

Strengths: _____

_____

Weaknesses: _____

_____

Addressing the social, emotional, and behavioral needs of children at-risk for behavior problems or who exhibit serious and chronic behavior problems.

Strengths: _____

_____

Weaknesses: _____

_____

Addressing the social, emotional, and behavioral needs of all students (please identify any groups of students whose needs are not being adequately met).

Strengths: _____

_____

Weaknesses: _____

_____

Guiding Questions to Help Determine Readiness for Change

- What is the school's primary mission with respect to schoolwide discipline?

- What are the school's strengths and needs? How do they relate to the school's mission?

- Why *should* we change?

- What changes are desirable? Feasible? Are such changes powerful enough to produce the desired outcomes reflected in our mission?

- What alternative evidence-based programs exist that best complement the school's assessed strengths and needs?

- What valued outcomes might be better realized by changing existing practices?

- Which programs or approaches are most compatible with the school's (and district's) mission and with the philosophy of the majority of stakeholders?

- What is the evidence that those programs are effective?

- How might the school look differently upon implementing the changes associated with other programs or approaches that are being considered?

- Do the positive outcomes presented as evidence of a program's effectiveness (e.g., reduced disciplinary referrals) truly reflect the school's mission (e.g., development of social and moral responsibility)?

- What do the programs being considered require with respect to resources, space, funding, training, and time?

- Does the new program overlap with existing programs (e.g., bullying prevention, DARE)? If so, how might the programs be integrated in order to avoid overlap and program fragmentation?

- How might the roles and expectations of the staff change? How might changes be perceived by those involved?

- Who will be primarily responsible for leadership during the change process?

- To what extent are we willing to do everything necessary to ensure the program's success?

- What obstacles should be anticipated in implementing the program? How might those obstacles be avoided or minimized?

- How long will the new program need to be implemented before seeing any evidence of its effectiveness? When the program is fully developed, what are realistic timelines for its implementation?

- What will be training requirements of stakeholders? When and where will training be provided? Who will provide it? Will it be mandatory?

- How is the program related to our school improvement plan?

- How will we know whether the program is effective? In general, what will be evaluated?

- How might features of the program (or programs) be adapted to best fit the needs and strengths of our school? Or, are all schools expected to be equally amenable to the program elements to be implemented?

Checklist of Items for Initial Implementation of the Program

Check each item that currently describes the program.

_____ Leaders are well trained in the practices to be implemented and are viewed by their peers as enthusiastically valuing the program's goals and able to offer practical strategies and techniques for achieving them.

_____ Efforts are made to create a schoolwide norm that reflects the school's shared vision and goals. Most members of the school community believe that the goals are important and can be achieved.

_____ Institutional support is actively sought for adequate funding, space, and the allocation of sufficient time for the full participation of stakeholders.

_____ Consultation from experts is sought, as needed. Maximum use is made of consultants and supervisors who are internal to the system, but external experts are also consulted, as needed.

_____ Staff development and training are scheduled or provided that match the school's needs to the project's goals.

_____ Staff development and training are ongoing rather than one-shot and piecemeal.

_____ If new positions are required, project staff members are hired who are well trained and qualified, who are culturally competent, and who understand and share the project's vision and goals.

_____ Deliberate steps are in place to help ensure that all action steps are being implemented as planned and with fidelity.

_____ There is ongoing communication among stakeholders. The project's goals and activities are routinely communicated to everyone involved, including teachers, parents, and students.

_____ All stakeholders are given ample opportunities to actively participate in program plans and implementation efforts.

_____ The majority of stakeholders *are* actively involved.

_____ To enhance fidelity of implementation, curriculum lessons, practices, and techniques are clear, specific, adequately detailed, and prescriptive. A system is provided for ongoing monitoring and supervision of the program's implementation.

_____ Committees are established and given specific responsibilities, roles, and assigned tasks. Most committees meet at least monthly and communicate frequently with all stakeholders.

Checklist of Items for Sustaining and Institutionalizing the Program

Check each item that currently describes the program.

____ The program is directly linked to the school's mission as well as the school district's goals.

____ Key goals or elements of the program (e.g., developing self-discipline and promoting a positive school climate) are highlighted as priorities in the school's improvement plan.

____ When appropriate, the program is directly linked to other school reform efforts at the school, district, or state level (e.g., response to intervention, bullying and violence prevention, character education, social and emotional learning).

____ Critical elements of the program are included in school policies (e.g., code of conduct) and the curriculum.

____ Where appropriate, the program is linked to state standards, such as standards for social and emotional learning and character education (see *www.CASEL.org* for examples). (Although not all states have standards specific to SEL or character education, most have multiple aspects of SEL and character education embedded in standards on health education, social studies, or guidance and counseling.)

____ Activities for achieving project goals are manifest throughout the curriculum, policies, practices, and professional training.

____ Ongoing staff development and training are provided, including booster sessions for previous training. This commitment includes provisions for addressing the common problem of turnover in trained staff. For example, new staff are given individual mentoring and are required to view video tapes of previous training sessions or complete instructional modules.

____ Action steps are implemented as planned and with full fidelity.

____ There is minimal reliance on external experts and trainers and greater reliance on ones who are internal to the school or district. (External experts and trainers are most important during Phases 1, 2, and 3, when alternative programs are being evaluated and the program is planned and first implemented.)

____ Recognition and incentives are provided to those implementing the program with fidelity or success (e.g., have students vote on their favorite teachers and recognize the winners). (Recognize, however, that persuasion is more powerful and lasting than incentives.)

____ The program is visible to parents and the community (e.g., via school newsletters, a project website linked to the school's website, articles in the local newspaper, brochures, and annual reports and presentations to the school board, PTA, and other groups).

____ Widespread support exists for the program, including support outside of the school, such as from parents, businesses, and community leaders.

____ Program-related responsibilities are included in the job descriptions of those implementing the program (e.g., they highlight the importance of establishing supportive teacher–student and teacher-parent relationships, developing self-discipline).

____ Continued institutional support, including funding, resources, and charismatic leaders, is in place.

Schoolwide and Classroom
Strengths-and-Needs Assessment
From Schoolwide Discipline to Self-Discipline

This assessment tool is designed to help educators identify strengths and needs in their implementation of important research-based elements of comprehensive schoolwide discipline, including social and emotional learning (SEL) and positive behavior interventions and supports (PBIS). It can be used at both the classroom and schoolwide levels for (1) self- or schoolwide assessment and reflection, (2) action planning for classroom or school improvement, and (3) professional development planning (e.g., to target specific areas for professional training). Research-based elements of schoolwide discipline are grouped under four interrelated components: (1) Developing Self-Discipline, (2) Preventing Behavior Problems with Effective Classroom and Schoolwide Management Systems, (3) Correcting Behavior Problems, and (4) Addressing the Needs of Students Who Are Currently Exhibiting Serious and Chronic Behavior Problems (or who are at risk of such). Ten items assess each of those four components and an additional 10 items assess program development and evaluation efforts related to the four components of comprehensive school discipline.

It is recommended that the assessment be completed by all staff members (including all teachers, administrators, and support staff who have sufficient knowledge to evaluate the majority of the items) and that individual responses be tallied and later discussed in a series of meetings with those who completed the assessment.

A guide for administering this assessment tool and using the results for classroom and schoolwide improvements can be downloaded from *www.delawarepbs.org*.

Please complete the following:

Name of school _____ Date _____

Your position: General Education Teacher   Special Education Teacher Administrator

Other Instructional or Certified Staff   Other: _____

Please rate each item as follows:

STRENGTH/WEAKNESS RATING: SCHOOLWIDE LEVEL

In the first column (SW), rate each item as to the extent to which you believe it is a Schoolwide strength or weakness. That is, think of the **school in general** (i.e., across classrooms at all grade levels and throughout the building). When the word "adults" appears, think of all school staff in general, including teachers, administrators, cafeteria workers, etc. Rate the item as follows:

> 5 = Major strength   4 = Strength   3 = Neither strength nor weakness   2 = Weakness
> 1 = Major weakness   DK = Don't know

For example, you should assign a 4 or 5 to those items that are currently in place, viewed as a strength, and not needing improvement. You would assign a 1 or 2 to those items that either do not exist or need much improvement.

(cont.)

STRENGTH/WEAKNESS RATING: CLASSROOM LEVEL

In the second column (CR), use the same 5-point scale to rate each item as to the extent to which you believe it is a strength or weakness in **your classroom**. This would include other settings in which students are taught as a class or group (e.g., library, gym, music). **If you do not have a class, do not complete this column.**
Note that items for Components 4 and 5 do not apply at the classroom level. Thus, you are asked to respond only at the schoolwide level for those items.

Please rate each item as follows:

IMPORTANCE RATING

Next, rate the item as to how important **you** think it is to comprehensive schoolwide discipline. That is, ask "Is this something that **should** be important in this school?"

$$5 = \text{Very important} \quad 4 = \text{Important} \quad 3 = \text{Neutral}$$
$$2 = \text{Not important} \quad 1 = \text{Not important at all} \quad DK = \text{Don't know}$$

For example, you should assign a 4 or 5 to those items that you believe should be important or very important. Assign a 1 or 2 to those items that you do not believe should be important (e.g., not appropriate at your grade level, not valued by the faculty, etc.).

Do not feel compelled to respond to every item. You should not rate items for which you feel uncomfortable making an "educated guess." For those items, please respond "don't know" (DK).

COMMENTS

After each item, provide any comments, as appropriate, that might help explain or qualify your ratings. For example, in explaining a low rating for strengths/needs, you might note, "This is done in some grades but not all." "Some of these things are done well, but not others, such as. . . . " Comments should always be provided for items receiving a rating of 3 or lower in any column.

COMPONENT I: DEVELOPING SELF-DISCIPLINE

Traditionally, the primary aim of school discipline is the long-term development of thoughts, feelings, and behaviors associated with self-discipline. Self-discipline entails students assuming responsibility for their actions, understanding right and wrong, showing empathy, respecting others, and inhibiting socially inappropriate behavior. It involves knowing what's right, desiring to do what is right, and most importantly *doing* what is right. In promoting self-discipline, schools adopt a variety of direct and indirect techniques for developing thoughts, feelings, and behaviors such that the behavior of students is not motivated *solely* by use of the techniques for prevention and correction, including the use of external rewards and punishment.

(cont.)

Reminders: SW = Schoolwide, CR = Classroom 5 = Major strength, 4 = Strength, 3 = Neither strength nor weakness, 2 = Weakness, 1 = Major weakness 5 = Very important, 4 = Important, 3 = Neutral, 2 = Not important, 1 = Not important at all DK = Don't know	Strength/ weakness rating		Importance rating
	SW	CR	
I.1	*Self-discipline is reflected in the school's mission statement and policies and in classroom rules.* The long-term aim of developing self-discipline is included or reflected in the school's mission statement and policies and in classroom rules. For example, in addition to school rules, the classroom rules emphasizes self-discipline, responsible citizenship, or such social and emotional competencies as responsibility, caring, and respect for others.		
	Comments:		
I.2	*Positive relationships with others.* Positive relationships with others, including student–student and teacher–student relationships, are expected, taught, and encouraged. This includes planned opportunities to develop positive relationships. For example, students are taught to resolve conflicts peacefully and to demonstrate respect for others, and they are provided ample opportunities as appropriate for the grade level, to develop and practice positive relationships in clubs, cooperative learning activities, sports, on field trips, etc.		
	Comments:		
I.3	*Lessons infused throughout the school curriculum.* Lessons designed to promote the development of thoughts, feelings, and behaviors associated with responsible behavior or self-discipline are infused in one or more areas of the curriculum. For example, curriculum activities in language arts and social studies highlight the general importance of empathy, perspective taking, and social and moral problem solving.		
	Comments:		

(cont.)

		Strength/ weakness rating		Importance rating
		SW	CR	
I.4	*Curriculum lessons specific to one or more areas of prevention and self-discipline.* Lessons are taught that target a specific problem behavior (such as bullying, school violence, or drug use) or one or more specific social competencies (e.g., conflict resolution, resisting peer pressure, managing anger). For example, teachers, or the school counselor, teach weekly lessons from a "packaged" evidence-based program on preventing school violence or bullying, conflict resolution, or empathy, *or* lessons in the general curriculum are taught that have been systematically aligned with targeted social and emotional competencies.			
	Comments:			
I.5	*Schoolwide and classroom activities.* A variety of schoolwide and classroom activities designed to promote self-discipline are provided. For example, schoolwide assemblies, morning announcements, posters, and bulletin boards highlight character traits and positive role models.			
	Comments:			
I.6	*Service learning.* Students are presented with service learning activities, such as mentoring younger children, assisting at a senior citizens center or Head Start program, coordinating a food drive for the needy, etc.			
	Comments:			
I.7	*Adult modeling of self-discipline.* School staff members provide models of the social, emotional, and behavioral qualities they expect of students. For example, they exhibit caring and kindness, regulate their emotions (i.e., refrain from yelling, inappropriately expressing anger), show respect for all others, and follow school rules (e.g., are not late for class).			
	Comments:			

(cont.)

		Strength/ weakness rating		Importance rating
		SW	CR	
I.8	*Student decision making.* Where appropriate for the school's grade level, classroom management and schoolwide practices include students in the decision-making process, especially decisions pertaining to socially responsible behavior. For example, students are given choices regarding classroom assignments, cooperative learning is emphasized, and class meetings are used to discuss rules, consequences, and behavior problems. At the schoolwide level, students participate in student government or other small groups that foster social and emotional learning (e.g., a student council that is involved in decisions about promoting a positive school climate).			
	Comments:			
I.9	*Student responsibility and choice.* Although teachers/schools are primarily responsible for all components of comprehensive school discipline. responsibility for student behavior is viewed as a shared responsibility (shared by teachers/staff, students, and parents). Teachers, administrators, and other school staff communicate clearly to students that students are responsible for their behavior—that they can make good or bad choices and should be held accountable for those choices.			
	Comments:			
I.10	*Strategic use of praise and rewards.* Praise and rewards are used strategically to recognize and reinforce social and emotional competencies that underlie prosocial behavior (even when rewards are not salient). For example, students are routinely recognized with praise and occasionally with rewards for demonstrating empathy, caring, responsibility, and respect. Although managing student behavior is important, it is understood that developing self-discipline is the primary aim of the use of praise and rewards.			
	Comments:			

(cont.)

General Comments for Component I:

COMPONENT II: PREVENTING BEHAVIOR PROBLEMS WITH EFFECTIVE CLASSROOM AND SCHOOLWIDE MANAGEMENT SYSTEMS

Effective teachers focus on the prevention of behavior problems, relying on evidence-based strategies and techniques of effective classroom management. Effective schools use similar techniques but apply them schoolwide (e.g., in the cafeteria, hallways, playground, and in all the classrooms). Effective teachers and schools foster a positive school climate while also reducing the need to correct misbehavior.

Reminders: SW = Schoolwide CR = Classroom 5 = Major strength, 4 = Strength, 3 = Neither strength nor weakness, 2 = Weakness, 1 = Major weakness 5 = Very important, 4 = Important, 3 = Neutral, 2 = Not important,	Strength/ weakness rating		
1 = Not important at all DK = Don't know	SW	CR	Importance rating
II.1 *Caring and supportive adult–student relationships.* Adults demonstrate warmth, respect, support, and caring toward *all* students (irrespective of gender, race, ethnicity, socioeconomic background, disabilities, previous history of behavior, etc.).			
Comments:			
II.2 *High expectations for all.* Adults convey a general attitude that *all* children can succeed both academically and socially. High academic and behavioral expectations permeate the classroom and school atmosphere, as reflected in both policies and practices.			
Comments:			

(cont.)

		Strength/ weakness rating		Importance rating
		SW	CR	
II.3	*Physical environment.* The physical environments of the classrooms and the school building are pleasant and conducive to academic, social, and emotional learning.			
	Comments:			
II.4	*Clear and fair behavioral expectations and rules.* Behavioral expectations and classroom and school rules (and their consequences) are clear, fair, and consistently enforced. They are taught early in the school year and are reviewed as often as needed; schoolwide expectations are worded positively and posted in classrooms and hallways; students and parents are presented with classroom expectations/rules and the code of conduct.			
	Comments:			
II.5	*Procedures, routines, and schedules.* Students are taught to follow procedures and routines for common tasks and school functions (e.g., procedures for leaving the classroom to go to the bathroom, to get on and off buses, for transitioning between classes, emergency drills, etc.). Scheduling (including lunch and dismissal times) minimizes time in the hallways and other locations where adequate supervision may be lacking.			
	Comments:			
II.6	*Monitoring and supervision.* Adults frequently monitor and supervise student behavior throughout the building and campus (including classrooms, hallways, cafeteria, playground, parking lot, bus area, etc.), and respond immediately to signs of misbehavior.			
	Comments:			

(cont.)

		Strength/ weakness rating		Importance rating
		SW	CR	
II.7	*Recognition of desired behaviors.* Students are frequently praised or otherwise acknowledged for desirable behaviors (including desirable thinking skills and emotional competencies). Students are recognized for appropriate behavior much more often than they are corrected for inappropriate behavior.			
	Comments:			
II.8	*Motivating instruction and curriculum.* Students are provided with academic instruction and curriculum materials that are motivating and engaging, thus helping to prevent many behavior problems from occurring. For example, teaching includes a variety of methods, clear directions, explicit instructions, and appropriate pacing, repetition, and practice. Instructional and curricular adaptations are made, as needed, for individual students.			
	Comments:			
II.9	*Home communications and collaboration.* Clear and open communications are maintained with the parents of students. Parental involvement in classrooms and the school is actively sought (e.g., parents are invited to visit often and to volunteer to help; newsletters are sent home; a school website keeps parents abreast of school activities; an active parent–school organization exists, etc.). The number of positive contacts with the home is greater than the number of negative contacts.			
	Comments:			
II.10	*Authoritative approach to prevention and correction.* In general, the classroom and schoolwide approach to discipline is authoritative, not authoritarian (overly harsh and controlling) and not permissive. This is seen in a healthy blend of responsiveness (support, caring, warmth, respect) and demandingness (structure, high expectations, close monitoring and supervision).			
	Comments:			

(cont.)

General Comments for Component II:

COMPONENT III: CORRECTING MISBEHAVIOR

Effective school officials view the development of self-discipline and the prevention of misbehavior as priorities in their comprehensive school discipline plan; however, they also recognize that behavior problems are to be expected, and corrected, and that in the process of correcting misbehavior they can also help develop student self-discipline. Behavior is viewed as a *joint responsibility* of students, the entire school staff, and the home.

Reminders: SW = Schoolwide CR = Classroom 5 = Major strength, 4 = Strength, 3 = Neither strength nor weakness, 2 = Weakness, 1 = Major weakness 5 = Very important, 4 = Important, 3 = Neutral, 2 = Not important, 1 = Not important at all DK = Don't know	Strength/ weakness rating		Importance rating
	SW	CR	
III.1 *Fairness of rules and written policies.* Disciplinary policies (e.g., the code of conduct and classroom rules) contain specific rules and consequences that are clear and fair, as viewed by school staff, students, and parents.			
Comments:			
III.2 *Awareness of rules and policies.* All school staff, students, and parents are informed of school rules, expectations, consequences, and due process rights. At the schoolwide and/or classroom level, they are reminded of such, as appropriate, throughout the school year.			
Comments:			

(cont.)

		Strength/ weakness rating		Importance rating
		SW	CR	
III.3	*Recognition of limitations of punishment.* School staff recognize, and are responsive to, the limitations and negative effects of punishment (ranging from verbal reprimands and taking away privileges to suspension). This is seen in the more frequent use of praise than punishment in preventing misbehavior. It also is seen in the use of punishment only in combination with other more positive techniques when correcting misbehavior (e.g., desired behaviors are reinforced, teacher guidance and support are provided, preventive techniques are emphasized).			
	Comments:			
III.4	*Consistent, fair, and judicious enforcement of rules.* Rules and disciplinary procedures are followed consistently but also in a flexible, fair, and judicious manner that allows for consideration of the circumstances involved, where appropriate (e.g., consideration for the student's age, intentions, and history of behavior problems). There is a continuum of consequences, and the harshness of those consequences corresponds proportionally to the nature of the offenses (e.g., students are not removed from the classroom for minor behavior problems, and suspension is used only for the most serious behavior problems).			
	Comments:			
III.5	*Self-discipline in correction.* Disciplinary encounters are viewed as opportunities to help students develop self-discipline, not simply as occasions to punish misbehavior. Strategies and techniques for correction promote individual responsibility for one's behavior. For example, when correcting misbehavior, teachers ask themselves, "What am I doing to help develop thoughts, feelings, and social skills associated with more appropriate behavior?" Students are taught problem-solving strategies that they can use to help prevent the behavior from recurring and are encouraged to reflect upon the impact of their behavior on themselves and others.			
	Comments:			

(cont.)

		Strength/ weakness rating		Importance rating
		SW	CR	
III.6	*Supports and modifications.* Adults in school reflect upon what they might provide or change in the classroom and the school to improve student behavior. For example, as needed, curriculum adaptations are made; seating arrangements are modified; increased monitoring, supervision, guidance, and reinforcement of positive behavior are provided; and parental and/or peer support is solicited.			
	Comments:			
III.7	*Individual behavior intervention and support plans.* As needed, such as when behavior problems are resistant to routine classroom interventions, individualized behavior intervention and support plans are developed that target individual and environmental factors contributing to the misbehavior. Such plans are implemented as designed, evaluated as to their effectiveness, and modified as needed.			
	Comments:			
III.8	*Principle of minimal sufficiency.* The least amount of external control as necessary and appropriate, either punitive or positive, is used to change behavior. For example, where appropriate, physical proximity and verbal warnings are used before taking away privileges or sending a student to the office. Suspension and expulsion are last resorts and in most cases are used only after all other positive techniques for preventing and correcting misbehavior have already been implemented. When intrinsic motivation for desired behavior is evident, tangible rewards are used sparingly and not in a controlling manner.			
	Comments:			
III.9	*Parental involvement.* Parents are informed immediately when their children's behavior becomes problematic and are included in developing interventions and positive behavior supports.			
	Comments:			

(cont.)

215

		Strength/ weakness rating		Importance rating
		SW	CR	
III.10	*Nondiscriminatory.* In correcting misbehavior, students are not treated differently and unfairly based on culture, race, ethnicity, gender, or disability. For example, data show that African American and Hispanic students do not experience more frequent or harsher consequences than other students for the same behaviors.			
	Comments:			
General Comments for Component III:				

COMPONENT IV: ADDRESSING THE NEEDS OF STUDENTS WHO ARE CURRENTLY EXHIBITING SERIOUS AND CHRONIC BEHAVIOR PROBLEMS (OR ARE AT RISK OF SUCH)

For most students, and most misbehavior, the techniques for developing self-discipline and for preventing and correcting problem behavior are sufficient. However, some students require additional services either because they are currently exhibiting serious or chronic behavior problems or because they are highly at risk of such (as evidenced by early signs of serious and chronic behavior problems, such as frequent referrals to the office). Effective schools are responsive to the needs of students with serious and chronic behavior problems. They also are well prepared in advance for any potential crisis or violent act that is committed by any student or by others.

(cont.)

Reminders: SW = Schoolwide 5 = Major strength, 4 = Strength, 3 = Neither strength nor weakness, 2 = Weakness, 1 = Major weakness 5 = Very important, 4 = Important, 3 = Neutral, 2 = Not important, 1 = Not important at all DK = Don't know	Strength/ weakness rating SW	Importance rating
IV.1 *Universal screening.* A system is in place for screening students who need educational and mental health services (in addition to those services provided to all students). The system includes use of *multiple* measures or methods, such as a close examination of office disciplinary referrals; teacher rankings of students with suspected emotional, social, and academic problem behaviors; teacher ratings of student behavior; and formal observations by support staff of students suspected of having behavior problems.		
Comments:		
IV.2 *Tier 2 interventions.* Evidence-based interventions are provided *early* to those students identified as at risk for behavior problems. *Early* refers to extra resources in the early grades as well as when signs of problem behavior are first observed. Interventions might include anger management training, social skills training (including communication, conflict resolution), individual counseling, mentoring or a "check-in" program, parent management training, and empathy training.		
Comments:		
IV.3 *Tier 3 interventions.* Evidence-based interventions are provided to those students identified as having serious or chronic behavior problems. Such interventions are likely to include those provided for students at Tier 2 but are generally more intensive, individualized, coordinated with outside agencies, and sustained over time than those for students at Tier 2. Eligibility for placement in special education, alternative education, or mental health services would be necessary for some but not all students at Tier 3.		
Comments:		

(cont.)

		Strength/ weakness rating	Importance rating
		SW	
IV.4	*Behavioral intervention and support team.* A team with expertise and skills in the area of behavior problems (e.g., general and special education teachers, school administrators, school psychologist, school counselor, school resource officer, school social worker) meets regularly to help plan and support interventions for students with behavior problems, especially those at Tiers 2 and 3. This includes conducting functional behavioral assessments, as needed, and helping develop individualized behavioral intervention and support plans. A simple, well-defined process exists for school staff to request the team's assistance, and all teachers are familiar with that process. The process is reviewed by teachers and staff as to its effectiveness.		
	Comments:		
IV.5	*Coordination and collaboration.* In providing services, school officials work collaboratively with the student's parents and with community agencies, as needed. These might include social service agencies, police and juvenile justice systems, mental health specialists, businesses, and faith and ethnic leaders. Families (and students, where appropriate) are actively involved in decision making and interventions.		
	Comments:		
IV.6	*Continuum of services and supports.* Students with serious and chronic behavior problems are provided a continuum of academic and behavioral supports and placements. These would include assistance to classroom teachers via collaborative consultation teams and individuals (e.g., school psychologists and other mental health specialists), student counseling, remedial reading, special education, and alternative education classes.		
	Comments:		

(cont.)

		Strength/ weakness rating	Importance rating
		SW	
IV.7	*School safety.* Buildings and grounds have appropriate lighting, alarm systems, fences, locks, etc. Only where appropriate and necessary, surveillance cameras, metal detectors, and locker inspections are used (e.g., in high schools where safety is a clear and substantial problem).		
	Comments:		
IV.8	*Crisis planning.* There is a school crisis plan, and staff are educated as to how to follow it. This requirement includes school staff being aware of early warning signs of potential violence and knowing how to respond appropriately.		
	Comments:		
IV.9	*Peer vigilance in threats of violence.* Students are taught and encouraged to recognize early warning signs of potential violence and to share any concerns they might have about potential school violence.		
	Comments:		
IV.10	*Laws and regulations.* School staff members are knowledgeable of, and follow, all laws and regulations pertaining to schoolwide discipline, particularly those referring to serious and chronic behavior problems. These include laws and regulations pertaining to bullying and criminal acts and the provisions in the Individuals with Disabilities Education Act that govern discipline and children with disabilities (e.g., the need to address behavior problems on a student's individualized education program, limitations to the number of days students with disabilities may be suspended without changing the IEP, the purposes and requirements of manifestation determinations, FBAs, positive behavioral supports and interventions, and behavior intervention plans).		
	Comments:		

(cont.)

General Comments for Component IV:

COMPONENT V. PROGRAM DEVELOPMENT AND EVALUATION

Effective schools continually assess their needs by identifying and acknowledging problems and collecting information regarding the progress toward solutions. Evaluation is ongoing and involves multiple measures. Staff professional development and program changes are responsive to evaluation results.

Reminders: SW = Schoolwide 5 = Major strength, 4 = Strength, 3 = Neither strength nor weakness, 2 = Weakness, 1 = Major weakness 5 = Very important, 4 = Important, 3 = Neutral, 2 = Not important, 1 = Not important at all DK= Don't Know	Strength/ weakness rating SW	Importance rating
V.1 *Representative schoolwide discipline team.* A schoolwide discipline or PBIS team, consisting of a variety of teachers (e.g., general and special education, all grade levels), one or more administrators (preferably the school principal), support staff (e.g., school psychologist, school counselor), and others as appropriate (e.g., students in upper grades, parents) meets regularly to plan, develop, monitor, evaluate, and modify all four components of comprehensive school discipline.		
Comments:		
V.2 *Schoolwide discipline team leadership.* This team provides leadership that is effective in engaging and motivating others to implement all components of comprehensive school discipline. Adequate opportunities are provided for the team to meet and for the faculty to provide input.		
Comments:		

(cont.)

		Strength/ weakness rating	Importance rating
		SW	
V.3	*Integrity of implementation.* Efforts are made via ongoing supervision, monitoring, and/or staff development to ensure that the strategies, techniques, and program components are implemented as planned and with integrity. For example, lessons are taught on self-discipline, staff use positive reinforcement more than punishment, and staff demonstrate support and caring.		
	Comments:		
V.4	*Strengths-and-needs assessment.* A strengths-and-needs assessment, such as this one, is conducted at least annually.		
	Comments:		
V.5	*Individual intervention plans.* Individual intervention and support plans are sufficiently comprehensive, monitored, evaluated as to their effectiveness, and modified as needed.		
	Comments:		
V.6	*Multiple evaluation measures.* Multiple measures of demonstrated reliability and validity are used to evaluate the effectiveness of all the components of comprehensive school discipline. Those measures include office disciplinary referrals, suspensions/expulsions, and surveys of perceptions of school climate by students, teachers, and parents.		
	Comments:		
V.7	*Ongoing evaluation.* The school's evaluation is not stagnant but rather is ongoing. It includes a comparison of measures (listed in V.6) over multiple points in time to gauge improvement.		
	Comments:		

(cont.)

		Strength/ weakness rating	Importance rating
		SW	
V.8	*Use of evaluation results.* Results of a strengths-and-needs assessment and other evaluation measures (including indicators of discipline problems and school climate) are shared with all school staff, parents, and students (as appropriate) as they become available throughout the school year. Results indicating weaknesses are incorporated into the school improvement plan or other plans to improve school discipline.		
	Comments:		
V.9	*Staff development.* Staff development and training are provided, based on program evaluation results and tailored to both individual staff members and schoolwide needs. As needed, staff development and training is provided for all four components of comprehensive school discipline and is sustained (as opposed to one-time workshops on selected topics with no follow-up or evidence of application of what was learned).		
	Comments:		
V.10	*Resource and logistical support.* Adequate resources (i.e., personnel, funding, supervision, training) and time (e.g., time for team meetings and planning) are provided to help achieve each of the components of comprehensive school discipline, as well as program development and evaluation.		
	Comments:		
General Comments for Component V:			

Delaware School Climate Survey
Student Version

1. School name or code: _____

2. Mark your grade: __ 3 __ 4 __ 5 __ 6 __ 7 __ 8 __ 9 __ 10 __ 11 __ 12

3. Mark which you are: ____ Boy or ____ Girl

4. Mark your race: ____ Black ____ White ____ Hispanic ____ Asian ____ Other (includes mixed race)

This survey is about how you feel about your school. Please check the one box that best shows how you feel about each item. Do NOT give your name. No one will know who answered this survey. Please answer every item.

IN THIS SCHOOL. . . .	Disagree A LOT	Disagree	Agree	Agree A LOT
1. Students treat each other with respect.				
2. Teachers treat students of all races with respect.				
3. The school rules are fair.				
4. This school is safe.				
5. The rules in this school are clear.				
6. Students get along with each other.				
7. Teachers care about their students.				
8. The consequences of breaking school rules are fair.				
9. Students threaten and bully others in this school.				
10. Students know how they are expected to act.				
11. Students are friendly with each other.				
12. Adults in this school care about students of all races.				
13. The rules in this school are too harsh.				
14. Students worry about others hurting them in this school.				
15. Students know what the rules are.				
16. Students care about each other.				
17. Teachers listen to students when they have problems.				
18. The school's Code of Conduct is fair.				
19. Students feel safe in this school.				
20. This school makes it clear how students are expected to act.				
21. Students get along with those of other races.				
22. Adults who work in this school care about the students.				
23. The rules in this school are unfair.				
24. Students know they are safe in this school.				

(cont.)

	Disagree A LOT	Disagree	Agree	Agree A LOT
25. The rules in this school are unclear.				
26. The color of your skin doesn't matter to *students* in this school.				
27. The color or your skin doesn't matter to *teachers* in this school.				
28. Adults in this school treat students fairly.				
29. Most students like this school.				

Please check the box that best shows how much you think the following happens *in this school.*	Disagree A LOT	Disagree	Agree	Agree A LOT
1. In this school students are punished a lot.				
2. Students are praised often.				
3. Students are taught to feel responsible for how they act.				
4. Students are often sent out of class for breaking rules.				
5. Students are often given rewards for being good.				
6. Students are taught to understand how others think and feel.				
7. Students are often yelled at by adults.				
8. Teachers let students know when they are being good.				
9. Students are taught they can control their own behavior.				
10. Many students are sent to the office for breaking rules.				
11. Classes get rewards for good behavior.				
12. Students are taught how to solve conflicts with others.				
13. Students are taught they should care about how others feel.				

Delaware School Climate Survey
Teacher and Staff Version

1. School Code: _____

2. Position:

    _____ Classroom teacher   _____ Administrator   _____ Other: _____

    _____ Support staff (e.g., school counselor, school psychologist, intervention specialist, school nurse, etc.)

3. Grade(s) taught. If you teach or support more than one grade level, check all that apply for this school

    __Preschool __K __1 __2 __3 __4 __5 __6 __7 __8 __9 __10 __11 __12

This survey is about how you feel about your school. To make sure that results are confidential, please do not write your name. Your score will be added by a computer with the scores of other staff members to see how all staff members, as a group, feel about the school. Please complete all items.

IN THIS SCHOOL. . . .	Disagree A LOT	Disagree	Agree	Agree A LOT
1. Students treat each other with respect.				
2. Teachers treat students of all races with respect.				
3. The school rules are fair.				
4. This school is safe.				
5. The rules in this school are clear.				
6. Students get along with each other.				
7. Teachers care about their students.				
8. The consequences of breaking school rules are fair.				
9. Students threaten and bully others in this school.				
10. Students know how they are expected to act.				
11. Students are friendly with each other.				
12. Adults in this school care about students of all races.				
13. The rules in this school are too harsh.				
14. Students worry about others hurting them in this school.				
15. Students know what the rules are.				
16. Students care about each other.				
17. Teachers listen to students when they have problems.				
18. The school's Code of Conduct is fair.				
19. Students feel safe in this school.				
20. This school makes it clear how students are expected to act.				
21. Students get along with those of other races.				
22. Adults who work in this school care about the students.				

(cont.)

Delaware School Climate Survey—Teacher and Staff Version *(page 2 of 2)*

IN THIS SCHOOL. . . .	Disagree A LOT	Disagree	Agree	Agree A LOT
23. The rules in this school are unfair.				
24. Students know they are safe in this school.				
25. The rules in this school are unclear.				
26. The color of a student's skin doesn't matter to other *students* in this school.				
27. The color of a student's skin doesn't matter to *teachers* in this school.				
28. Adults in this school treat students fairly.				
29. Most students like this school.				
30. Teachers listen to the concerns of parents.				
31. Teachers do a good job communicating with parents.				
32. Teachers show respect toward parents.				
33. Teachers work closely with parents to help students when they have problems.				
34. Parents are informed not only about their child's misbehavior, but also about good behavior.				

Please check how often each item has happened during the PAST WEEK.	Never	1–2 times	3–5 times	6 or more times
1. I corrected one or more students for violating the school's Code of Conduct.				
2. I praised an individual student for good behavior.				
3. I raised my voice in the classroom to correct the behavior of one or more students.				
4. I gave a token, such as a ticket or a coupon, to one or more students to reward good behavior.				
5. I sent one or more students out of the classroom for misbehavior.				
6. I contacted a parent of a student to tell him/her how well the student was doing.				
7. I sent one or more students to the office for misbehavior.				
8. I rewarded one or more students for good behavior.				
9. I rewarded my class for good behavior.				

Please indicate the extent to which you generally use techniques *other than* reinforcement and consequences to teach students the following. Such techniques would include curriculum lessons, direct teaching, a student conference, class discussion, etc.

	Never	Sometimes	Often	Very often
10. To feel responsible for how they act.				
11. To understand how others think and feel.				
12. That they can control their own behavior.				
13. How to solve conflicts with others.				
14. They should care about how others feel.				

Delaware School Climate Survey
Home Version

School name or code: _____

Your child's grade:

__PreK/K __1 __2 __3 __4 __5 __6 __7 __8 __9 __10 __11 __12

Yourchild'sgender: ____ Boy ____ Girl

Yourchild'srace: ____ Black ____ White ____ Hispanic ____ Asian ____ Other
(includes mixed race)

This survey is about how you feel about your child's school. Please check the box that best shows how you feel about each item. Do NOT give your name. No one will know who answered this survey. Please answer every item.

IN THIS SCHOOL. . . .	Disagree A LOT	Disagree	Agree	Agree A LOT
1. Students treat each other with respect.				
2. Teachers treat students of all races with respect.				
3. The school rules are fair.				
4. This school is safe.				
5. The rules in this school are clear.				
6. Students get along with each other.				
7. Teachers care about their students.				
8. The consequences of breaking school rules are fair.				
9. Students threaten and bully others in this school.				
10. Students know how they are expected to act.				
11. Students are friendly with each other.				
12. Adults in this school care about students of all races.				
13. The rules in this school are too harsh.				
14. Students worry about others hurting them in this school.				
15. Students know what the rules are.				
16. Students care about each other.				
17. Teachers listen to students when they have problems.				
18. The school's Code of Conduct is fair.				
19. Students feel safe in this school.				
20. This school makes it clear how students are expected to act.				
21. Students get along with those of other races.				
22. Adults who work in this school care about the students.				
23. The rules in this school are unfair.				

(cont.)

IN THIS SCHOOL. . . .	Disagree A LOT	Disagree	Agree	Agree A LOT
24. My child feels safe in this school.				
25. The rules in this school are unclear.				
26. The color of a student's skin doesn't matter to other *students* in this school.				
27. The color of a student's skin doesn't matter to *teachers* in this school.				
28. Adults in this school treat students fairly.				
29. My child likes this school.				
30. Teachers listen to the concerns of parents.				
31. Teachers do a good job communicating with parents.				
32. Teachers show respect toward parents.				
33. Teachers work closely with parents to help students when they have problems.				
34. Parents are informed not only about their child's misbehavior, but also about good behavior.				

Please check the box that best shows how much you think the following happens *in this school*.	Disagree A LOT	Disagree	Agree	Agree A LOT
1. In this school students are punished a lot.				
2. Students are praised often.				
3. Students are taught to feel responsible for how they act.				
4. Students are often sent out of class for breaking rules.				
5. Students are often given rewards for being good.				
6. Students are taught to understand how others think and feel.				
7. Students are often yelled at by adults.				
8. Teachers often let students know when they are being good.				
9. Students are taught they can control their own behavior.				
10. Many students are sent to the office for breaking rules.				
11. My child gets a lot of praise from adults.				
12. Students are taught how to solve conflicts with others.				
13. Students are taught they should care about how others feel.				

References

Adelman, H. S., & Taylor, L. (2006). *The school leader's guide to student learning supports: New directions for addressing barriers to learning.* Thousand Oaks, CA: Corwin Press.

Advancement Project/Civil Rights Project. (2000). *Opportunities suspended: The devastating consequences of zero tolerance and school discipline policies.* Cambridge, MA: Harvard University Press.

Ahmed, E. (2006). Understanding bullying from a shame management perspective: Findings from a three-year follow-up study. *Educational and Child Psychology, 23,* 26–40.

Ainsworth, M. D. S. (1989). Attachments beyond infancy. *American Psychologist, 44,* 709–716.

Akin-Little, K. A., Eckert, T. L., Lovett, B. J., & Little, S. G. (2004). Extrinsic reinforcement in the classroom: Bribery or best practice? *School Psychology Review, 33,* 344–362.

Albee, G. W., & Gullotta, T. P. (1997). *Primary prevention's evolution.* In G. W. Albee & T. P. Gullotta (Eds.), *Primary prevention works* (pp. 3–32). New York: Sage.

Albert, L. (1996). *Cooperative discipline.* Circle Pines, MN: American Guidance Service.

Alberto, P. A., & Troutman, A. C. (2006). *Applied behavior analysis for teachers* (7th ed.). Upper Saddle River, NJ: Merrill Prentice-Hall.

American Academy of Pediatrics, Committee on Public Education. (2001). Media violence. *Pediatrics, 108,* 1222–1226.

American Federation of Teachers. (2000). *Building on the best, learning from what works: Five promising discipline and violence prevention programs.* Retrieved March 10, 2009, from *www.aft.org/pubs-reports/downloads/teachers/wwdiscipline.pdf.*

American Psychological Association Zero Tolerance Task Force. (2008). Are zero tolerance policies effective in the schools?: An evidentiary review and recommendations. *American Psychologist, 63,* 852–862.

Ames, C. (1992). Classrooms: Goals, structures, and student motivation. *Journal of Educational Psychology, 84,* 261–271.

Anderson, C. S. (1982). The search for school climate: A review of the research. *Review of Educational Research, 52,* 368–420.

Anderson, J. (2002). Individualized behavior contracts. *Intervention in School and Clinic, 37,* 168–175.

Appleton, J. J., Christenson, S. L., & Furlong, M. J. (2008). Student engagement with school: Critical conceptual and methodological issues of the construct. *Psychology in the Schools, 45,* 369–386.

Ardoin, S. P., & Martens, B. K. (2004). Training children to make accurate self-evaluations: Effects on behavior and the quality of self-ratings. *Journal of Behavioral Education, 13,* 1–23.

Arsenio, W. F., Gold, J., & Adams, E. (2004). Adolescents' emotion expectancies regarding aggressive and nonaggressive events: Connections with behavior problems. *Journal of Experimental Child Psychology, 89,* 338–355.

Arsenio, W. F., & Lemerise, E. A. (2001). Varieties of childhood bullying: Values, emotion processes, and social competence. *Social Development, 10,* 59–73.

Arsenio, W. F., & Lemerise, E. A. (2004). Aggression and moral development: Integrating social information processing and moral domain models. *Child Development, 75,* 987–1002.

Arum, R. (2003). *Judging school discipline: The crisis of moral authority.* Cambridge, MA: Cambridge University Press.

Astor, R. A., Benbenishty, R., Marachi, R., & Meyer, H. A. (2006). In S. R. Jimerson & M. J. Furlong (Eds.), *Handbook of school violence and school safety: From research to practice* (pp. 221–233). Mahwah, NJ: Erlbaum.

Axelrod, S. (1996). What's wrong with behavior analysis? *Journal of Behavioral Education, 6,* 247–256.

Baer, D. M., Wolf, M. M., & Risley, T. R. (1968). Some current dimensions of applied behavior analysis. *Journal of Applied Behavior Analysis, 1,* 91–97.

Bagley, W. C. (1908). *Classroom management: Its principles and technique.* New York: Macmillan.

Balfanz, R., Herzog, L., & Mac Iver, D. J. (2007). Preventing student disengagement and keeping students on the graduation path in urban middle-grades schools: Early identification and effective interventions. *Educational Psychologist, 42,* 223–235.

Bambara, L. M. (2005). Evolution of positive behavior support. In L. M. Bambara & L. Kern (Eds.), *Individualized supports for students with problem behaviors: Designing positive behavior plans* (pp. 1–24). New York: Guilford Press.

Bandura, A. (1986). *Social foundations of thought and action: A social cognitive theory.* Upper Saddle River, NJ: Prentice-Hall.

Bandura, A. (1991). Social cognitive theory of moral thought and action. In W. M. Kurtines & J. L. Gewirtz (Eds.), *Handbook of moral behavior and development* (pp. 45–103). Mahwah, NJ: Erlbaum.

Bandura, A. (1997). *Self-efficacy: The exercise of control.* New York: Freeman.

Bandura, A. (2001). Social cognitive theory: An agentic perspective. *Annual Review of Psychology. 52,* 1–26.

Bandura, A. (2002). Selective moral disengagement in the exercise of moral agency. *Journal of Moral Education. 31,* 101–119.

Bandura, A., Caprara, G. V., Barbaranelli, C., Pastorelli, C., & Regalia, C. (2001). Sociocognitive self-regulatory mechanisms governing transgressive behavior. *Journal of Personality and Social Psychology, 80,* 125–135.

Barber, B. L., Eccles, J. S., & Stone, M. R. (2001). Whatever happened to the jock, the brain, and the princess?: Young adult pathways linked to adolescent activity involvement and social identity. *Journal of Adolescent Research, 16,* 429–455.

Barker, G. P., & Graham, S. (1987). Developmental study of praise and blame as attributional cues. *Journal of Educational Psychology, 79,* 62–66.

Barkley, R. A., Shelton, T. L., Crosswait, C., Moorehouse, M., Fletcher, K., Barrett, S., et al. (2002). Preschool children with disruptive behavior: Three-year outcome as a function of adaptive disability. *Development and Psychopathology, 14,* 45–67.

Barriga, A. Q., Landau, J. R., Stinson, B. L., Liau, A. K., & Gibbs, J. C. (2000). Cognitive distortion and problem behaviors in adolescents. *Criminal Justice and Behavior, 27,* 36–56.

Barrish, H. H., Saunders, M., & Wolf, M. M. (1969). Good behavior game: Effects of individual contingencies for group consequences on disruptive behavior in a classroom. *Journal of Applied Behavior Analysis, 2,* 119–124.

Barton, L. E., Brulle, A. R., & Repp, A. C. (1983). Aversive techniques and the doctrine of the least restrictive alternative. *Exceptional Education Quarterly, 3,* 1–8.

Batsche, G. M., & Porter, L. J. (2006). Bullying. In G. G. Bear & K. M. Minke (Eds.), *Children's needs III: Development, prevention, and intervention* (pp. 135–148). Bethesda, MD: National Association of School Psychologists.

Battistich, V., & Hom, A. (1997). The relationship between students' sense of their school as a community and their involvement in problem behaviors. *American Journal of Public Health, 87,* 1997–2001.

Battistich, V., Schaps, E., Watson, M., Solomon, D., & Lewis, C. (2000). Effects of the Child Development Project on students' drug use and other problem behaviors. *Journal of Primary Prevention, 21,* 75–99.

Battistich, V., Solomon, D., Watson, M., & Schaps, E. (1997). Caring school communities. *Educational Psychologist, 32.* 137–151.

Baumrind, D. (1968). Authoritarian vs. authoritative parental control. *Adolescence, 3,* 255–272.

Baumrind, D. (1971). Current patterns of parental authority. *Developmental Psychology Monographs, 4*(2).

Baumrind, D. (1996). The discipline controversy revisited. *Family Relations, 45,* 405–414.

Beaman, R., & Wheldall, K. (2000). Teachers' use of approval and disapproval in the classroom. *Educational Psychology, 20,* 431–446.

Bear, G. G. (1998). School discipline in the United States: Prevention, correction, and long-term social development. *School Psychology Review, 27,* 14–32.

Bear, G. G. (with A. Cavalier & M. Manning). (2005). *Developing self-discipline and preventing and correcting misbehavior.* Boston: Allyn & Bacon.

Bear, G. G. (2007). School-wide approaches to behavior problems. In B. Doll & J. Cummings (Eds.), *Transforming school mental health services: Population-based approaches to promoting the competency and wellness in children* (pp. 103–141). Thousand Oaks, CA: Corwin Press.

Bear, G. G. (2008). Best practices in classroom discipline. In A. Thomas & J. Grimes (Eds.), *Best practices in schools psychology* (5th ed.; Vol. 4, pp. 1403–1420). Bethesda, MD: National Association of School Psychologists.

Bear, G. G. (2009). The positive in positive models of discipline. In R. Gilman, E. S. Huebner, & M. Furlong (Eds.), *Handbook of positive psychology* (pp. 305–321). New York: Routledge.

Bear, G. G., Blank, J., & Pell, M. (2009, February). *What's positive about school-wide positive behavioral supports?* Paper presented at the meeting of the National Association of School Psychologists, Boston.

Bear, G. G., Giancola, S. P., Veach, J., & Goetz, L. (2006). Beyond face validity: When less is more. In S. Jimerson & M. J. Furlong (Eds.), *The handbook of school violence and school safety: From research to practice* (pp. 537–552). Mahwah, NJ: Erlbaum.

Bear, G. G., Manning, M. A., & Izard, C. (2003). Responsible behavior: The importance of social cognition and emotion. *School Psychology Quarterly, 18,* 140–157.

Bear, G. G., Manning, M. A., & Shiomi, K. (2006). Children's reasoning about aggression: Differences between Japan and the United States and implications for school discipline. *School Psychology Review, 35,* 62–77.

Bear, G. G., Quinn, M., & Burkholer, S. (2002). *Interim alternative educational settings and children with disabilities.* Bethesda, MD: National Association of School Psychologists.

Bear, G. G., & Rys, G. (1994). Moral reasoning, classroom behavior, and sociometric status among elementary school children. *Developmental Psychology, 30,* 633–638.

Bear, G. G., Smith, C., Blank, J., & Chen, F. F. (under review). *The Delaware School Climate Survey— Student: Evidence of confirmatory and concurrent validity.*

Bear, G. G., & Watkins, J. M. (2006). Developing self-discipline. In G. G. Bear & K. M. Minke (Eds.), *Children's needs III: Development, prevention, and intervention* (pp. 29–44). Bethesda, MD: National Association of School Psychologists.

Bear, G. G., Webster-Stratton, C., Furlong, M., & Rhee, S. (2000). Preventing aggression and violence. In K. M. Minke & G. G. Bear (Eds.), *Preventing school problems—promoting school success: Strategies and programs that work* (pp. 1–69). Bethesda, MD: National Association of School Psychologists.

Benner, A. D., Graham, S., & Mistry, R. S. (2008). Discerning direct and mediated effects of ecological structures and processes on adolescents' educational outcomes. *Developmental Psychology, 44,* 840–854.

Berkowitz, L. (1989a). Situational influences on aggression. In J. Groebel & R. A. Hinde (Eds.), *Aggression and war: Their biological and social bases* (pp. 91– 100). Thousand Oaks, CA: Sage.

Berkowitz, L. (1989b). Frustration–aggression hypothesis: Examination and reformulation. *Psychology Bulletin, 106,* 59–73.

Berkowitz, M. W., & Bier, M. C. (2004). Research-based character education. *Annals of the American Academy of Political and Social Science, 591,* 72–85.

Berkowitz, M. W., & Schwartz, M. (2006). Character education. In G. G. Bear & K. M. Minke (Eds.), *Children's needs III: Development, prevention, and intervention* (pp. 15–27). Bethesda, MD: National Association of School Psychologists.

Berkowitz, M. W., Sherblom, S., Bier, M., & Battistich, V. (2006). Educating for positive youth development. In M. Killen & J. Smetana (Eds.), *Handbook of moral development* (pp. 683–701). Mahwah, NJ: Erlbaum.

Bierman, K. L., Coie, J. D., Dodge, K. A., Foster, E. M., Greenberg, M. T., Lochman, J. E., et al. (2007). Fast track randomized controlled trail to prevent externalizing psychiatric disorders: Findings from grades 3 to 9. *Journal of the American Academy of Child and Adolescent Psychiatry, 46,* 1250–1262.

Birnbaum, P. (1962). *A treasury of Judaism.* New York: Hebrew Publishing.

Birch, S. H., & Ladd, G. W. (1998). Children's interpersonal behaviors and the teacher–child relationship. *Developmental Psychology, 34,* 934–946.

Blair, R. J. R., Monson, J., & Frederickson, N. (2001). Moral reasoning and conduct problems in children with emotional and behavioural difficulties. *Personality and Individual Differences, 31,* 799–811.

Bohanon, H., Fenning, P., Carney, K. L., Minnis-Kim, M. J., Anderson-Harriss, S., Moroz, K. B., et al. (2006). Schoolwide application of positive behavior support in an urban high school: A case study. *Journal of Positive Behavior Interventions, 8,* 131–145.

Bowlby, J. (1982). *Attachment and loss: Vol. 1. Attachment* (2nd ed.). New York: Basic Books.

Bradshaw, C. P., Koth, C. W., Bevans, K. B., Ialongo, N., & Leaf, P. (2008). The impact of school-wide positive behavioral interventions and supports (PBIS) on the organizational health of elementary schools. *School Psychology Quarterly, 23,* 462–473.

Brand, S., Felner, R., Shim, S., Seitsinger, A., & Dumas, T. (2003). Middle school improvement and reform: Development and validation of a school-level assessment of climate, cultural pluralism, and school safety. *Journal of Educational Psychology, 95,* 570–588.

Briesch, A. M., & Cahfouleas, S. M. (2009). Review and analysis of literature on self-management interventions to promote appropriate classroom behaviors (1988–2008). *School Psychology Quarterly, 24,* 106–118

Brock, L. L., Nishida, T. K., Chiong, C., Grimm, K., & Rimm-Kaufman, S. E. (2008). Children's perceptions of the classroom environment and social and academic performance: A longitudinal analysis of the contribution of the Responsive Classroom approach. *Journal of School Psychology, 46*, 129–149.

Bronfenbrenner, U. (1979). *The ecology of human development*. Cambridge, MA: Harvard University Press.

Brophy, J. E. (1981). On praising effectively. *Elementary School Journal, 81*, 269–278.

Brophy, J. E. (1996). *Teaching problem students*. New York: Guilford Press.

Brophy, J. E. (2004). *Motivating students to learn*. Mahwah, NJ: Erlbaum.

Brophy, J. E., & McCaslin, M. (1992). Teachers' reports of how they perceive and cope with problem students. *Elementary School Journal, 93*, 3–68.

Brown, A. L., & Palincsar, A. (1989). Guided cooperative learning and individual knowledge acquisition. In L. Resnick (Ed.), *Knowing, learning, and procedure* (pp. 393–452). Hillsdale, NJ: Erlbaum.

Brownell, M. T., Ross, D. D., Colón, E. P., & McCallum, C. L. (2005). Critical features of special education teacher preparation: A comparison with general teacher education, *Journal of Special Education, 38*, 242–252.

Bru, E., Murberg, T. A., & Stephens, P. (2001). Social support, negative life events and pupil misbehavior among young Norwegian adolescents. *Journal of Adolescence, 24*, 715–727.

Bru, E., Stephens, P., & Torsheim, T. (2002). Students' perceptions of class management and reports of their own misbehavior. *Journal of School Psychology, 40*, 287–307.

Buhs, E. S., & Ladd, G. W. (2001). Peer rejection as an antecedent of young children's school adjustment: An examination of the mediating process. *Developmental Psychology, 37*, 550–560.

Buhs, E. S., Ladd, G. W., & Herald, S. L. (2006). Peer exclusion and victimization: Processes that mediate the relation between peer group rejection and children's classroom engagement and achievement. *Journal of Educational Psychology, 98*, 1–13.

Bullis, M., Walker, H., & Sprague, J. R. (2001). A promise unfulfilled: Social skills training with at-risk and antisocial children and youth. *Exceptionality, 9*, 67–90.

Burchard, J., Burns, E., & Burchard, S. (2002). The wraparound approach. In B. Burns & K. Hoagwood (Eds.), *Community treatment for youth: Evidence-based interventions for severe emotional and behavioral disorders* (pp. 69–90). New York: Oxford University Press.

Burks, V. S., Laird, R. D., Dodge, K. A., Pettit, G. S., & Bates, J. E. (1999). Knowledge structures, social information processing, and children's aggressive behavior. *Social Development, 8*, 220–236.

Burnett, P. C. (2002). Teacher praise and feedback and students' perceptions of the classroom environment. *Educational Psychology, 22*, 1–16.

Burrell, N., Zirbel, C. S., & Allen, M. (2003). Evaluating peer mediation outcomes in educational settings: A meta-analytic review. *Conflict Resolution Quarterly, 21*, 7–26.

Caldarella, P., Christensen, L., Kramer, T. J., & Kronmiller, K. (2009). The effects of Strong Start on second grade students' emotional and social competence. *Early Childhood Education Journal, 37*, 51–56.

California Task Force to Promote Self-Esteem and Personal and Social Responsibility. (1990). *Toward a state of esteem: The final report of the California Task Force to Promote Self-Esteem and Personal and Social Responsibility*. Sacramento, CA: Author.

Cameron, J. (2001). Negative effects of reward on intrinsic motivation—a limited phenomenon: Comment on Deci, Loestner, and Ryan. *Review of Educational Research, 71*, 29–42.

Cameron, J., & Pierce, W. D. (1994). Reinforcement, reward, and intrinsic motivation: A meta-analysis. *Review of Educational Research, 64*, 363–423.

Camodeca, M., & Goossens, F. A. (2005). Aggression, social cognitions, anger and sadness in bullies and victims. *Journal of Child Psychology and Psychiatry, 46*, 186–197.

Cangelosi, J. S. (2007). *Classroom management strategies: Gaining and maintaining students' cooperation* (6th ed.). Hoboken, NJ: Wiley.

Canter, L. (1976). *Assertive discipline: A take charge approach for today's educator.* Santa Monica, CA: Canter and Associates.

Canter, L., & Canter, M. (2001). *Assertive discipline: Positive behavior management for today's classroom.* Los Angeles, CA: Canter and Associates.

Caprara, G. V., Barbaranelli, C., Pastorelli, C., Bandura, A., & Zimbardo, P. G. (2000). Prosocial foundations of children's academic achievement. *Psychological Science, 11,* 302–306.

Catalano, R. F., Berglund, M. L., Ryan, J. A. M., Lonczak, H. S., & Hawkins, J. D. (2004). Positive youth development in the United States: Research findings on evaluations of positive youth development programs. *Annals of the American Academy of Political and Social Science, 591,* 98–124.

Center for Effective Discipline. (2009). *Discipline and the law.* Retrieved July 13, 2009, from *www.stophitting.com/index.php?page=statesbanning.*

Center for Mental Health in Schools. (2008). *Mental health in schools and school improvement: Current status, concerns, and new directions.* Los Angeles, CA: Author.

Character Education Partnership. (2004). *Character education: Questions and answers.* Washington, DC: Author.

Charles, C. M. (2008a). *Building classroom discipline* (9th ed.). Boston: Pearson.

Charles, C. M. (2008b). *Today's best classroom management strategies: Paths to positive discipline.* Boston: Pearson.

Charney, R. S. (2002). *Teaching children to care: Classroom management for ethical and academic growth, K–8* (rev. ed.). Greenfield, MA: Northeast Foundation for Children.

Chinman, M., Imm, P., & Wandersman, A. (2004). *Getting to outcomes: Promoting accountability through methods and tools for planning, implementation, and evaluation.* Santa Monica, CA: RAND Corporation.

Christenson, S. L., & Sheridan, S. M. (2001). *Schools and families: Creating essential connections for learning.* New York: Guilford Press.

Clever, A., Bear, G. G., & Juvonen, J. (1992). Discrepancies between competence and importance in self-perceptions of children in integrated classrooms. *Journal of Special Education, 26,* 125–138.

Cohen, R., Kincaid, D., & Childs, K. E. (2007). Measuring school-wide positive behavior support implementation: Development and validation of the benchmarks of quality. *Journal of Positive Behavior Interventions, 9,* 203–213.

Cohen, J., McCabe, E. M., Michelli, N. M., & Pickeral, T. (2009). School climate: Research, policy, practice, and teacher education. *Teachers College Record, 111,* 180–213.

Cohen, D., & Strayer, J. (1996). Empathy in conduct-disordered and comparison youth. *Developmental Psychology, 32,* 988–998.

Colby, A., & Damon, W. (1999). The development of extraordinary moral commitment. In M. Killen & D. Hart (Eds.), *Morality in everyday life: Developmental perspectives* (pp. 342–370). New York: Cambridge University Press.

Collaborative for Academic, Social, and Emotional Learning. (2005). *Safe and sound: An educational leader's guide to evidence-based social and emotional learning programs—Illinois edition.* Retrieved February 28, 2009, from *www.casel.org.*

Comer, J. P., Haynes, N. M., Joyner, E. T., & Ben-Avie, M. (Eds.). (1996). *Rallying the whole village: The Comer process for reforming education.* New York: Teachers College Press.

Committee for Children. (2001). *Steps to Respect: A bullying prevention program.* Seattle, WA: Author.

Committee for Children. (2003). *Second Step: A violence prevention curriculum.* Seattle, WA: Author.

Coogan, B. A., Kehle, T. J., Bray, M. A., & Chafouleas, S. M. (2007). Group contingencies, randomization of reinforcers, and criteria for reinforcement, self-monitoring, and peer feedback on reducing inappropriate classroom behavior. *School Psychology Quarterly, 22,* 540–556.

Corcoran, J., & Pillai, V. K. (2007). Effectiveness of secondary pregnancy prevention programs: A meta-analysis. *Research on Social Work Practice, 17,* 5–18.

Corporation for National and Community Service. (n.d.). *What is service-learning?* Retrieved July 20, 2009, from *www.servicelearning.org/what-service-learning*.

Covington, M. V. (1984). The self-worth theory of achievement motivation: Findings and implications. *The Elementary School Journal, 85,* 5–20.

Covington, M. V. (2000). Goal theory, motivation, and school achievement: An integrative review. *Annual Review of Psychology, 51,* 171–200.

Crick, N. R., & Dodge, K. A. (1994). A review and reformulation of social information-processing mechanisms in children's social adjustment. *Psychological Bulletin, 115,* 74–101.

Crick, N. R., & Ladd, G. W. (1990). Children's perceptions of the outcomes of aggressive strategies: Do the ends justify being mean? *Developmental Psychology, 26,* 612–620.

Crone, D. A., & Horner, R. H. (2003). *Building positive behavior support systems in schools: Functional behavioral assessment.* New York: Guilford Press.

Crone, D. A., Horner, R. H., & Hawken, L. S. (2004). *Responding to problem behavior in schools: The Behavior Education Program.* New York: Guilford Press.

Croninger, R. G., & Lee, V. E. (2001). Social capital and dropping out of high school: Benefits to at-risk students of teachers' support and guidance. *Teachers College Record, 103,* 548–581.

Crozier, J. C., Dodge, K. A., Fontaine, R. G., Lansford, J. E., Bates, J. E., Pettit, G. S., et al. (2008). Social information processing and cardiac predictors of adolescent antisocial behavior. *Journal of Abnormal Psychology, 117,* 253–267.

Curtis, M. J., Batsche, G. M., & Mesmer, E. M. (2000). Implementing the IDEA 1997 amendments: A compelling argument for systems change. In C. F. Telzrow & M. Tankersley (Eds.), *IDEA amendments of 1997: Practice guidelines for school-based teams* (pp. 383–410). Bethesda, MD: National Association of School Psychologists.

Curtis, J. C., Castillo, J. M., & Cohen, R. M. (2008). Best practices in system-level change. In A. Thomas and J. Grimes (Eds.), *Best practices in school psychology* (5th ed., Vol. 3, pp. 887–902). Bethesda, MD: National Association of School Psychologists.

Curwin, R. L., Mendler, A. N., & Mendler, B. D. (2008). *Discipline with dignity: New challenges, new solutions.* Alexandria, VA: Association for Supervision and Curriculum Development.

Daly, M. D., Jacob, S., King, D. W., & Cheramie, G. (1984). The accuracy of teacher predictions of student reward preferences. *Psychology in the Schools, 21,* 520–524.

Damon, W. (2004). What is positive youth development? *Annals of the American Academy of Political and Social Science, 591,* 13–24.

Davidson, L. M., & Demaray, M. K. (2007). Social support as a moderator between victimization and internalizing–externalizing distress from bullying. *School Psychology Review, 36,* 383–405.

Day, H. M., Horner, R. H., & O'Neill, R. E. (1994). Multiple functions or problem behaviors: Assessment and intervention. *Journal of Applied Behavior Analysis. Special Issue: Functional analysis approaches to behavioral assessment and treatment, 27,* 279–289.

de Castro, B. O., Merk, W., Koops, W., Veerman, J. W., & Bosch, J. D. (2005). Emotions in social information processing and their relations with reactive and proactive aggression in referred aggressive boys. *Journal of Clinical Child and Adolescent Psychology, 34,* 105–116.

de Castro, B. O., Veerman, J. W., Koops, W., Bosch, J., & Monshouwer, J. J. (2002). Hostile attribution of intent and aggressive behavior: A meta-analysis. *Child Development, 73,* 916–934.

Deci, E. L., Koestner, R., & Ryan, R. M. (1999). A meta-analytic review of experiments examining the effects of extrinsic rewards on intrinsic motivation. *Psychological Bulletin, 125,* 627–668.

Deci, E. L., Koestner, R., & Ryan, R. M. (2001). Extrinsic rewards and intrinsic motivation in education: Reconsidered once again. *Review of Educational Research, 71,* 1–27.

Deming, A. M., & Lochman, J. E. (2008). The relation of locus of control, anger, and impulsivity to boys' aggressive behavior. *Behavioral Disorders, 33,* 108–119.

Desimone, L. (2002). How can comprehensive school reform models be successfully implemented? *Review of Educational Research, 72,* 433–479.

Dewey, J. (1960). *Theory of the moral life.* New York: Holt, Rinehart & Winston. (Original work published 1908)

DiBiase, A., Gibbs, J. C., & Potter, G. B. (2005). *EQUIP for educators: Teacher youth to think and act responsibility.* Champaign, IL: Research Press.

Dixon, R. A., & Lerner, R. M. (1999). History and systems in developmental psychology. In M. H. Bornstein & M. E. Lamb (Eds.), *Developmental psychology: An advanced textbook* (2nd ed., pp. 3–45). Hillsdale, NJ: Erlbaum.

Dodge, K. A., Coie, J. D., & Lynam, D. (2006). Aggression and antisocial behavior in youth. In W. Damon & R. M. Learner (Series Ed.), & N. Eisenberg (Vol. Ed.), *Handbook of child psychology: Vol. 3. Social, emotional, and personality development* (6th ed., pp. 719–788). New York: Wiley.

Dolan, L., Turkan, J., Werthamer-Larsson, L., & Kellam, S. (1989). *The Good Behavior Game training manual.* Baltimore: Johns Hopkins Prevention Research Center. Retrieved June 27, 2009, from *www.jhsph.edu/prevention/Publications/gbg.pdf.*

Dolan, L. J., Kellam, S. G., Brown, C. H., Werthamer-Larsson, L., Rebok, G. W., Mayer, L. S., et al. (1993). The short-term impact of two classroom-based preventive interventions on aggressive and shy behaviors and poor achievement. *Journal of Applied Developmental Psychology, 14,* 165–176.

Doll, B., & Cummings, J. A. (2007). Why population-based services are essential for school mental health, and how to make them happen in your school. In B. Doll & J. Cummings (Eds.), *Transforming school mental health services: Population-based approaches to promoting competency and wellness in children* (pp. 1–19). Thousand Oaks, CA: Corwin Press.

Doll, B., Kurien, S., LeClair, C., Spies, R., Champion, A., & Osborn, A. (2009). The ClassMaps Survey: A framework for promoting positive classroom environments. In R. Gilman, S. Huebner, & M. Furlong (Eds.), *Handbook of positive psychology in the schools* (pp. 213–227). New York: Routledge.

Doll, B., Zucker, S., & Brehm, K. (2004). *Resilient classrooms: Creating healthy environments for learning. Practical intervention in the schools series.* New York: Guilford Press.

Doyle, W. (1986). Classroom management techniques and student discipline. Washington, DC: Office of Educational Research and Improvement.

Dreikurs, R., & Grey, L. (1968). *Logical consequences: A handbook of discipline.* New York: Meredith Press.

Duckworth, A. L., & Seligman, M. E. P. (2005). Self-discipline outdoes IQ in predicting academic performance of adolescents. *Psychological Science, 16,* 939–944.

Duke, D. L. (2002). *Creating safe schools for all children.* Boston: Allyn & Bacon.

Dunlap, G., Sailor, W., Horner, R. H., & Sugai, G. (2009). Overview and history of positive behavior support. In W. Sailor, G. Dunlap, G. Sugai, & R. Horner (Eds.), *Handbook of positive behavior support* (pp. 3–16). New York: Springer.

DuPaul, G. J., & Eckert, T. L. (1994). The effects of social skills curricula: Now you see them, now you don't. *School Psychology Quarterly, 9,* 113–132.

Durlak, J. A., & Dupre, E . P. (2008). Implementation matters: A review of research on the influence of implementation on program outcomes and the factors affecting implementation. *American Journal of Community Psychology, 41,* 327–350.

Durlak, J. A., Taylor, R. D., Kawashima, K., Pachan, M. K., DuPre, E. P., Celio, C. I., et al. (2007). Effects of positive youth development programs on school, family, and community systems. *American Journal of Community Psychology, 39,* 269–286.

Durlak, J. A., & Weissberg, R. P., & Pachan, M. (in press). A meta-analysis of after-school programs that seek to promote personal and social skills in children and adolescents. *American Journal of Community Psychology.*

Durlak, J. A., & Wells, A. M. (1997). Primary prevention mental health programs for children and adolescents: A meta-analytic review. *American Journal of Community Psychology, 25,* 115–152.

Dweck, C. S. (1999, Spring). Caution—praise can be dangerous. *American Educator, 23*(1), 1–5.

Eisenberg, N. (2006). Introduction. In W. Damon & R. M. Learner (Series Ed.), & N. Eisenberg (Vol. Ed.), *Handbook of child psychology: Vol. 3. Social, emotional, and personality development* (6th ed., pp. 1–23). New York: Wiley.

Eisenberg, N., Cialdini, R. B., McCreath, H., & Shell, R. (1989). Consistency-based compliance in children: When and why do consistency procedures have immediate effects? *Journal of Behavioral Development, 12,* 351–367.

Eisenberg, N., Fabes, R. A., & Spinrad, T. L. (2006). Prosocial behavior. In W. Damon & R. M. Learner (Series Ed.), & N. Eisenberg (Vol. Ed.), *Handbook of child psychology: Vol. 3. Social, emotional, and personality development* (6th ed., pp. 646–718). New York: Wiley.

Elias, M. J., Zins, J. E., Weissberg, R. P., Frey, K. S., Greenberg, M. T., Haynes, N. M., et al. (1997). *Promoting social and emotional learning: Guidelines for educators.* Alexandria, VA: Association for Supervision and Curriculum Development.

Elwell, W. C., & Tiberio, J. (1994). Teacher praise: What students want. *Journal of Instructional Psychology, 21,* 322–328.

Embry, D. D. (2002). The Good Behavior Game: A best practice candidate as a universal behavioral vaccine. *Clinical Child and Family Psychology Review, 5,* 273–297.

Epstein, M., Atkins, M., Cullinan, D., Kutash, K., & Weaver, R. (2008). *Reducing behavior problems in the elementary school classroom: A practice guide* (NCEE No. 2008-012). Washington, DC: National Center for Education Evaluation and Regional Assistance, Institute of Education Sciences, U. S. Department of Education. Retrieved from *ies.ed.gov/ncee/wwc/publications/practiceguides.*

Epstein, M. H., Nordness, P. D., Gallagher, K., Nelson, J. R., Lewis, L., & Schrepf, S. (2005). School as the entry point: Assessing adhering to the basic tenets of the wraparound approach. *Behavioral Disorders, 30,* 85–93.

Erdley, C. A., & Asher, S. R. (1999). A social goals perspective on children's social competence. *Journal of Emotional and Behavioral Disorders, 7,* 156–167.

Ervin, R. A., Schaughency, E., Matthews, A., Goodman, S. D., & McGlinchey, M. T. (2007). Primary and secondary prevention of behavior difficulties: Developing a data-informed problem-solving model to guide decision making at a school-wide level. *Psychology in the Schools, 44,* 7–18.

Espelage, D. L., & Swearer, S. M. (Eds.). (2004). *Bullying in American schools: A social-ecological perspective on prevention and intervention.* Mahwah, NJ: Erlbaum.

Evertson, C. M., & Emmer, E. T. (2008). *Classroom management for elementary teachers* (8th ed.). Boston: Allyn & Bacon.

Evertson, C. M., Emmer, E. T., & Worsham, M. E. (2006). *Classroom management for elementary teachers* (7th ed.). Boston: Allyn & Bacon.

Evertson, C. M., & Weinstein, C. S. (Eds.). (2006). *Handbook of classroom management: Research, practice, and contemporary issues.* Mahwah, NJ: Erlbaum.

Fantuzzo, J., & Ginsburg-Block, M. (1998). Reciprocal peer tutoring: Developing and testing effective peer collaborations for elementary school students. In K. J. Topping & S. Ehly (Eds.), *Peer assisted learning* (pp. 121–144). Hillsdale, NJ: Erlbaum.

Fantuzzo, J. W., & Rohrbeck, C. A. (1991). Teachers' use and children's preferences of rewards in elementary school. *Psychology in the Schools, 28,* 175–181.

Fay, J., & Funk, D. (1995). *Teaching with love and logic: Taking control of the classroom.* Golden, CO: Love and Logic Press.

Fitzgerald, P. D., & Van Schoiack-Edstrom, L. (2006). Second Step: A violence prevention curriculum. In S. R. Jimerson & M. J. Furlong (Eds.), *Handbook of school violence and school safety: From research to practice* (pp. 383–395). Mahwah, NJ: Erlbaum.

Fontaine, R. G., Yang, C., Dodge, K. A., Pettit, G. S., & Bates, J. E. (2009). Development of response evaluation and decision (red) and antisocial behavior in childhood and adolescence. *Developmental Psychology, 45,* 447–459.

Ford, M. E., Wentzel, K. R., Wood, D., Stevens, E., & Sisfield, G. A. (1989). Processes associated with integrative social competence: Emotional contextual influences on adolescent social responsibility. *Journal of Adolescent Research, 4,* 405–425.

Fredricks, J. A., Blumenfeld, P. C., & Paris, A. H. (2004). School engagement: Potential of the concept, state of the evidence. *Review of Educational Research, 74,* 59–109.

Fredricks, J. A., & Eccles, J. S. (2006a). Is extracurricular participation associated with beneficial outcomes: Concurrent and longitudinal relations? *Developmental Psychology, 42,* 698–713.

Fredricks, J. A., & Eccles, J. S. (2006b). Extracurricular involvement and adolescent adjustment: Impact of duration, number of activities, and breadth of participation. *Applied Developmental Science, 10,* 132–146.

Fredricks, J. A., & Eccles, J. S. (2008). Participation in extracurricular activities in the middle school years: Are there developmental benefits for African American and European American youth? *Journal of Youth and Adolescence, 37,* 1029–1043.

Freiberg, H. J. (1999). Beyond behaviorism. In H. J. Freiberg (Ed.), *Beyond behaviorism: Changing the classroom management paradigm* (pp. 3–20). Needham Heights, MA: Allyn & Bacon.

Freiberg, H. J., & Lapointe, J. M. (2006). In research-based programs for preventing and solving discipline problems. In C. M. Evertson & C. S. Weinstein (Eds.), *Handbook of classroom management: Research, practice, and contemporary issues* (pp. 735–786). Mahwah, NJ: Erlbaum.

French, D. C., & Conrad, J. (2001). School dropout as predicted by peer rejection and antisocial behavior. *Journal of Research on Adolescence, 11,* 225–244.

Frick, P. J., & White, S. F. (2008). Research review: The importance of callous–unemotional traits for developmental models of aggressive and antisocial behavior. *Journal of Child Psychology and Psychiatry, 49,* 359–375.

Fullan, M. (2007). *The new meaning of educational change* (4th ed.). New York: Teachers College Press.

Gable, R. A., Hester, P. H., Rock, M. L., & Hughes, K. G. (2009). Back to basics: Rules, praise, ignoring, and reprimands, revisited. *Intervention in School and Clinic, 44,* 195–205.

Gathercoal, F. (2001). *Judicious discipline* (5th ed.). San Francisco: Caddo Gap Press.

George, H. P., Harrower, J. K., & Knoster, T. (2003). School-wide prevention and early intervention: A process for establishing a system of school-wide behavior support. *Preventing School Failure, 47,* 170–176.

George, M. P., White, G. P., & Schlaffer, J. J. (2007). Implementing school-wide behavior change: Lessons from the field. *Psychology in the Schools, 44,* 41–51.

Geunyoung, K., Walden, T., Harris, V., Karrass, J., & Catron, T. (2007). Positive emotion, negative emotion, and emotion control in the externalizing problems of school aged children. *Child Psychiatry and Human Development, 37,* 221–239.

Giancola, S. P., & Bear, G. G. (2003). Face validity: Perspectives from a local evaluator. *Psychology in the Schools, 40,* 515–529.

Gibbs, J. C., Potter, G. B., & Goldstein, A. P. (1995). *The EQUIP program: Teaching youth to think and act responsibly through a peer-helping approach.* Champaign, IL: Research Press.

Gilman, R., Huebner, E. S., & Furlong, M. (Eds.). (2009). *Handbook of positive psychology.* New York: Routledge.

Gina, G. (2006). Social cognition and moral cognition in bullying: What's wrong? *Aggressive Behavior, 32,* 528–539.

Ginsburg-Block, M. D., Rohrbeck, C. A., & Fantuzzo, J. W. (2006). A meta-analytic review of social, self-concept, and behavioral outcomes of peer-assisted learning. *Journal of Educational Psychology, 98,* 732–749

Ginsburg-Block, M., Rohrbeck, C., Fantuzzo, J., & Lavigne, N. (2006). Peer-assisted learning strategies. In G. G. Bear & K. M. Minke (Eds.), *Children's needs III: Development, prevention, and intervention* (pp. 631–645). Bethesda, MD: National Association of School Psychologists.

Glasser, W. (1965). *Reality therapy.* New York: Harper & Row.

Glasser, W. (1969). *Schools without failure.* New York: Harper & Row.

Glasser, W. (1986). *Control theory in the classroom.* New York: Harper & Row.

Glasser, W. (1998). *The quality school: Managing students without coercion.* New York: Harper & Row.

Goldstein, A. P., Harootunian, B., & Conoley, J. C. (1994). *Student aggression: Prevention, management, and replacement training.* New York: Guilford Press.

Goleman, D. (1995). *Emotional intelligence.* New York: Bantam.

Gonzales, N., Cauce, A., Friedman, R., & Mason, C. (1996). Family, peer and neighborhood influences on academic achievement among African-American adolescents: One-year prospective effects. *American Journal of Community Psychology, 24,* 365–387.

Good, T. L., & Brophy, J. E. (2007). *Looking in classrooms* (10th ed.). Boston: Allyn & Bacon.

Gordon, T. (2003). *TET: Teacher effectiveness training.* New York: Three Rivers Press.

Gorman-Smith, D., Tolan, P. H., & Henry, D. B. (2000). Patterns of family functioning and adolescent outcomes among urban African American and Mexican American families. *Journal of Family Psychology, 14,* 436–457.

Gottfredson, D. C. (2001). *Schools and delinquency.* New York: Cambridge University Press.

Gottfredson, D. C., Gottfredson, G. D., & Hybl, L. G. (1993). Managing adolescent behavior: A multiyear, multischool study. *American Educational Research Journal, 30,* 179–215.

Gottfredson, D. C., Gottfredson, G. D., Skroban, S. (1996). A multimodel school-based prevention demonstration. *Journal of Adolescent Research, 11,* 97–115.

Gottfredson, G. D., Gottfredson, D. C., Payne, A. A., & Gottfredson, N. C. (2005). School climate predictors of school disorder: Results from a national study of delinquency prevention in schools. *Journal of Research in Crime and Delinquency, 42,* 412–444.

Greenberg, M. T., Domitrovich, C., & Bumbarger, B. (2001). The prevention of mental disorders in school-aged children: Current state of the field. *Prevention and Treatment, 4,* 1–62.

Greenberg, M. T., & Kusche, C. A. (2006). Building social and emotional competence: The PATHS curriculum. In S. R. Jimerson & M. J. Furlong (Eds.), *Handbook of school violence and school safety: From research to practice* (pp. 395–412). Mahwah, NJ: Erlbaum.

Greenwood, C. R., Maheady, L., & Delquadri, J. (2002). Classwide peer tutoring programs. In M. R. Shinn, H. M. Walker, & G. Stoner (Eds.), *Interventions for academic and behavior problems II: Preventive and remedial approaches* (pp. 611–649). Bethesda, MD: National Association of School Psychologists.

Gregory, A., Cornell, D., Fan, X., Sheras, P., Shih, T., & Huang, F. (in press). High school practices associated with lower student bullying and victimization. *Journal of Educational Psychology.*

Gregory, A., & Weinstein, R. S. (2004). Connection and regulation at home and in school: Predicting growth in achievement for adolescents. *Journal of Adolescent Research, 19,* 405–427.

Gregory, A., & Weinstein, R. S. (2008). A window on the discipline gap: Cooperation or defiance in the classroom. *Journal of School Psychology, 46,* 455–475.

Gresham, F. M. (2002). Social skills assessment and instruction for students with emotional and behavioral disorders. In K. L. Lane, F. M. Gresham & T. E. O'Shaughnessy (Eds.), *Interventions for children with or at risk for emotional and behavioral disorders* (pp. 242–258). Boston: Allyn & Bacon.

Gresham, F. M. (2004). Current status and future directions of school-based behavioral interventions. *School Psychology Review, 33*, 326–343.

Gresham, F. M., McIntyre, L. L, Olson-Tinker, H., Dolstra, L., McLaughlin, V., & Van, M. (2004). Relevance of functional behavioral assessment research for school-based interventions and positive behavioral support. *Research in Developmental Disabilities, 25*, 19–37.

Gresham, F. M., Sugai, G., & Horner, R. H. (2004). Interpreting outcomes of social skills training for students with high-incidence disabilities. *Exceptional Children, 67*, 331–344.

Grusec, J. E., & Goodnow, J. J. (1994). Impact of parental discipline methods on the child's internalization of values: A reconceptualization of current points of view. *Developmental Psychology, 30*, 4–19.

Grusec, J. E., & Redler, E. (1980). Attribution, reinforcement, and altruism: A developmental analysis. *Developmental Psychology, 16*, 525–534.

Gun-Free Schools Act of 1994. Public Law 103–382. 108 Statute 3907. Title 14.

Guerra, N. G. (1989). Consequential thinking and self-reported delinquency in high-school youth. *Criminal Justice and Behavior, 16*, 440–454.

Guerra, N. G., Huesmann, L. R., & Hanish, L. (1995). The role of normative beliefs in children's social behavior. In N. Eisenberg (Ed.), *Social development: Review of personality and social psychology* (pp. 140–158). Thousand Oaks, CA: Sage.

Guerra, N. G., & Slaby, R. G. (1989). Evaluative factors in social problem solving by aggressive boys. *Journal of Abnormal Child Psychology, 17*, 277–289.

Hahn, R., Fuqua-Whitley, D., Wethington, H., Lowy, J., Crosby, A., Fullilove, M., et al. (2007). Effectiveness of universal school-based programs to prevent violent and aggressive behavior: A systematic review. *American Journal of Preventive Medicine, 33*(Suppl. 2S), 114–129.

Hamre, B., & Pianta, R. (2001). Early teacher–child relationships and the trajectory of children's school outcomes through eighth grade. *Child Development, 72*, 625–638.

Hamre, B. K., & Pianta, R. C. (2006). Student–teacher relationships. In G. G. Bear & K. M. Minke (Eds.), *Children's needs III: Development, prevention, and intervention* (pp. 59–71). Bethesda, MD: National Association of School Psychologists.

Hamre, B. K., Pianta, R. C., Downer, J. T., & Mashburn, A. J. (2008). Teachers' perceptions of conflict with young students: Looking beyond problem behaviors. *Social Development, 17*, 115–136.

Hardy, S. A., & Carlo, G. (2005). Identity as a source of moral motivation. *Human Development, 48*, 232–256.

Hart, D., Atkins, R., & Donnelly, T. M. (2006). Community service and moral development. In M. Killen & J. Smetana (Eds.), *Handbook of moral development* (pp. 633–656). Mahwah, NJ: Erlbaum.

Hart, D., Matsuba, M. K., & Atkins, R. (2008). The moral and civic effects of learning to serve. In L. P. Nucci & D. Narvaez (Eds.), *Handbook of moral and character education* (pp. 484–499). New York: Routledge.

Harter, S. (1999). *The construction of the self: A developmental perspective*. New York: Guilford Press.

Harter, S. (2006). The self. In W. Damon & R. M. Learner (Series Ed.), & N. Eisenberg (Vol. Ed.), *Handbook of child psychology: Vol. 3. Social, emotional, and personality development* (6th ed., pp. 505–570). New York: Wiley.

Hartshorne, H., & May, M. A. (1928). *Studies in the nature of character: Vol. I. Studies in deceit*. New York: Macmillan.

Hattie, J., & Timperley, H. (2007). The power of feedback. *Review of Educational Research, 77*, 81–112.

Henderlong, J., & Lepper, M. R. (2002). The effects of praise on children's intrinsic motivation. A review and synthesis. *Psychological Bulletin, 128*, 774–795.

Henrich, C. C., Brookmeyer, K. A., & Shahar, G. (2005). Weapon violence in adolescence: Parent and school connectedness as protective factors. *Journal of Adolescent Health, 37,* 306–312.

Hirschstein, M., & Frey, K. S., (2006). Promoting behavior and beliefs that reduce bullying: The Steps to Respect program. In S. R. Jimerson & M. J. Furlong (Eds.), *Handbook of school violence and school safety: From research to practice* (pp. 309–323). Mahwah, NJ: Erlbaum.

Hirischi, T. (1969). *Causes of delinquency.* Berkeley: University of California Press.

Hoff, K. E., & Sawka-Miller, K. D. (2010). Self-management interventions. In G. Gimpel Peacock, R. A. Ervin, E. J. Daly, III, & K. W. Merrell (Eds.), *Practical handbook of school psychology: Effective practices for the 21st century* (pp. 337–352). New York: Guilford Press.

Hoffman, M. L. (2000). *Empathy and moral development: Implications for caring and justice.* Cambridge, UK: Cambridge University Press.

Hoglund, W. L. G., Lalonde, C. E., & Leadbeater, B. J. (2008). Social-cognitive competence, peer rejection and neglect, and behavioral and emotional problems in middle childhood. *Social Development, 17,* 528–553.

Horner, R. H. (2000). Positive behavior supports. *Focus on Autism and other Developmental Disabilities, 15,* 97–105.

Horner, R. (2009, March). *Expanding the science, values, and vision of positive behavior support.* Keynote address presented at the sixth annual International Conference on Positive Behavior Support. Retrieved June 16, 2009, from *www.pbis.org.*

Horner, R. H., Sugai, G., Smolkowski, K., Eber, L., Nakasato, J., Todd, A. W., et al. (2009). A randomized, wait-list controlled effectiveness trial assessing School-Wide Positive Behavior Support in elementary schools. *Journal of Positive Behavior Interventions, 11,* 133–144.

Horner, R. H., Sugai, G., Todd, A. W., & Lewis-Palmer, T. (2005). Schoolwide behavior support. In L. M. Bambara & L. Kern (Eds.), *Individualized supports for students with problem behaviors: Designing positive behavior plans* (pp. 359–390). New York: Guilford Press.

Horner, R. H., Todd, A. W., Lewis-Palmer, T., Irvin, L. K., Sugai, G., & Boland, J. B. (2004). The Schoolwide Evaluation Tool (SET): A research instrument for assessing school-wide positive behavior support. *Journal of Positive Behavior Interventions, 6,* 3–12.

Hoy, W., & Feldman, J. (1987). Organizational health: The concept and its measure. *Journal of Research and Development in Education, 20,* 30–38.

Hubbard, J. A., Dodge, K. A., Cillessen, A., H. N., Coie, J. D., & Schwartz, D. (2001). The dyadic nature of social information processing in boys' reactive and proactive aggression. *Journal of Personality and Social Psychology, 80,* 268–280.

Huesmann, L. R. (1988). An information processing model for the development of aggression. *Aggressive Behavior, 14,* 13–24.

Hughes, C., & Lloyd, J. W. (1993). An analysis of self-management. *Journal of Behavioral Education, 3,* 405–425.

Hughes, J. N., Cavell, T. A., & Willson, V. (2001). Further support for the developmental significance of the quality of the teacher–student relationship. *Journal of School Psychology, 39,* 289–301.

Hughes, J. N., & Hill, C. R. (2006). Lying. In G. G. Bear & K. M. Minke (Eds.), *Children's needs III: Development, prevention, and intervention* (pp. 159–169). Bethesda, MD: National Association of School Psychologists.

Hunley, S. (2008). Best practices for preparing learning space to increase engagement. In A. Thomas & J. Grimes (Eds.), *Best practices in school psychology V* (pp. 813–826). Bethesda: National Association of School Psychologists.

Hyman, I. A., & Perone, D. C. (1998). The other side of school violence: Educator policies and practices that may contribute to student misbehavior. *Journal of School Psychology, 3,* 7–27.

Ialongo, N., Poduska, J., Werthamer, L., & Kellam, S. (2001). The distal impact of two first-grade preventive interventions on conduct problems and disorder in early adolescence. *Journal of Emotional and Behavioral Disorders, 9,* 146–160.

Ialongo, N. S., Werthamer, L., Kellam, S. G., Brown, C. H., Wang, S., & Lin, Y. (1999). Proximal impact of two first-grade preventive interventions on the early risk behaviors for later substance abuse, depression, and antisocial behavior. *American Journal of Community Psychology, 27,* 599–641.

Izard, C. E. (1991). *The psychology of emotions.* New York: Plenum Press.

Izard, C. E. (2002). Translating emotion theory and research into preventive interventions. *Psychological Bulletin, 128,* 796–824.

Jekielek, S., Kristin, M. A., Moore, A., & Hair, E. C. (2002). *Mentoring programs and youth development: A synthesis.* Washington, DC: Child Trends.

Johnson, D. W., & Johnson, R. T. (1999). Making cooperative learning work. *Theory into Practice, 38,* 67–73.

Johnson, D. W., & Johnson, R. T. (2005). *Teaching students to be peacemakers.* Edina, MN: Interaction Book Company.

Johnson, D. W., & Johnson, R. T. (2006). Conflict resolution, peer mediation, and peacemaking. In C. M. Evertson & C. S. Weinstein (Eds.), *Handbook of classroom management: Research, practice, and contemporary issues* (pp. 803–832). Mahwah, NJ: Erlbaum.

Johnson, R. T., & Johnson, D. W. (2002). Teaching students to be peacemakers: A meta-analysis. *Journal of Research in Education, 12,* 25–39.

Jolliffe, D., & Farrington, D. P. (2004). Empathy and offending: A systematic review and meta–analysis. *Aggressive and Violent Behavior, 9,* 441–476.

Jones, V., & Jones, L. (2010). *Comprehensive classroom management: Creating communities of support and solving problems* (9th ed.). Upper Saddle River, NJ: Merrill.

Juvonen, J. (2007). Reforming middle schools: Focus on continuity, social connectedness, and engagement. *Educational Psychologist, 42,* 197–208.

Kanouse, D. E., Gumpert, P., & Canavan-Gumpert, D. (1981). The semantics of praise. In J. H. Harvey, W. Ickes, & R. F. Kidd (Eds.), *New directions in attribution research* (Vol. 3, pp. 97–115). Hillsdale, NJ: Erlbaum.

Kauffman, J. M., & Brigham, F. J. (2000). Editorial: Zero tolerance and bad judgment in working with students with emotional or behavioral disorders. *Behavioral Disorders, 25,* 277–279.

Kauffman, J. M., Conroy, M., Gardner, R., & Oswald, D. (2008). Cultural sensitivity in the application of behavior principles to education. *Education and Treatment of Children, 31,* 239–262.

Kauffman, J. M., & Landrum, T. J. (2008). *Characteristics of emotional and behavioral disorders of children and youth* (8th ed.). Columbus, OH: Merrill.

Kavale, K. A., Mathur, S. R., & Mostert, M. P. (2004). Social skills training and teaching social behavior to students with emotional and behavioral disorders. In R. B. Rutherford, M. M. Quinn, & S. R. Mathur (Eds.), *Handbook of research in emotional and behavioral disorders* (pp. 446–461). New York: Guilford Press.

Kazdin, A. E. (1981). Behavior modification in education: Contributions and limitations. *Developmental Review, 1,* 34–57.

Kazdin, A. E. (2003). Problem-solving skills training and parent management training for conduct disorder. In A. E. Kazdin & J. R. Weisz (Eds.), *Evidence-based psychotherapies for children and adolescents* (pp. 241–262). New York: Guilford Press.

Kellam, S. G., & Anthony, J. C. (1998). Targeting early antecedents to prevent tobacco smoking: Findings from an epidemiologically based randomized field trial. *American Journal of Public Health, 88,* 1490–1495.

Kellam, S. G., Brown, C. H., Poduska, J., Ialongo, N., Wang, W., Toyinbo, P., et al. (2008). Effects of a universal classroom behavior management program in first and second grades on young adult behavioral, psychiatric, and social outcomes. *Drug and Alcohol Dependence, 95,* S5–S28.

Kellam, S. G., Ling, X., Merisca, R., Brown, C. H., & Ialongo, N. (1998). The effect of the level of aggression in the first grade classroom on the course and malleability of aggressive behavior into middle school. *Development and Psychopathology, 10,* 165–185.

Kellam, S. G., Rebok, G. W., Ialongo, N., & Mayer, L. S., (1994). The course and malleability of aggressive behavior from early first grade into middle school: Results of a developmental epidemiologically-based preventive trial. *Journal of Child Psychology and Psychiatry, 35,* 259–282.

Kelley, M. L., Power, T. G., & Winbush, D. D. (1992). Determinants of disciplinary practices in low-income Black mothers. *Child Development, 63,* 573–582.

Kern, L., & Clemens, N. H. (2007). Antecedent strategies to promote appropriate classroom behavior. *Psychology in the Schools, 44,* 65–75.

Kerr, M. M., & Nelson, C. M. (2009). *Strategies for addressing behavior problems in the classroom* (4th ed.). Upper Saddle River, NJ: Pearson.

Knoff, H. M. (2005). *Student discipline, positive behavior supports and management, and school safety: A conceptual blueprint for schools and school districts.* Little Rock, AR: Project Achieve Press.

Knoff, H. M. (2008). Best practices in implementing statewide positive behavioral support systems. In A. Thomas & J. Grimes (Eds.), *Best practices in schools psychology* (5th ed., Vol. 3, pp. 749–763). Bethesda, MD: National Association of School Psychologists.

Kochanska, G. (2002). Committed compliance, moral self, and internalization: A mediational model. *Developmental Psychology, 38,* 339–351.

Kohlberg, L. (with R. Mayer). (1981). Development as the aim of education: The Dewey view. In L. Kohlberg, *Essays on moral development: Vol. 1. The philosophy of moral development* (pp. 49–100). New York: Harper & Row.

Kohlberg, L. (1984). *Essays on moral development: Vol. 2. The psychology of moral development.* New York: Harper & Row.

Kohn, A. (1996). *Beyond discipline: From compliance to community.* Alexandria, VA: Association for Supervision and Curriculum.

Kohn, A. (1999). *Punished by rewards: The trouble with gold stars, incentive plans, A's, praise, and other bribes.* Boston: Houghton Mifflin.

Koth, C. W., Bradshaw, C. P., & Leaf, P. J. (2008). A multilevel study of predictors of student perceptions of school climate: The effect of classroom-level factors. *Journal of Educational Psychology, 100,* 96–104.

Kounin, J. (1970). *Discipline and group management in classrooms.* New York: Holt, Rinehart & Winston.

Kounin, J. S., & Gump, P. (1974). Signal systems of lesson settings and the task-related behavior of preschool children. *Journal of Educational Psychology, 66,* 554–562.

Kratchowill, T. R. (2008). Best practices in school-based problem-solving consultation: Applications in prevention and intervention systems. In A. Thomas & J. Grimes (Eds.), *Best practices in schools psychology* (5th ed., Vol. 5, pp. 1673–1688). Bethesda, MD: National Association of School Psychologists.

Kurdek, L. A., & Fine, M. A. (1994). Family acceptance and family control as predictors of adjustment in young adolescents: Linear, curvilinear, or interactive effects? *Child Development, 65,* 1137–1146.

Kusche, C. A., & Greenberg, M. T. (2000). *The PATHS (Promoting Alternative Thinking Strategies) curriculum.* South Deerfield, MA: Channing-Bete.

Kuther, T. L. (2000). Moral reasoning, perceived competence, and adolescent engagement in risky activity. *Journal of Adolescence, 23*, 599–604.

Laible, D., Eye, J., & Carlo, G. (2008). Dimensions of conscience in mid-adolescence: Links with social behavior, parenting, and temperament. *Journal of Youth and Adolescence, 37*, 875–887

Lamborn, S. D., Mounts, N. S., Steinberg, L., & Dornbusch, S. M. (1991). Patterns of competence and adjustment among adolescents from authoritative, authoritarian, indulgent, and neglectful families. *Child Development, 62*, 1049–1065.

Landrum, T. J., & Kauffman, J. M. (2006). Behavioral approaches to classroom management. In C. M. Evertson & C. S. Weinstein (Eds.), *Handbook of classroom management: Research, practice, and contemporary issues* (pp. 47–71). Mahwah, NJ: Erlbaum.

Lansford, J. E., Malone, P. S., Dodge, K. A., Crozier, J. C., Pettit, G. S., & Bates, J. E. (2006). A 12-year prospective study of patterns of social information processing problems and externalizing behaviors. *Journal of Abnormal Child Psychology, 34*, 715–724.

Lassen, S. R., Steele, M. M., & Sailor, W. (2006). The relationship of school-wide positive behavior support to academic achievement in an urban middle school. *Psychology in the Schools, 43*, 701–712.

Lepper, M. (1983). Social-control processes and the internalization of social values: An attributional perspective. In E. T. Higgins, D. Ruble, & W. Hartup (Eds.), *Social cognition and social development: A socio-cultural perspective* (pp. 294–330). New York: Cambridge University Press.

Lepper, M. R., Corpus, J. H., & Iyengar, S. S. (2005). Intrinsic and extrinsic motivational orientations in the classroom: Age differences and academic correlates. *Journal of Educational Psychology, 97*, 184–196.

Lepper, M. R., & Woolverton, M. (2002). The wisdom of practice: Lessons learned from the study of highly effective tutors. In J. Aronson (Ed.), *Improving academic achievement: Contributions of social psychology* (pp. 135–158). Orlando, FL: Academic Press.

Lewis, T. J., Newcomer, L. L., Trussell, R., & Richter, M. (2006). Schoolwide Positive Behavior Support: Building systems to develop and maintain appropriate social behavior. In C. M. Evertson & C. S. Weinstein (Eds.), *Handbook of classroom management: Research, practice, and contemporary issues* (pp. 833–854). Mahwah, NJ: Erlbaum.

Lewis, T. J., Sugai, G., & Colvin, G. (1998). Reducing problem behavior through a school-wide system of effective behavioral support: Investigation of a school-wide social skills training program and contextual interventions. *School Psychology Review, 27*, 446–459.

Lickona, T. (2004). *Character matters: How to help our children develop good judgment, integrity, and other essential virtues.* New York: Touchstone.

Lochman, J. E., Powell, N. R., Clanton, N., & McElroy, H. K. (2006). Anger and aggression. In G. G. Bear & K. M. Minke (Eds.), *Children's needs III: Development, prevention, and intervention* (pp. 115–133). Bethesda, MD: National Association of School Psychologists.

Lohrmann-O'Rourke, S., Knoster, T., Sabatine, K., Smith, D., Horvath, B., & Llewellyn, G. (2000). School-wide application of PBS in the Bangor Area School District. *Journal of Positive Behavior Interventions, 2*, 238–240.

Lösel, F., & Beelman, A. (2003). Effects of child skills training in preventing antisocial behavior: A systematic review of randomized evaluations. *Annals of the American Academy of Political and Social Science, 587*, 84–109.

Lösel, F., Bliesener, T., & Bender, D. (2007). Social information processing, experiences of aggression in social contexts, and aggressive behavior in adolescents. *Criminal Justice and Behavior, 34*, 330–347.

Lovegrove, M. N., Lewis, R., Fall, C., & Lovegrove, H. (1985). Students' preferences for discipline practices in schools. *Teaching and Teacher Education, 1*, 325–333.

Lovett, B. J., & Sheffield, R. A. (2007). Affective empathy deficits in aggressive children and adolescents: A critical review. *Clinical Psychology Review, 27,* 1–13.

Luiselli, J. K., Putnam, R. F., & Sunderland, M. (2002). Longitudinal evaluation of behavior support intervention in a public middle school. *Journal of Positive Behavior Interventions, 4,* 182–188.

Lynam, D. R., Milich, R., Zimmerman, R., Novak, S. P., Logam, T. K., Martin, C., et al. (1999) Project DARE: No effects at 10-year follow-up. *Journal of Consulting and Clinical Psychology, 67,* 590–593.

Maag, J. W. (2001). Rewarded by punishment: Reflections on the disuse of positive reinforcement in schools. *Exceptional Children, 67,* 173–186.

Mahoney, J. L. (2000). School extracurricular activity participation as a moderator in the development of antisocial patterns. *Child Development, 71,* 502–516.

Mahoney, J. L., & Cairns, R. B. (1997). Do extracurricular activities protect against early school dropout? *Developmental Psychology, 33,* 241–253.

Mahoney, J. L., Schweder, A. E., & Stattin, H. (2002). Structured after-school activities as a moderator of depressed mood for adolescents with detached relations to their parents. *Journal of Community Psychology, 30,* 69–86.

Malecki, C. K., & Elliott, S. (2002). Children's social behaviors as predictors of academic achievement: A longitudinal analysis. *School Psychology Quarterly, 17,* 1–23.

Malti, T., Gasser, L., & Buchmann, M. (2009). Aggressive and prosocial children's emotion attributions and moral reasoning. *Aggressive Behavior, 35,* 90–102.

Mandara, J., & Murray, C. B. (2002). Development of an empirical typology of African American family functioning. *Journal of Family Psychology, 16,* 318–337.

Manning, M. A., & Bear, G. G. (2002). Are children's concerns about punishment related to their aggression? *Journal of School Psychology, 40,* 523–539.

Marquis, J. G., Horner, R. H., Carr, E. G., Turnbull, A. P., Thompson, M., Behrens, G. A., et al. (2000). A meta-analysis of positive behavior support. In R. M. Gersten, E. P. Schiller, & S. Vaughn (Eds.), *Contemporary special education research: Syntheses of the knowledge base on critical instructional issues. The LEA series on special education and disability* (pp. 137–178). Mahwah, NJ: Erlbaum.

Martella, R. C., Nelson, J. R., & Marchand-Martella, N. E. (2003). *Managing disruptive behaviors in the schools: A schoolwide, classroom, and individualized social learning approach.* Boston, MA: Allyn & Bacon.

Martens, B. K., Peterson, R. L., Witt, J. C., & Cirone, S. (1986). Teacher perceptions of school-based interventions. *Exceptional Children, 53,* 213–223.

Martens, B. K., Witt, J. C., Daly, E. J., III, & Vollmer, T. R. (1999). Behavior analysis: Theory and practice in educational settings. In C. R. Reynolds & T. B. Gutkin (Eds.), *Handbook of school psychology* (pp. 638–663). New York: Wiley.

Marzano, R. J. (2003). *Classroom management that works: Research-based strategies for every teacher.* Alexandria, VA: Association for Supervision and Curriculum Development.

Mayer, M. J., & Leone, P. E. (1999). A structural analysis of school violence and disruption: Implications for creating safer schools. *Education and Treatment of Children, 22,* 333–356.

McClellan, B. E. (1999). *Moral education in America: Schools and the shaping of character from colonial times to the present.* New York: Teachers College Press.

McIntosh, K., Chard, D. J., Boland, J. B., & Horner, R. H. (2006). Demonstration of combined efforts in school-wide academic and behavioral systems and incidence of reading and behavior challenges in early elementary grades. *Journal of Positive Behavior Interventions, 8,* 146–154.

McKevitt, B. C., & Braaksma, A. D. (2008). Best practices in developing a positive behavior support system at the school level. In A. Thomas & J. Grimes (Eds.), *Best practices in school psychology* (5th ed., Vol. 3, pp. 735–747). Bethesda, MD: National Association of School Psychologists.

McLaughlin, T. F. (1975). The applicability of token reinforcement systems in public school systems. *Psychology in the Schools, 12,* 84–89.

Meehan, B. T., Hughes, J. N., & Cavell, T. A. (2003). Teacher–student relationships as compensatory resources for aggressive children. *Child Development, 74,* 1145–1157.

Menesini, E., & Camodeca, M. (2008). Shame and guilt as behaviour regulators: Relationships with bullying, victimization, and prosocial behaviour. *British Journal of Developmental Psychology, 26,* 183–196.

Menesini, E., Sanchez, V., Fonzi, A., Ortega, R., Costabile, A., & Lo Feudo, G. (2003). Moral emotions and bullying: A cross-national comparison of differences between bullies, victims and outsiders. *Aggressive Behavior, 29,* 515–530.

Merrell, K. W., & Gueldner, B. A. (2010). *Social and emotional learning in schools: Promoting mental health and academic success.* New York: Guilford Press.

Merrell, K. W., Gueldner, B. A., Ross, S. W., & Isava, D. M. (2008). How effective are school bullying intervention programs?: A meta-analysis of intervention research. *School Psychology Quarterly, 23,* 26–42.

Meyers, J., Meyers, A. B., Proctor, S. L., & Graybill, E. C. (2009). Organizational consultation and systems intervention. In T. B. Gutkin & C. R. Reynolds (Eds.). *The handbook of school psychology* (4th ed., pp. 821–940). Hoboken, NJ: Wiley.

Mikami, A. Y., Lee, S. S., Hinshaw, S. P., & Mullin, B. C. (2008). Relationships between social information processing and aggression among adolescent girls with and without ADHD. *Journal of Youth and Adolescence, 37,* 761–771.

Minke, K. M. (2006). Parent–teacher relationships. In G. G. Bear & K. M. Minke (Eds.), *Children's needs III: Development, prevention, and intervention* (pp. 73–85). Bethesda, MD: National Association of School Psychologists.

Minke, K. M., & Bear, G. G. (2000). *Preventing school problems—promoting school success: Strategies and programs that work.* Bethesda, MD: National Association of School Psychologists.

Mitchell, J. M., Johnson, D. W., & Johnson, R. T. (2002). Are all types of cooperation equal?: Impact of academic controversy versus concurrence-seeking on health education. *Social Psychology of Education, 5,* 329–344.

Montessori, M. (1974). Disciplining children. In R. C. Oren (Ed.), *Montessori: Her method and the movement. What you need to know* (pp. 136–154). New York: G. P. Putnam's Sons. (Original work published 1912)

Morrison, G. M., Redding, M., Fisher, E., & Peterson, R. (2006). Assessing school discipline. In S. R. Jimerson & M. J. Furlong (Eds.), *Handbook of school violence and school safety: From research to practice* (pp. 211–220). Mahwah, NJ: Erlbaum.

Morrone, A. S., & Pintrich, P. R. (2006). Achievement motivation. In G. G. Bear & K. M. Minke (Eds.), *Children's needs III: Development, prevention, and intervention* (pp. 431–442). Bethesda, MD: National Association of School Psychologists.

Murdock, T. B. (1999). The social context of risk: Predictors of alienation in middle school. *Journal of Educational Psychology, 91,* 62–75.

Murdock, T. B., Hale, N. M., & Weber, M. J. (2001). Predictors of cheating among early adolescents: Academic and social motivations. *Contemporary Educational Psychology, 26,* 96–115.

Muscott, H. S., Mann, E. L., & LeBrun, M. R. (2008). Positive behavioral interventions and supports in New Hampshire: Effects of a large-scale implementation of schoolwide positive behavior support on student discipline and academic achievement. *Journal of Positive Behavior Interventions, 10,* 190–205.

Myers, B. K., & Holland, K. L. (2000). Classroom behavioral interventions: Do teachers consider the function of the behavior? *Psychology in the Schools, 37,* 271–280.

Natasi, B. K., & Clements, D. H. (1991). Research on cooperative learning: Implications for practice. *School Psychology Review, 20,* 110–137.

Nelsen, J., Lott, L., & Glenn, H. (2000). *Positive discipline in the classroom.* Rocklin, CA: Prima.

Nelson, R. J., Smith, D. J., Young, R. K., & Dodd, J. M. (1991). A review of self-management outcome research conducted with students who exhibit behavioral disorders. *Behavioral Disorders, 16,* 169–179.

Noddings, N. (2002). *Educating moral people: A caring alternative to character education.* New York: Teachers College Press.

O'Brennan, L. M., Bradshaw, C. P., & Sawyer, A. L. (2009). Examining developmental differences in the social-emotional problems among frequent bullies, victims, and bully/victims. *Psychology in the Schools, 46,* 100–115.

O'Leary, K. D., & Drabman, R. (1971). Token reinforcement programs in the classroom: A review. *Psychological Bulletin, 75,* 379–398.

O'Leary, K. D., & O'Leary. S. G. (Eds.). (1977). *Classroom management: The successful use of behavior modification* (2nd ed.). New York: Pergamon Press.

Osher, D., Bear, G. G., Sprague, J. R., & Doyle, W. (2010). How can we improve school discipline? *Educational Researcher, 39,* 48–58.

Osterman, K. F. (2000). Students' need for belonging in the school community. *Review of Educational Research, 70,* 323–367.

Palmer, E. J., & Hollin, C. R. (2001). Sociomoral reasoning, perceptions of parenting, and self-reported delinquency in adolescents. *Applied Cognitive Psychology, 15,* 85–100.

Parke, R. D., & Buriel, R. (2006). Socialization in the family: Ethnic and ecological perspectives. In W. Damon & R. M. Learner (Series Ed.), & N. Eisenberg (Vol. Ed.), *Handbook of child psychology: Vol. 3. Social, emotional, and personality development* (6th ed., pp. 429–504). New York: Wiley.

Parker, J. G., & Asher, S. R. (1993). Friendship and friendship quality in middle childhood: Links with peer group acceptance and feelings of loneliness and social dissatisfaction. *Developmental Psychology, 29,* 611–621.

Peterson, C., & Seligman, M. E. P. (2004). *Character strengths and virtues: A handbook and classification.* Washington, DC: American Psychological Association.

Peterson, L. D., Young, K. R., Salzberg, C. L., West, R. P., & Hill, M. (2006). Using self-management procedures to improve classroom social skills in multiple general education settings. *Education and Treatment of Children, 29,* 1–21.

Petras, H., Kellam, S. G., Brown, C. H., Muth´en, B. O., Ialongo, N. S., Poduska, J. M. (2008). Developmental epidemiological courses leading to ASPD and violent and criminal behavior: Effects by young adulthood of a universal preventive intervention in first- and second-grade classrooms. *Drug and Alcohol Dependence, 95,* S45–S59.

Piaget, J. (1965). *The moral judgment of the child.* New York: Free Press. (Original work published 1932)

Pianta, R. C. (1999). *Enhancing relationships between children and teachers.* Washington, DC: American Psychological Association.

Pintrich, P. R. (2000). Multiple goals, multiple pathways: The role of goal orientation in learning and achievement. *Journal of Educational Psychology, 92,* 544–555.

Planty, M., Hussar, W., Synder, T., Kena, G., Kewal Ramani, A., Kemp, J., et al. (2009). The Condition of Education 2009 (NCES 2009-081). Washington, DC: National Center for Education Statistics, Institute of Education Statistics, U.S. Department of Education.

Poduska, J., Kellam, S., Wang,W., Brown, C. H., Ialongo, N., Toyinbo, P., (2008). Impact of the good behavior game, a universal classroom-based behavior intervention, on young adult service use for problems with emotions, behavior, or drugs or alcohol. *Drug and Alcohol Dependence, 95,* S29–S44.

Power, F. C., Higgins, A., & Kohlberg, L. (1989). *Lawrence Kohlberg's approach to moral education.* New York: Columbia University Press.

Quiggle, N. L., Garber, J., Panak, W. F., & Dodge, K. A. (1992). Social information processing in aggressive and depressed children. *Child Development, 63,* 1305–1320.

Raths, L., Harmin, M., & Simon, S. (1966). *Values and teaching.* Columbus, OH: Merrill.

Raub, A. N. (1882). *School management.* Lock Haven, PA: Wescott & Thompson.

Reeve, R. E., & Weiss, M. R. (2006). Sports and physical activities. In G. G. Bear & K. M. Minke (Eds.), *Children's needs III: Development, prevention, and intervention* (pp. 485–498). Bethesda, MD: National Association of School Psychologists.

Reimers, T. M., Wacker, D. P., & Koeppl, G. (1987). Acceptability of behavioral interventions: A review of the literature. *School Psychology Review, 16,* 212–227.

Reschly, A., & Christenson, S. L. (2006). School completion. In G. G. Bear & K. M. Minke (Eds.), *Children's needs III: Development, prevention, and intervention* (pp. 103–113). Bethesda, MD: National Association of School Psychologists.

Riley-Tillman, T. C., Chafouleas, S. M., & Briesch, A. M. (2007). A school practitioner's guide to using daily behavior report cards to monitor student behavior. *Psychology in the Schools, 44,* 77–89.

RMC Research Corporation. (2009). *K–12 Service-Learning Project planning toolkit.* Scotts Valley, CA: National Service-Learning Clearinghouse. Retrieved July 20, 2009, from: *www.servicelearning. org/filemanager/download/K12_ServiceLearning_Project_Planning_Toolkit.pdf*

Rose, L. C., & Gallup, A. M. (2000). The 32nd annual Phi Delta Kappa/Gallup Poll of the public's attitudes toward the public schools. *Phi Delta Kappan, 82,* 41–66.

Rosén, L. A., Taylor, S. A., O'Leary, S. G., & Sanderson, W. (1990). A survey of classroom management practices. *Journal of School Psychology, 28,* 257–269.

Rubin, K. H., Bukowski, W. M., & Parker, J. G. (2006). Peer interactions, relationships, and groups. In W. Damon & R. M. Learner (Series Ed.), & N. Eisenberg (Vol. Ed.), *Handbook of child psychology: Vol. 3. Social, emotional, and personality development* (6th ed., pp. 571–645). New York: Wiley.

Rueger, S. Y., Malecki, C. K., & Demaray, M. K. (2008). Gender differences in the relationship between perceived social support and student adjustment during early adolescence. *School Psychology Quarterly, 23,* 496–514.

Ryan, R. M., & Deci, E. L. (2000). Self-determination theory and the facilitation of intrinsic motivation, social development, and well-being. *American Psychologist, 55,* 68–78.

Ryan, R. M., & Deci, E. L. (2006). Self-regulation and the problem of human autonomy: Does psychology need choice, self-determination, and will? *Journal of Personality, 74,* 1557–1585.

Ryan, R. M., Deci, E. L., Grolnick, W. S., & LaGuardia, J. G. (2006). The significance of autonomy and autonomy support in psychological development and psychopathology. In D. Cicchetti & D. Cohen (Eds.), *Developmental psychopathology: Vol. 1. Theory and methods* (2nd ed., pp. 795–849). New York: Wiley.

Ryan, A. M., & Patrick, H. (2001). The classroom social environment and changes in adolescents' motivation and engagement during middle school. *American Educational Research Journal, 38,* 437–460.

Saarni, C. (1999). *The development of emotional competence.* New York: Guilford Press.

Sadler, C. (2000). Effective behavior support implementation at the district level: Tigard–Tualatin School District. *Journal of Positive Behavior Interventions, 2,* 241–243.

Sasso, G. M., Conroy, M. A., Stichter, J. P., & Fox, J. J. (2001). Slowing down the bandwagon: The misapplication of functional assessment for students with emotional and behavioral disorders. *Behavioral Disorders, 26,* 282–296.

Scheuermann, B. K., & Hall, J. A. (2008). *Positive behavioral supports for the classroom.* Upper Saddle River, NJ: Pearson.

Schill, M. T., Kratochwill, T. R., & Elliott, S. N. (1998). Functional assessment in behavioral consultation: A treatment utility study. *School Psychology Quarterly, 13,* 116–140.

Schultz, D., Izard, C. E., & Ackerman, B. P. (2000). Children's anger attribution bias: Relations to family environment and social adjustment. *Social Development, 9,* 284–301.

Scott, T. M., & Barrett, S. B. (2004). Using staff and student time engaged in disciplinary procedures to evaluate the impact of school-wide PBS. *Journal of Positive Behavior Interventions, 6,* 21–27.

Scott, T. M., & Caron, D. B. (2005). Conceptualizing functional behavior assessment as prevention practice within positive behavior support systems. *Preventing School Failure, 50,* 13–20.

Scott, T. M., McIntyre, J., Liaupsin, C., Nelson, C. M., Conroy, M., & Payne, L. D. (2005). An examination of the relation between functional behavior assessment and selected intervention strategies with school-based teams. *Journal of Positive Behavior Interventions, 7,* 205–215.

Seligman, M. E. P., & Csikszentmihalyi, M. (2000). Positive psychology: An introduction. *American Psychologist, 55,* 5–14.

Seligman, M. E. P., Steen, T. A., Park, N., & Peterson, C. (2005). Positive psychology progress: Empirical validation of interventions. *American Psychologist, 60,* 410–421.

Shapiro, E. S., & Cole, C. L. (1994). *Behavior change in the classroom: Self-management interventions.* New York: Guilford Press.

Shapiro, E. S., Durnan, S. L., Post, E. E., & Levinson, T. S. (2002). Self-monitoring procedures for children and adolescents. In M. R. Shinn, H. M. Walker, & G. Stoner (Eds.), *Interventions for academic and behavior problems II: Preventive and remedial approaches* (pp. 433–454). Bethesda, MD: National Association of School Psychologists.

Sheridan, S. M., & Kratochwill, T. R. (2008). *Conjoint behavioral consultation: Promoting family-school connections and interventions* (2nd ed.). New York: Springer.

Shumow, L., Vandell, D. L., & Posner, J. (1999). Risk and resilience in the urban neighborhood: Predictors of academic performance among low-income elementary school children. *Merrill–Palmer Quarterly, 45,* 309–331.

Shure, M. (2001). I can problem solve (ICPS): An interpersonal cognitive problem solving program for children. *Residential Treatment for Children and Youth* [Special issue] *Innovative mental health interventions for children: Programs that work, 18,* 3–14.

Sijtsema, J. J., Veenstra, R., Lindenberg, S., & Salmivalli, C. (2009). Empirical test of bullies' status goals: Assessing direct goals, aggression, and prestige. *Aggressive Behavior, 35,* 57–67.

Skiba, R. J., & Noam, G. G. (2002). *Zero tolerance: Can suspension and expulsion keep schools safe?: New directions for youth development.* San Francisco: Jossey-Bass.

Skinner, B. F. (1953). *Science and human behavior.* New York: Macmillan.

Skinner, B. F. (1966). Contingencies of reinforcement in the design of a culture. *Behavioral Science, 11,* 159–166.

Skinner, C. H., Cashwell, T. H., & Dunn, M. S. (1996). Independent and interdependent group contingencies: Smoothing the rough waters. *Special Services in the Schools, 12,* 61–78.

Skinner, C. H., Cashwell, T. H., & Skinner, A. L. (2000). Increasing tootling: The effects of a peer monitored group contingency program on students' reports of peers' prosocial behaviors. *Psychology in the Schools, 37,* 263–270.

Skinner, C. H., Neddenriep, C. E., Robinson, S. L., Ervin, R., & Jones, K. (2002). Altering educational environments through positive peer reporting: Prevention and remediation of social problems associated with behavior disorders. *Psychology in the Schools, 39,* 191–202.

Solomon, D., Battistich, V., Watson, M., Schaps, E., & Lewis, C. (2000). A six-district study of educational change: Direct and mediated effects of the Child Development Project. *Social Psychology of Education, 4,* 3–51.

Spirito, A., Stark, L. J., Grace, N., & Stamoulis, D. (1991). Common problems and coping strategies reported in childhood and early adolescence. *Journal of Youth and Adolescence, 20,* 531–544.

Spivack, G., Platt, J. J., & Shure, M. B. (1976). *The problem-solving approach to adjustment.* San Francisco: Jossey-Bass.

Sprague, J., Colvin, G., & Irvin, L. (1996). *The Oregon School Safety Survey.* Eugene: University of Oregon.

Sprague, J., Walker, H., Golly, A., White, K., Myers, D. R., & Shannon, T. (2001). Translating research into effective practice: The effects of a universal staff and student intervention on indicators of discipline and school safety. *Education and Treatment of Children, 24,* 495–511.

Stage, S. A., & Quiroz, D. R. (1997). A meta-analysis of interventions to decrease disruptive classroom behavior in public education settings. *School Psychology Review, 26,* 333–368.

Stams, G. J., Brugman, D., Dekovic, M., van Rosmalen, L., van der Laan, P., & Gibbs, J. C. (2006). The moral judgment of juvenile delinquents: A meta-analysis. *Journal of Abnormal Child Psychology, 34,* 697–713.

Stearns, E., Dodge, K. A., & Nicholson, M. (2008). Peer contextual influences on the growth of authority-acceptance problems in early elementary school, *Merrill–Palmer Quarterly, 54,* 208–231.

Steinberg, L. (1996). *Beyond the classroom: Why school reform has failed and what parents need to do.* New York: Simon & Schuster.

Steinberg, L., Elmen, J. D., & Mounts, N. S. (1989). Authoritative parenting, psychosocial maturity, and academic success among adolescents. *Child Development, 60,* 1424–1436.

Stipek, D. (2002). *Motivation to learn: Integrating theory and practice* (4th ed.) Boston, MA: Allyn & Bacon.

Stoiber, K. C. (2004). *Functional assessment and intervention system.* San Antonio, TX: PsychCorp.

Stone, C. A. (1998). The metaphor of scaffolding: Its utility for the field of learning disabilities. *Journal of Learning Disabilities, 31,* 344–364.

Storr, C. L., Ialongo, N. S., Kellam, S. G., & Anthony, J. C. (2002). A randomized controlled trial of two primary school intervention strategies to prevent early onset tobacco smoking. *Drug and Alcohol Dependence, 66,* 51–60. .

Sugai, G., & Horner, R. H. (2002). Introduction to the special series on positive behavior support in schools. *Journal of Emotional and Behavioral Disorders, 10,* 130–135.

Sugai, G., & Horner, R. H. (2008). What we know and need to know about preventing problem behavior in schools. *Exceptionality, 16,* 67–77.

Sugai, G., & Horner, R. H. (2009). Defining and describing schoolwide positive behavior support. In W. Sailor, G. Dunlap, G. Sugai & R. Horner (Eds.), *Handbook of positive behavior support* (pp. 307–326). New York: Springer.

Sugai, G., Horner, R., Dunlap, G., Hieneman, M., Lewis, T. J., Nelson, C. M., et al. (2000). Applying positive behavior support and functional behavioral assessment in schools. *Journal of Positive Behavior Interventions, 2,* 131–143.

Sugai, G., Horner, R., & McIntosh, K. (2008). Best practices in developing a broad-scale system of schoolwide positive behavior support. In A. Thomas & J. Grimes (Eds.), *Best practices in school psychology* (5th ed., Vol. 3, pp. 765–779). Bethesda, MD: National Association of School Psychologists.

Sugai, G., Lewis-Palmer, T., Todd, A., & Horner, R. H. (2001). *School-wide evaluation tool.* Eugene: University of Oregon.

Sugai, G., Sprague, J. R., Horner, R. H., & Walker, H. M. (2000). Preventing school violence: The use of office discipline referrals to assess and monitor school-wide discipline interventions. *Journal of Emotional and Behavioral Disorders, 8,* 94–101.

Tangney, J. P., Stuewig, J., & Mashek, D. J. (2007). Moral emotions and moral behavior. *Annual Review of Psychology, 58*, 345–372.

Taylor, L. C., Hinton, I. D., & Wilson, M. N. (1995). Parental influences on academic performance in African-American students. *Journal of Child and Family Studies, 4*, 293–302.

Taylor-Greene, S., Brown, D., Nelson, L., Longton, J., Gassman, T., Cohen, J., et al. (1997). School-wide behavioral support: Starting the year off right. *Journal of Behavioral Education, 7*, 99–112.

Taylor-Greene, S. J., & Kartub, D. T. (2000). Durable implementation of school-wide behavior support: The High Five Program. *Journal of Positive Behavior Interventions, 2*, 233–235.

Thomas, D. E., Bierman, K. L., Thompson, C., & Powers, C. J. (2008). Double jeopardy: Child and school characteristics that predict aggressive–disruptive behavior in first grade. *School Psychology Review, 37*, 516–532.

Thorndike, E. L. (1920). *Educational psychology: Vol. 1. The original nature of man.* New York: Teachers College Press.

Tingstrom, D. H., Sterling-Turner, H. E., & Wilczynski, S. M. (2006). The Good Behavior Game: 1969–2002. *Behavior Modification, 30*, 225–253.

Tobin, T., & Sugai, G. M. (1999). Using sixth-grade school records to predict school violence, chronic discipline problems, and high school outcomes. *Journal of Emotional and Behavioral Disorders, 7*, 40–53.

Tyler, T. (2006). Psychological perspectives on legitimacy and legitimation. *Annual Review of Psychology, 57*, 375–400.

Tyler, T. R., & Degoey, P. (1995). Collective restraint in social dilemmas: Procedural justice and social identification effects on support for authorities. *Journal of Personality and Social Psychology, 69*, 482–497.

Unnever, J. D., & Cornell, D. G. (2004). Middle school victims of bullying: Who reports being bullied? *Aggressive Behavior, 30*, 373–388.

U.S. Department of Justice, Office of Justice Programs. (2006). *Reentry trends in the U.S.* Retrieved July 18, 2009, from *www.ojp.usdoj.gov/bjs/reentry/recidivism.htm.*

U.S. Surgeon General (2001). *Surgeon general's report on youth violence.* Department of Health and Human Services. Rockville, MD: Author.

Valdez, C. R., Carlson, C., & Zanger, D. (2005). Evidence-based parent training and family interventions for school behavior change. *School Psychology Quarterly.* [Special issue]. *Evidence-Based Parent and Family Interventions in School Psychology, 20*, 403–433.

van Lier, P. A. C., Muthén, B. O., van der Sar, R. M., & Crijnen, A. A. M. (2004). Preventing disruptive behavior in elementary schoolchildren: Impact of a universal classroom-based intervention. *Journal of Consulting and Clinical Psychology, 72*, 467–478.

van Lier, P. A. C., Vuijk, P., & Crijnen, A. M. (2005). Understanding mechanisms of change in the development of antisocial behavior: The impact of a universal intervention. *Journal of Abnormal Child Psychology, 33*, 521–535.

Vieno, A., Perkins, D. D., Smith, T. M., & Santinello, M. (2005). Democratic school climate and sense of community in school: A multilevel analysis. *American Journal of Community Psychology, 36*(3&4), 327–341.

Vygotsky, L. (1987). Thinking and speech. In L. S. Vygotsky, R. Rieber, & A. Carton (Eds.), *The collected works of L. S. Vygotsky: Vol. 1. Problems of general psychology* (pp. 37–285). New York: Plenum Press. (Original work published 1934)

Waas, G. (2006). Peer relationships. In G. G. Bear & K. M. Minke (Eds.), *Children's needs III: Development, prevention, and intervention* (pp. 325–340). Bethesda, MD: National Association of School Psychologists.

Wald, J., & Losen, D. J. (2003). Defining and redirecting a school-to-prison pipeline. In J. Wald & D. J.

Losen (Eds.), *New directions for youth development, No. 99: Deconstructing the school-to-prison pipeline* (pp. 9–15). San Francisco: Jossey-Bass.

Walker, H. M., Ramsey, E., & Gresham, F. M. (2004). *Antisocial behavior in schools: Evidence-based practices* (2nd ed.). Belmont, CA: Wadsworth/Thomson Learning.

Watson, J. B. (1913). *Psychology from the standpoint of a behaviorist.* Philadelphia: Lippincott.

Watson, M., & Battistich, V. (2006). Building and sustaining caring communities. In C. M. Evertson & C. S. Weinstein (Eds.), *Handbook of classroom management: Research, practice, and contemporary issues* (pp. 253–279). Mahwah, NJ: Erlbaum.

Watson, T. S., & Sterling-Turner, H. (2008). Best practices in direct behavioral consultation. In A. Thomas & J. Grimes (Eds.), *Best Practices in Schools Psychology* (5th ed., Vol. 4, pp. 903–916). Bethesda, MD: National Association of School Psychologists.

Weiner, B. (2006). *Social motivation, justice, and the moral emotions: An attributional approach.* Mahwah, NJ: Erlbaum.

Weinstein, C. S. (2006). *Secondary classroom management: Lessons from research and practice* (3rd ed.). New York: McGraw-Hill.

Weinstein, C. S., & Mignano, A. J. (2007). *Elementary classroom management: Lessons from research and practice* (4th ed.). Boston: McGraw-Hill.

Welsh, W. N. (2000). The effects of school climate on school disorder. *Annals of the American Academy of Political and Social Science, 567,* 88–107.

Welsh, W. N. (2003). Individual and institutional predictors of school disorder. *Youth Violence and Juvenile Justice, 1,* 346–368.

Welsh, M., Parke, R. D., Widaman, K., & O'Neil, R. (2001). Linkages between children's social and academic competence: A longitudinal analysis. *Journal of School Psychology, 39,* 463–482.

Wentzel, K. R. (1994). Relations of social goal pursuit to social acceptance, classroom behavior, and perceived social support. *Journal of Educational Psychology, 86,* 173–182.

Wentzel, K. R. (1996). Social and academic motivation in middle school: Concurrent and long-term relations to academic effort. *Journal of Early Adolescence, 16,* 390–406.

Wentzel, K. R. (1997). Student motivation in middle school: The role of perceived pedagogical caring. *Journal of Educational Psychology, 89,* 411–419.

Wentzel, K. R. (2002). Are effective teachers like good parents?: Teaching styles and student adjustment in early adolescence. *Child development, 73,* 287–301.

Wentzel, K.. R. (2004). Understanding classroom competence: The role of social-motivational and self-processes. In R. V. Kail (Ed.), *Advances in child development and behavior* (Vol. 32, pp. 213–241). San Diego: Elsevier.

Wentzel, K. R. (2006). A social motivation perspective for classroom management. In C. M. Evertson & C. S. Weinstein (Eds.), *Handbook of classroom management: Research, practice, and contemporary issues* (pp. 619–643). Mahwah, NJ: Erlbaum.

Wentzel, K. R., & Wigfield, A. (2007). Motivational interventions that work: Themes and remaining issues. *Educational Psychologist, 42,* 261–271.

Werner, E. E. (1982). *Vulnerable but invincible: A longitudinal study of resilient children and youth.* New York: McGraw-Hill.

Werner, N., & Nixon, C. L. (2005). Normative beliefs and relational aggression: An investigation of the cognitive bases of adolescent aggressive behavior. *Journal of Youth and Adolescence, 34,* 229–243.

Wilson, D. (2004). The interface of school climate and school connectedness and relationships with aggression and victimization. *Journal of School Health, 74,* 293–299.

Wilson, D. B., Gottfredson, D. C., & Najaka, S. S. (2001). School-based prevention of problem behaviors: A meta-analysis. *Journal of Quantitative Criminology, 17,* 247–272.

Wilson, S. J., & Lipsey, M. W. (2007). School-based interventions for aggressive and disruptive behavior: Update of a meta-analysis. *American Journal of Preventive Medicine, 33*(Suppl. 2S), 130–143.

Wilson, S. J., Lipsey, M. W., & Derzon, J. H. (2003). The effects of school-based intervention programs on aggressive behavior: A meta-analysis. *Journal of Consulting and Clinical Psychology, 71,* 136–149.

Winett, R. A., & Winkler, R. C. (1972). Current behavior modification in the classroom: Be still, be quiet, be docile. *Journal of Applied Behavior Analysis, 5,* 499–504.

Wright, J. A., & Dusek, J. B., 1998). Compiling school base rates for disruptive behaviors from student disciplinary referral data. *School Psychology Review, 27,* 138–147.

Wubbels, T., Brekelmans, M., van Tartwijk, J., & Admiral, W. (1999). Interpersonal relationships between teachers and students in the classroom. In H. C. Waxman & H. J. Walberg (Eds.), *New directions for teaching, practice, and research* (pp. 151–170). Berkeley, CA: McCutchan.

Yates, M., & Youniss, J. (2001). Promoting identity development: Ten ideas for school-based service-learning programs. In J. Claus & C. Ogden (Eds.), *Service learning for youth empowerment and social change* (pp. 43–67). New York: Peter Lang.

Youniss, J., Yates, M., & Su, Y. (1997). Social integration: Community service and marijuana use in high school seniors. *Journal of Adolescent Research, 12,* 245–262.

Zelli, A., Dodge, K. A., Lochman, J. E., & Laird, R. D. (1999). The distinction between beliefs legitimizing aggression and deviant processing of social cues: Testing measurement validity and the hypothesis that biased processing mediates the effects of beliefs on aggression. *Journal of Personality and Social Psychology, 77,* 150–166.

Zins, J. E., & Elias, M. J. (2006). Social and emotional learning. In G. G. Bear & K. M. Minke (Eds.), *Children's needs III: Development, prevention, and intervention* (pp. 1–13). Bethesda, MD: National Association of School Psychologists.

Zins, J. E., Weissberg, R. P., Wang, M. C., & Walberg. H. J. (Eds.). (2004). *Building academic success on social and emotional learning: What does the research say?* New York: Teachers College Press.

Index

Page number followed by an *f* or *t* indicate figures or tables.